Reductive Metabolites of Curcuminoids

Editors
Muhammed Majeed, Ph. D.
Kalyanam Nagabhushanam, Ph. D.

Authors
Muhammed Majeed, Ph. D.
Kalyanam Nagabhushanam, Ph. D.
Narayanan K. Narayanan, Ph. D.
Ambar K. Choudhury, Ph. D.
Lakshmi Mundkur, Ph. D.
Mahadeva Nayak, Ph. D.
Smitha Thazhathidath, M. Sc.

Graphic Designer
K. G. Girish, MVA

First Printing
NutriScience Publishers, LLC
East Windsor, NJ 08520, The United States of America

Disclaimer

The information contained in this book, **Reductive Metabolites of Curcuminoids** is intended to provide helpful and informative material for scientific and educational purposes only. It is not designed, in whole or in part, as an advice for self-diagnosis or self-treatment; nor is intended to serve as a replacement for professional medical advice.

NutriScience Publishers, LLC
20 Lake Drive,
East Windsor, NJ 08520,
The United States of America

Copyright © 2019 NutriScience Publishers, LLC

All rights reserved, including the right of reproduction in whole or in part in any form.

NutriScience Publishers, LLC, First Edition, 2019
ISBN: 978-0-9883209-4-9

Prologue:

*"For every drug that benefits a patient,
there is a natural substance that can achieve the same effect."*
—Carl Pfeiffer

The traditional uses of turmeric as a household nutrient over time immemorial coronate it as a gift from nature to human beings. In our previous book, the emphasis was placed heavily on the clinical use of curcumin and the related health benefits. It is evident that curcumin, or diferuloylmethane, isolated from turmeric (Curcuma longa) is known to exhibit pleiotropic activities and thus undoubtedly offers several health benefits. Primarily, the functional health benefits of curcumin when consumed as a diet or dietary supplement accrue through its antioxidant, anti-inflammatory, antiviral, antifungal, antibacterial, anticancer, antidiabetic, and neuroprotective activities.

In principle, the health benefits of any nutrient are the aggregate effects of the nutrient and possibly of its metabolites too. Curcumin/curcuminoids are known to be extensively metabolized to various compounds. The literature is replete with references documenting the pharmacological benefits of these metabolites. On sifting the contents of numerous papers and understanding the bioavailability pathways of curcumin led us to further unmask the importance, stability, and mechanisms of the key metabolites of curcuminoids that have been already identified. Although quantitative analysis of the benefits of curcumin and the associated curcuminoids from Curcuma longa rhizomes are well documented, it is important to assess the health benefits of the individual metabolites of curcumin.

The contents of this book in great depth enlighten the potential health benefits of reductive metabolites of curcumin/curcuminoids in particular.

When administered orally/intraperitoneally/intravenously, curcumin gets biotransformed into numerous metabolites and degradants. Besides the major metabolite tetrahydrocurcumin (THC), various other reductive metabolites identified are dihydrocurcumin (DHC), hexahydrocurcumin (HHC) and octahydrocurcumin (OHC), in addition to curcumin-glucuronide, DHC-glucuronide, THC-glucuronide, and curcumin sulfate. While the literature now extant clearly points to the biological inactivity of curcumin-glucuronides, it unmistakably points to the other curcumin reductive metabolites primarily exerting both anti-inflammatory and antioxidant properties at different degrees in different organ systems.

The central objective of this book is on detailing the role of the reductive metabolites in specific health conditions. It is noteworthy to mention here that all of the reductive metabolites also share key pharmacological activities (for instance, anti-inflammatory and antioxidant) with the parent compound curcumin, and thus could be accounting for the total health benefits synergistically with curcumin.

This book chapters highlights the importance of each reductive metabolite of curcumin that could function as a nutrient in promoting health benefits often in consort with each other.

We are greatly indebted to the innumerable number of scientists, who worked on these various reductive metabolites to understand their biological effects.

Wishing you and your loved ones the best of health today and always.

- Muhammed Majeed, Ph.D.
-Kalyanam Nagabhushanam, Ph.D.

ABOUT THE EDITORS

Muhammed Majeed, Ph. D.

Dr. Muhammed Majeed holds a doctorate in Industrial Pharmacy from St. John's University, New York. He has over 14 years of pharmaceutical research experience in the United States with leading pharma companies, such as Pfizer Inc., Carter-Wallace and Paco Research.

Subsequent to the formation of his company, Sabinsa Corporation in 1988, he pursued his interest in phytochemistry and pharmaceutical sciences. He leads a team of scientists, both in India and USA. He is an inventor in 210+ US and International patents so far. He is aggressively pursuing his interest in natural products and continues to develop new products for the world markets based on Ayurveda.

Kalyanam Nagabhushanam, Ph. D.

Dr. Kalyanam Nagabhushanam is the President of Sami-Sabinsa Group R&D. His research interests are in synthetic methodology, chiral chemistry and natural products. He obtained his M.Sc. in Chemistry from University of Madras and Ph. D. from Baylor, Texas. After a further two-year post-doctoral studies in the USA on chiral chemistry and chiro-optical methods, he returned to India to work with IPCL (now part of Reliance group), Ciba-Geigy (now known as Novartis) and SPIC Pharma. He has been with Sabinsa since 1999. Dr. Kalyanam's primary reponsibilities at Sabinsa include development of new products and exploration of new business areas.

ABOUT THE AUTHORS

Narayanan K. Narayanan, Ph. D.

Dr. Narayanan K. Narayanan is a Scientist at the Sabinsa Corporation. He obtained his Ph. D. degree from the University of Madras, Chennai and did his postdoctoral training at the Medical University South Carolina, Charleston, SC, USA. He worked as Scientist at the American Health foundation, an NCI-designated Comprehensive Cancer Prevention Center, Valhalla, NY and also as Assistant Professor at the New York University School of Medicine, NY before joining Sabinsa in the year 2017. He has more than 20 years of research experience in the areas of safety, efficacy and molecular mechanisms of several natural compounds using animal models against cancers and diseases associated with metabolic disorders. Currently, as a member of the R&D team at Sabinsa, Dr. Narayanan is evaluating the phytochemical and pharmacological properties of various plant-derived products for the prevention of various diseases.

Ambar K. Choudhury, Ph. D.

Dr. Ambar K. Choudhury has completed his Ph. D. (1997) in chemistry from IACS, Kolkata, India and postdoctoral studies from ISRAEL, USA and JAPAN. He worked with Professor Sidney M. Hecht (Associate Editor of JACS) at University of Virginia, USA on chemical biology. He was the recipients of prestigious JSPS-postdoctoral fellowship awarded by The Japan Society for the Promotion of Science and Visiting Fellowship approved by NSERC, CANADA. He worked as R&D-Head, SGL/JBL, Hyderabad. Presently he is working in Sami Labs, since 2008. He has about 25 years of research experiences on synthetic organic chemistry and chemical biology and is involved in the development of new products and methodologies, natural product synthesis and process development. He has published 20 research articles in peer-reviewed reputed journals.

Lakshmi Mundkur, Ph. D.

Dr. Lakshmi Mundkur obtained her M. Sc. and Ph. D. in Biotechnology, specializing in Immunology from Madurai Kamaraj University, Madurai. She started her career with Lupin Chemicals Ltd. (India) and moved on to Wockhardt Research Centre (India), Novartis Healthcare (India) and Thrombosis Research Institute (India) during her 20 years of experience in pharma and drug discovery research. Her research interests include immunology, molecular biology and mechanism of action of natural products. Presently, she is the Vice President of Biological Research at Sami Labs. Her major responsibilities at Sami-Sabinsa are to explore the biological efficacy and mechanism of action of new products.

Mahadeva Nayak, Ph. D.

Dr. Mahadeva Nayak obtained his Ph. D in Chemistry from the University of Mysore. He has been closely involved with research activities related to natural products and their biological activities for more than 17 years. Currently heading the Technical Marketing Department at Sami Labs, he is into development and management of innovative research projects. His current position in the company is an important bridge between the R&D team and the marketing team. He provides technical support to various Sami-Sabinsa representatives and clients for business development. He obtained his Masters degree in Pharmacy from Government College of Pharmacy (RGUHS) Bangalore and Bachelor degree in Pharmacy from College of Pharmaceutical Sciences, Manipal (Mangalore University).

Smitha Thazhathidath, M. Sc.

Smitha Thazhathidath holds Masters degree in Biochemistry from Bangalore University, Bangalore and has been with Sami Labs for over 10 years. Presently, she is a part of Technical Support of Sami Labs, which works as an important bridge between the global marketing/business development team and the R&D team. She provides overall technical and techno-marketing support to all business development teams of Sami-Sabinsa Group.

ABOUT GRAPHIC DESIGNER

K. G. Girish, MVA

Girish holds a Masters degree in Visual Arts from Jain University, Bangalore and Bachelor degree in Fine Art from College of Fine Arts (Karnataka Chitrakala Parishath). He has more than 18 years of experience in Graphic design (print & web), Web design and UI design. He has been with Sami-Sabinsa group for over 15 years, presently handling all creative design works for the group. He is also involved in new website design & development for the group.

© NutriScience Publishers, LLC. 2019

CONTENTS

Chapter 1
Curcuminoids and their Metabolites

- 01 Curcumin Metabolites — 3
  - Phase I Metabolites
  - Phase II Metabolites
  - Degradation Products of Curcumin
- 02 Conclusion — 8
- 03 References — 9

Chapter 2
Dihydrocurcumin (DHC)
A Transient Metabolite With Tangible Benefits

- 01 Introduction — 15
- 02 Natural Occurrence — 16
- 03 Crystal Structure — 17
- 04 Metabolic Biotransformation - In vivo — 18
- 05 Pharmacokinetics and Tissue Distribution - In vivo — 18
- 06 A Metabolic Product of Gut Microbiota — 19
- 07 Pharmacological Significance — 21
  - Cytotoxic Effects
  - Antioxidant Potential
  - Insulin Resistance
  - Anti-allergic Activity
  - Trypanocidal Activity
- 08 Conclusion — 27
- 09 References — 28

Chapter 3
Tetrahydrocurcumin (THC)
The Major Metabolite With Major Benefits

01	Introduction	31
02	Characteristics of Tetrahydrocurcumin	33
03	Natural Occurrence	34
04	Biotransformation of Curcumin to THC	35
05	Identification & Quantification	35
06	Preparation of THC by Hydrogenation	38
07	Crystal Structure	39
08	Microbial Transformation	41
09	Absorption Characteristics: Curcumin vs. THC	44
	Distribution of Curcumin vs. THC in Serum and Liver	
	Pharmacokinetics and Tissue Distribution of Curcumin and THC	
10	Pharmacological Significance	49
	Antioxidant Potential	
	Anti-inflammatory Potential	
	Anti-glycation Potential	
	Cardioprotective Potential	
	Nephroprotective Potential	
	Hepatoprotective Potential	
	Anti-hyperlipidemic Potential	
	Anticancer Activity	
	Anti-diabetic Potential	
	Anti-obesity Activity	
	Neuroprotective Potential	
	Anti-aging Potential	
	Anti-osteoarthritic Potential	
	Anti-allergic Activity	
	Anti-asthmatic Activity	
	Anti-viral Potential	
	Oral Health	
	Summary	

11	Cosmetic Applications	146
	THCs in Cosmetic Formulations	
	THC Against Skin Disorders	
12	*In vitro* Studies for Cosmetic Applications	153
	Antioxidant Assay Using Cell Lines by ROS Scavenging Method	
	Antioxidant Assay by Lipid Peroxidation Method	
	Antioxidant Assay by DPPH Method	
	Antioxidant Assay by ORAC Method	
	Antioxidant Assay by HORAC Method	
	Melanogenesis Inhibitory Activity	
	Cyclooxygenase (COX) Inhibitory Activity	
	Summary	
13	Toxicity Studies	160
14	Safety Study	163
15	Conclusion	165
16	References	166

Chapter 4
Hexahydrocurcumin (HHC)
The Unsung Metabolite of Curcumin

01	Introduction	183
02	Natural Occurrence and Biosynthesis	185
03	Cellular & Mammalian Metabolism of Curcumin & HHC	188
04	Preparation of HHC by Hydrogenation	192
05	Microbial Biotransformation of Curcumin to HHC	193
06	Gut Microbiota Influence the Fate of Curcumin to Produce HHC in the Colon	195

07	Pharmacological Significance
	    Antimicrobial Activity
	    Anthelmintic and Larvicidal Activities
	    Antioxidant Potential
	    Anti-inflammatory Potential
	    Anti-allergic Activity
	    Immunomodulatory Activity
	    Neuroprotective Potential
	    Cardioprotective Potential
	    Anticancer Activity
		197

08	Conclusion	215
09	References	217

Chapter 5

Octahydrocurcumin (OHC)
The Final Reductive Metabolite of Curcumin

01	Introduction	227
02	Natural Occurrence	228
03	Preparation of OHC by Hydrogenation	228
04	Biotransformation - In vivo	229
05	Microbial Transformation of Curcumin to OHC	231
06	Biotransformation of Curcumin to OHC by Gut Microbiota	233

07	Pharmacological Significance
	    Antioxidant Potential
	    Anti-inflammatory Potential
	    Immunosuppressive Effect
	    Hepatoprotective Potential
	    Anticancer Activity
		233

08	Conclusion	246
09	References	247

Epilogue   249

Glossary   251

Abstract

The transition of curcumin, despite its therapeutic potential against various health conditions in humans, from a phytonutrient to a drug is said to be hampered by its poor bioavailability, rapid metabolism, chemical instability under physiological conditions and rapid elimination. The major phase I (reductive) metabolites after oral ingestion of curcumin have been identified as dihydrocurcumin, tetrahydrocurcumin, hexahydrocurcumin and octahydrocurcumin together with phase II metabolites, such as curcumin glucuronides and curcumin sulfates. Other phase I metabolites have also been reported. This section briefs the relative pharmacological importance of these metabolites in lieu of curcumin and curcuminoids (a mixture of curcumin as the dominant constituent together with two naturally co-occurring molecules, demethoxycurcumin and bisdemethoxycurcumin). It is concluded that the reductive metabolites of phase I share very similar or surpass biological activity of curcumin while the importance of other phase I metabolites is yet to be proven.

© NutriScience Publishers, LLC. 2019

Chapter 1

Curcuminoids and their Metabolites

Turmeric (*Curcuma longa*), the golden colored curry ingredient, is one of the most consumed spices in India and Asia, and is also used as a traditional medicine over centuries often without the knowledge of its mechanistic aspect or its pharmacological action. Isolation of components present in turmeric commenced two centuries ago and curcumin was isolated in the year 1815 (Vogel and Pelletier, 1815). Curcumin, the main polyphenol, present in turmeric has a unique structure and exists in solution as keto-enol tautomer (Kocaadam and Sanlier, 2017). Pharmacological studies on curcumin exemplified its potential as an anti-inflammatory (Jurenka, 2009), antioxidant (Asouri *et al.*, 2013), antiviral (Mathew and Hsu, 2018) and antimicrobial (Moghadamtousi *et al.*, 2014) agent. Consequently, clinical trials demonstrate curcumin's safety and efficacy in various human diseases including cancer (Majeed *et al.*, 2015), diabetes (de Melo *et al.*, 2018), hepatoprotection, neuroprotection, and other ailments/disorders (Kunnumakkara *et al.*, 2017; Salehi *et al.*, 2019). It is thus necessary to review the pharmacological significance of metabolites for a complete understanding of

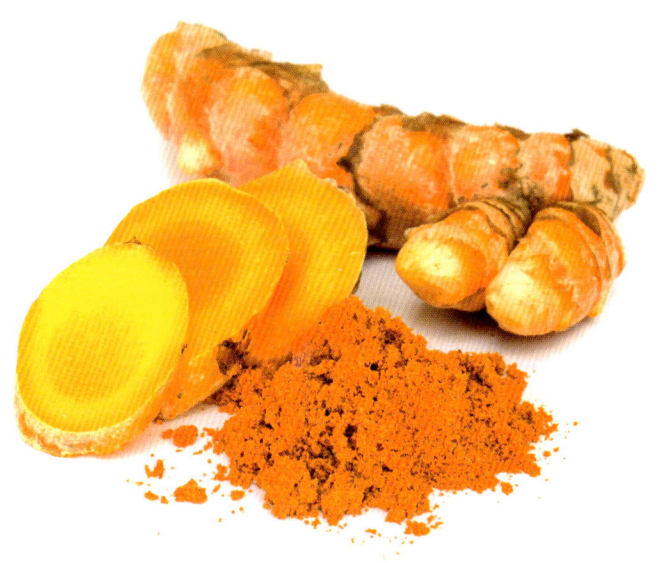

curcumin's molecular mechanisms in the biological system. Recent studies have been specifically designed to determine the role of metabolites in relationship with the therapeutic effect of curcumin. It is also believed that lone phytonutrient curcumin may not always produce optimum pleiotropic effects; however, a mixture of phytonutrients consisting of curcumin and the two naturally co-occurring demethoxycurcumin (DMC) and bisdemethoxycurcumin (BDMC) possessing synergistic and complementary actions could provide the best results. It is found that a mixture of three bioactive curcuminoids [Curcumin **(1)**, DMC **(2)** and BDMC **(3)** (Fig. 1)] showed better pharmacological efficacy than curcumin alone (Ahmed and Gilani, 2014). Recent studies demonstrate that curcumin-glucuronide metabolites are non-toxic in cancer cells and hence, ineffective as an anticancer agent and do not possess any bioactivity of curcumin. Phase I metabolites, namely, reductive ones such as dihydrocurcumin (DHC), tetrahydrocurcumin (THC), hexahydrocurcumin (HHC) and octahydrocurcumin (OHC) are garnering the attention of researchers due to their similar or superior efficacy compared to curcumin.

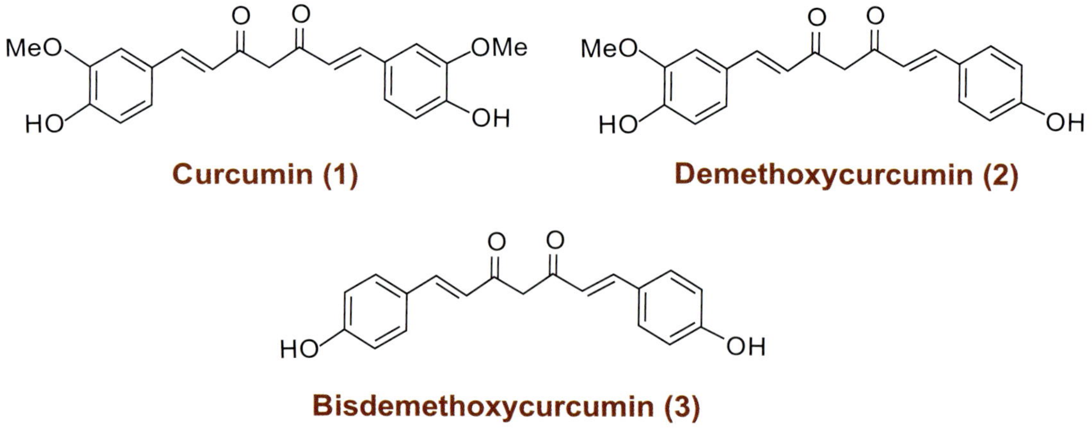

Curcumin (1)

Demethoxycurcumin (2)

Bisdemethoxycurcumin (3)

Fig. 1: Structures of Curcuminoids.

Curcumin Metabolites

Some of the major enzymes that metabolize curcumin into numerous metabolites are:

i) UDP glucuronosyl transferase (Pan *et al.*, 1999)
ii) Human phenol sulfotransferase isoenzymes (Ireson *et al.*, 2002)
iii) Alcohol dehydrogenase (Ireson *et al.*, 2002)
iv) NADPH-dependent curcumin/dihydrocurcumin reductase (Hassaninasab *et al.*, 2011)

The metabolism of curcumin into reduced metabolites was also detected in the gastrointestinal (GI) tract of mice (Li *et al.*, 2017). Thus, the metabolites of curcumin (Fig. 2) that are of interest are:

i) Phase I metabolites especially reductive ones such as DHC, THC, HHC and OHC (Hoehle *et al.*, 2006; Metzler *et al.*, 2013; Yu *et al.*, 2018)
ii) Phase II metabolites including glucuronides and sulfates (Hoehle *et al.*, 2007; Kunati *et al.*, 2018; Liu *et al.*, 2018; Mahale *et al.*, 2018)
iii) Degradative metabolites such as vanillin, ferulic acid, feruloylmethane, *trans*-6-(4'-hydroxy-3'-methoxyphenyl)-2,4-dioxo-5-hexenal (Shen *et al.*, 2016)

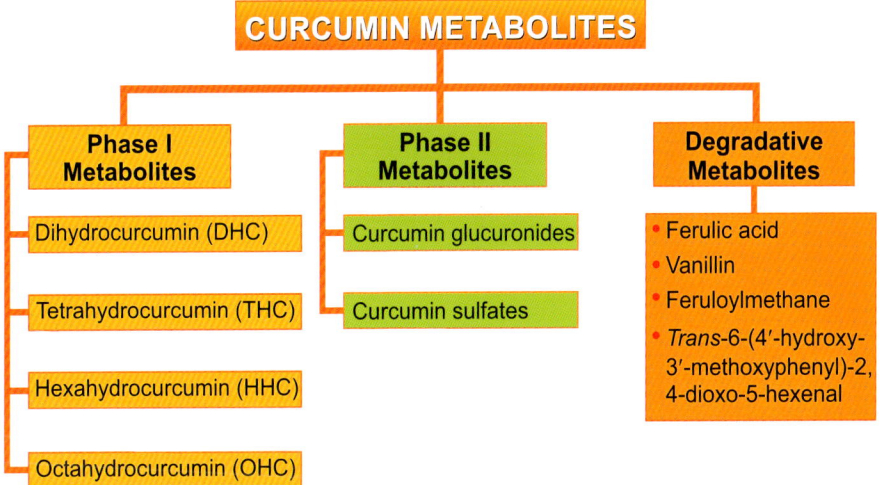

Fig. 2: Schematic representation of curcumin metabolic transformations.

Chapter 1
CURCUMINOIDS AND THEIR METABOLITES

Glucuronide metabolites are found to be in higher concentration in plasma compared to sulfates; however, no mixed conjugate such as curcumin glucuronide-sulfate was detected (Vareed et al., 2008). The metabolites that are detected after intraperitoneal administration of curcumin are not only curcumin-glucuronide but also dihydrocurcumin-glucuronide and tetrahydrocurcumin-glucuronide (Pan et al., 1999).

At least 23 phase I and phase II metabolites have been identified after metabolism of curcumin (Fig. 1) by human intestinal bacteria *in vitro* (Lou et al., 2015). Exclusive of these metabolites, a recent report describes yet another metabolism of curcuminoids by human intestinal microbiota in which the cleavage of aryl methyl ethers occurs forming the major demethylated products, demethylcurcumin **(4)** and bisdemethylcurcumin **(5)** (Fig. 3) (Burapan et al., 2017). It is to be noted here that the elaborative study on bisdemethylcurcumin indicated its anti-proliferative and anti-inflammatory activity comparable to curcumin (Ravindran et al., 2010).

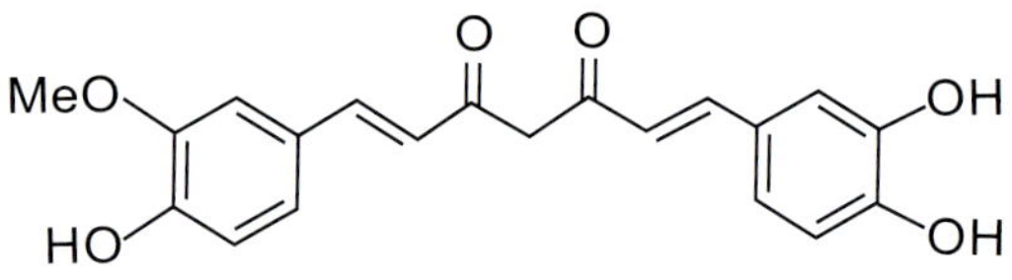

Demethylcurcumin (4) 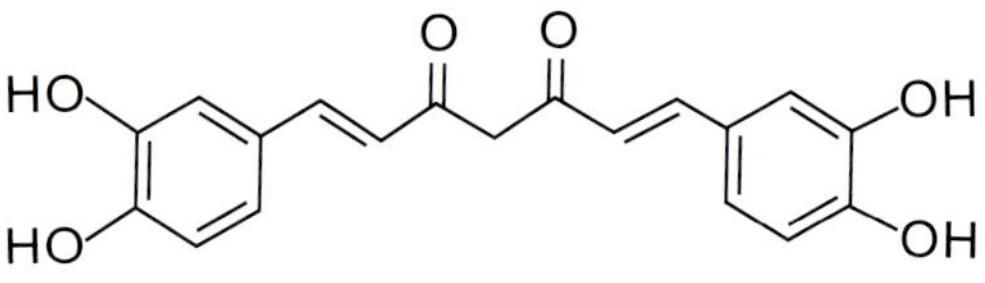   **Bisdemethylcurcumin (5)**

Fig. 3: Structures of Demethylcurcumin **(4)** and Bisdemethylcurcumin **(5)**.

Phase I Metabolites

Phase I metabolites of curcumin were identified especially as reductive ones such as DHC **(6)**, THC **(7)**, HHC **(8)** and OHC **(9)** (Fig. 4) (Jia et al., 2017). Unlike other metabolites such as glucuronides as well as degradative metabolites, the reductive metabolites are found to retain many of the pleiotropic actions of curcumin, including antioxidant, anti-inflammatory, anticancer, anti-diabetic etc (Sirijaroonwong et al., 2007; Somparn et al., 2007). Despite fourteen reductive metabolites of curcuminoids (Li et al., 2012) being identified in rats, the pharmacological importance of many of these metabolites is yet to be proven. Several of the reductive metabolites of curcumin are identified in nature (Han *et al.*, 2015; Ning *et al.*, 2012; Wei-Xin *et al.*, 2007); however, they are commonly biotransformed by the reductive enzymes (Mimura *et al.*, 1993; Pan *et al.*, 1999).

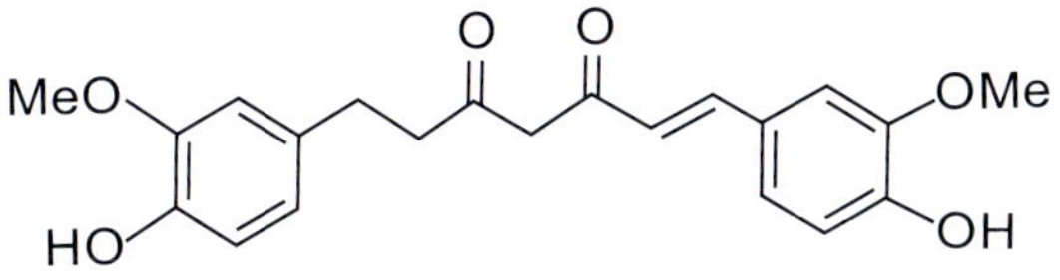

Dihydrocurcumin (6)

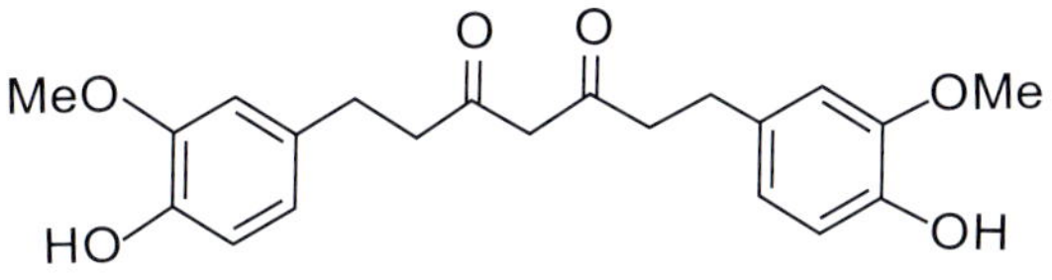

Tetrahydrocurcumin (7)

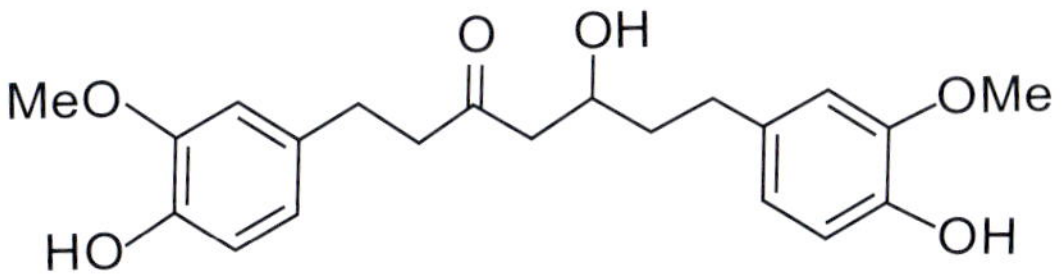

Hexahydrocurcumin (8)

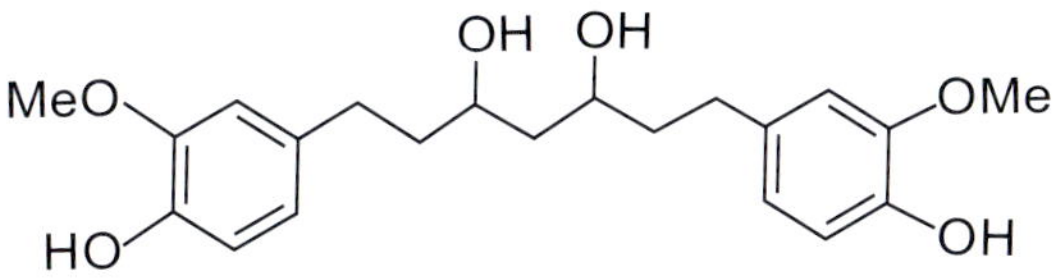

Octahydrocurcumin (9)

Fig. 4: Reductive metabolites of curcumin.

Phase II Metabolites

Phase II metabolites predominantly curcumin glucuronides rarely occur in plants. However, they form via biotransformation during the metabolism of curcumin by the enzyme UDP glucuronosyl transferase (Pan *et al.*, 1999) and were detected by LC-MS/MS from human plasma after oral ingestion of curcumin (Hoehle *et al.*, 2007; Kunati *et al.*, 2018; Liu *et al.*, 2018; Mahale *et al.*, 2018).

Despite its detection in human plasma, there were no reports on the availability of these molecules in reasonable quantity for further analysis. Recently, curcumin metabolites were synthesized both chemically as well as enzymatically and evaluated for their biological significance (Choudhury *et al.*, 2015; Pal *et al.*, 2014; Shoji *et al.*, 2014; Singh and Aggarwal, 1995).

Considering curcumin's poor bioavailability, curcumin glucuronides [monoglucuronide **(10)** and diglucuronide **(11)**] (Fig. 5), were assumed to be the indicators for bioavailability enhancement of curcumin and were hoped to retain curcumin's bioactivity as well. Curcumin glucuronides bioactivity could only be assessed recently (Choudhury *et al.*, 2015; Pal *et al.*, 2014; Shoji *et al.*, 2014; Singh and Aggarwal, 1995), while the pharmacological studies on curcumin sulfate **(12)** metabolite (Fig. 5) could rarely be seen in the literature. Curcumin monoglucuronide, when ingested orally, was not absorbed well in spite of its higher aqueous solubility (Ozawa *et al.*, 2017). These studies clearly demonstrated that glucuronide metabolites of curcumin are ineffective and do not contribute to any of the reported bioactivity of curcumin such as antioxidant, anti-inflammatory activity and anti-proliferative effects.

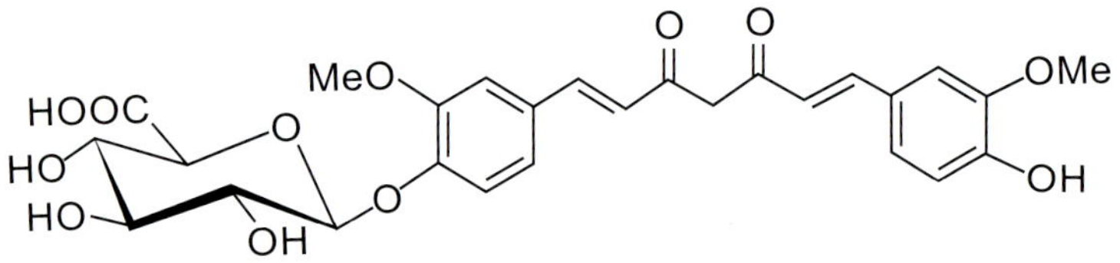

Curcumin monoglucuronide (10)

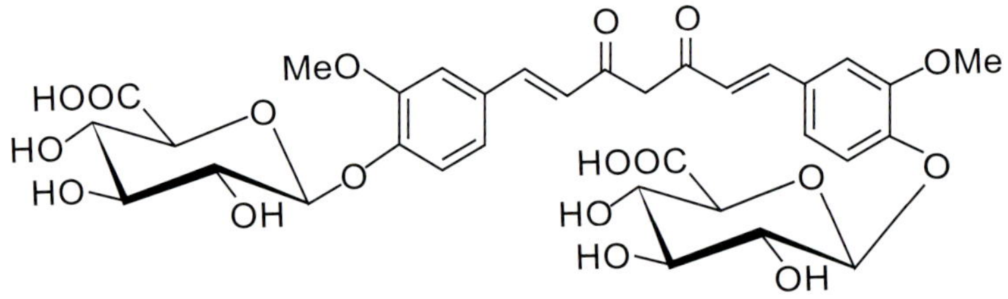

Curcumin diglucuronide (11)

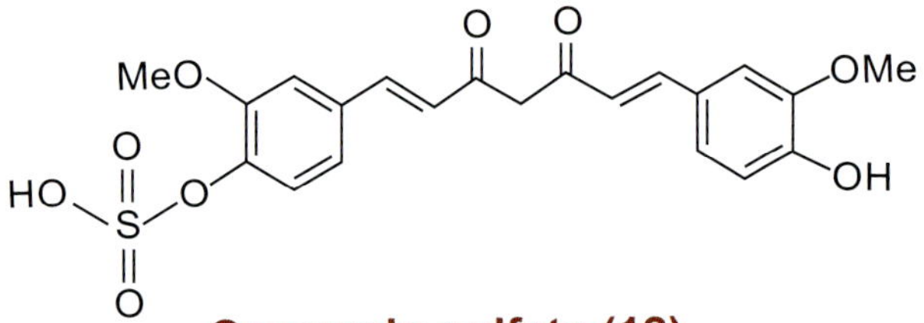

Curcumin sulfate (12)

Fig. 5: Phase II metabolites of curcumin.

Degradation Products of Curcumin

Poor stability of curcumin in physiological pH gives the speculation that curcumin's bioactivity might be attributed to its degradation products. The degradation products occurring in the biological system are the hydrolyzed products of curcumin. Curcumin is hydrolyzed to vanillin **(13)**, ferulic acid **(14)**, feruloyl methane **(15)**, *trans*-6-(4'-hydroxy-3'-methoxyphenyl)-2,4-dioxo-5-hexenal **(16)** (Fig. 6) and other feruloyl derivatives (Gordon and Schneider, 2012; Shen *et al.*, 2016; Shen and Ji, 2012a & 2012b; Wang *et al.*, 1997).

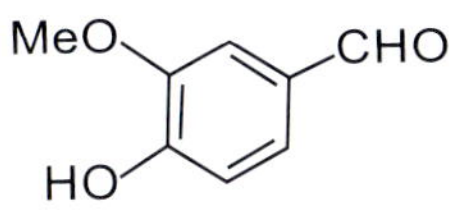

Vanillin (13) 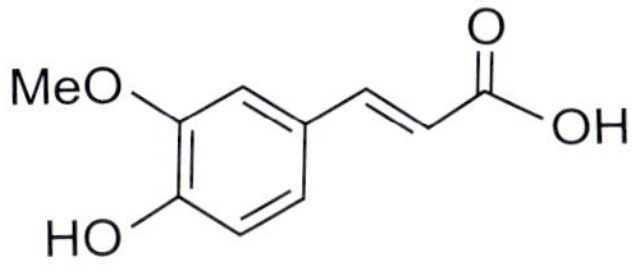   **Ferulic acid (14)** 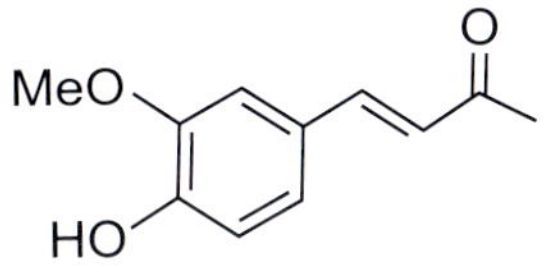   **Feruloyl methane (15)**

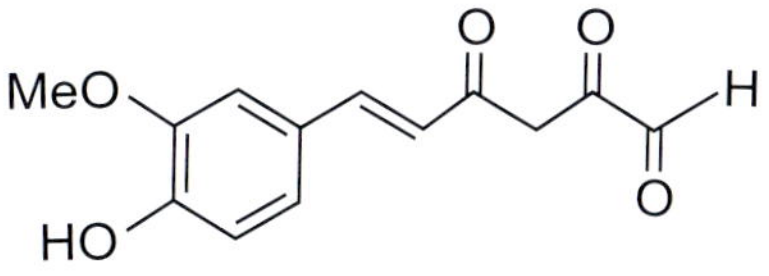

***Trans*-6-(4'-hydroxy-3'-methoxyphenyl)-2,4-dioxo-5-hexenal (16)**

Fig. 6: Degradation products of curcumin.

In few studies, it was reported that degradative products may have potential to contribute curcumin bioactivity (Gordon and Schneider, 2012; Schneider *et al.*, 2015; Shen and Ji, 2012a & 2012b). However, the present level of evidence (Sanidad *et al.*, 2016) points to the fact that the degradative metabolites may not account for the diverse activities of curcumin leading to the speculation that the activities of curcumin are attributable to the low levels of curcumin in circulation possibly bolstered by reductive phase I metabolites.

Conclusion

The studies prove that phase II metabolite of curcumin; especially curcumin-glucuronide metabolites do not possess antioxidant, anti-inflammatory activity, anti-proliferative effect, and any effect on mitotic catastrophe. They are non-toxic to cancer cells and ineffective as anticancer agents. Similarly, recent studies demonstrate that degradative metabolites of curcumin are highly ineffective and do not contribute to any of the reported bioactivity of curcumin. Curcumin phase I metabolites possess very similar biological activity as that of curcumin. The available evidence clearly indicates that future efforts should be directed in exploring the beneficial effects of the reductive metabolites of curcumin especially leading to tetrahydrocurcumin (THC).

References

Ahmed T, Gilani AH. 2014. Therapeutic potential of turmeric in Alzheimer's disease: curcumin or curcuminoids? *Phytother Res*. 28(4):517-525.

Asouri M, Ataee R, Ahmadi AA, Amini A, Moshaei MR. 2013. Antioxidant and free radical scavenging activities of curcumin. *Asian J Chem*. 25(13): 7593-7595.

Burapan S, Kim M, Han J. 2017. Curcuminoid demethylation as an alternative metabolism by human intestinal microbiota. *J Agric Food Chem*. 65(16): 3305-3310.

Choudhury AK, Raja S, Mahapatra S, Nagabhushanam K, Majeed M. 2015. Synthesis and evaluation of the antioxidant capacity of curcumin glucuronides, the major curcumin metabolites. *Antioxidants*. 4(4): 750-767.

de Melo ISV, Dos Santos AF, Bueno NB. 2018. Curcumin or combined curcuminoids are effective in lowering the fasting blood glucose concentrations of individuals with dysglycemia: Systematic review and meta-analysis of randomized controlled trials. *Pharmacol Res*. 128: 137-144.

Gordon ON, Schneider C. 2012. Vanillin and ferulic acid are not the major degradation products of curcumin. *Trends Mol Med*. 18(7): 361-364.

Han JS, Lee S, Kim HY, Lee CH. 2015. MS-Based metabolite profiling of above ground and root components of *Z. mioga* and *Z. officinale*. *Molecules*. 20: 16170-16185.

Hassaninasab A, Hashimoto Y, Tomita-Yokotani K, Kobayashi M. 2011. Discovery of the curcumin metabolic pathway involving a unique enzyme in an intestinal microorganism. *Proc Natl Acad Sci USA*. 108(16): 6615-6620.

Hoehle SI, Pfeiffer E, Solyom AM, Metzler M. 2006. Metabolism of curcuminoids in tissue slices and subcellular fractions from rat liver. *J Agric Food Chem*. 54(3): 756-764.

Hoehle SI, Pfeiffer E, Metzler M. 2007. Glucuronidation of curcuminoids by human microsomal and recombinant UDP-glucuronosyltransferases. *Mol Nutr Food Res*. 51(8): 932-938.

Ireson CR, Jones DJ, Orr S, Coughtrie MW, Boocock DJ, Williams ML *et al*. 2002. Metabolism of the cancer chemopreventive agent curcumin in human and rat intestine. *Cancer Epidemiol Biomarkers Prev*. 11: 105-111.

Jia S, Du Z, Song C, Jin S, Zhang Y, Feng Y *et al*. 2017. Identification and characterization of curcuminoids in turmeric using ultra-high performance liquid chromatography-quadrupole time of flight tandem mass spectrometry. *J Chromatogr A*. 1521: 110-122.

Jurenka JS. 2009. Anti-inflammatory properties of curcumin, a major constituent of *Curcuma longa*: a review of preclinical and clinical research. *Altern Med Rev*. 14(2): 141-153.

Kocaadam B, Sanlier N. 2017. Curcumin, an active component of turmeric (*Curcuma longa*), and its effects on health. *Crit Rev Food Sci Nutr*. 57(13): 2889-2895.

Kunati SR, Yang S, William BM, Xu Y. 2018. An LC-MS/MS method for simultaneous determination of curcumin, curcumin glucuronide and curcumin sulfate in a phase II clinical trial. *J Pharm Biomed Anal*. 156: 189-198.

Kunnumakkara AB, Bordoloi D, Padmavathi G, Monisha J, Roy NK, Prasad S, Aggarwal BB. 2017. Curcumin, the golden nutraceutical: Multitargeting for multiple chronic diseases. *Br J Pharmacol*. 174(11): 1325-1348.

Li J, Liu Y, Wei JQ, Wang K, Chen LX, Yao XS *et al*. 2012. Isolation and identification of phase I metabolites of curcuminoids in rats. *Planta Med*. 78(12): 1351-1356.

Li Z, Sun Y, Song M, Li F, Xiao H. 2017. Gut microbiota dictate metabolic fate of curcumin in the colon. *The FASEB J*. 31(1): Supplement 646.12.

Liu Y, Siard M, Adams A, Keowen ML, Miller TK, Garza F Jr *et al*. 2018. Simultaneous quantification of free curcuminoids and their metabolites in equine plasma by LC-ESI-MS/MS. *J Pharm Biomed Anal*. 154: 31-39.

Lou Y, Zheng J, Hu H, Lee J, Zeng S. 2015. Application of ultra-performance liquid chromatography coupled with quadrupole time-of-flight mass spectrometry to identify curcumin metabolites produced by human intestinal bacteria. *J Chromatogr B Analyt Technol Biomed Life Sci*. 985: 38-47.

Mahale J, Singh R, Howells LM, Britton RG, Khan SM, Brown K. 2018. Detection of plasma curcuminoids from dietary intake of turmeric-containing food in human volunteers. *Mol Nutr Food Res*. 62(16): e1800267.

Majeed M, Majeed A (Eds). 2015. Curry Powder to Clinical Significance. New Jersey: *NutriScience Publishers, LLC*. Part II: pp 63-183.

Mathew D, Hsu WL. 2018. Antiviral potential of curcumin. *J Funct Foods*. 40: 692-699.

Metzler M, Pfeiffer E, Schulz SI, Dempe JS. 2013. Curcumin uptake and metabolism. *Biofactors*. 39(1): 14-20.

Mimura A, Takahara Y, Osawa T. 1993. Method for making tetrahydrocurcumin and a substance containing the antioxidative substance tetrahydrocurcumin. US Patent 5266344.

Moghadamtousi SZ, Kadir HA, Hassandarvish P, Tajik H, Abubakar S, Zandi K. 2014. A review on antibacterial, antiviral, and antifungal activity of curcumin. *Biomed Res Int*. 2014:186864.

Ning L, Lingyu W, Lingbo Z, Kaijin W, Lei D, Zhi W. 2012. Antioxidant and cytotoxic diarylheptanoids isolated from *Zingiber officinale* rhizomes. *Chin J Chem*. 30: 1351-1355.

Ozawa H, Imaizumi A, Sumi Y, Hashimoto T, Kanai M, Makino Y *et al*. 2017. Curcumin β-D-glucuronide plays an important role to keep high levels of free-form curcumin in the blood. *Biol Pharm Bull*. 40(9): 1515-1524.

Pal A, Sung B, Bhanu Prasad BA, Schuber PT Jr, Prasad S, Aggarwal BB *et al*. 2014. Curcumin glucuronides: Assessing the proliferative activity against human cell lines. *Bioorg Med Chem*. 22(1): 435-439.

Pan MH, Huang TM, Lin JK. 1999. Biotransformation of curcumin through reduction and glucuronidation in mice. *Drug Metab Dispos*. 27(1): 486-494.

Ravindran J, Subbaraju GV, Ramani MV, Sung B, Aggarwal BB. 2010. Bisdemethylcurcumin and structurally related hispolon analogues of curcumin exhibit enhanced prooxidant, anti-proliferative and anti-inflammatory activities *in vitro*. *Biochem Pharmacol*. 79(11): 1658-1666.

Salehi B, Stojanovic-Radic Z, Matejic J, Sharifi-Rad M, Anil Kumar NV, Martins N, Sharifi-Rad J. 2019. The therapeutic potential of curcumin: A review of clinical trials. *Eur J Med Chem*. 163: 527-545.

Sanidad KZ, Zhu J, Wang W, Du Z, Zhang G. 2016. Effects of stable degradation products of curcumin on cancer cell proliferation and inflammation. *J Agric Food Chem*. 64(48): 9189-9195.

Schneider C, Gordon ON, Edwards RL, Luis PB. 2015. Degradation of curcumin: From mechanism to biological implications. *J Agric Food Chem*. 63(35): 7606-7614.

Shen L, Ji HF. 2012a. The pharmacology of curcumin: is it the degradation products? *Trends Mol Med*. 18(3): 138-144.

Shen L, Ji HF. 2012b. Low stability remedies the low bioavailability of curcumin. *Trends Mol Med*. 18(7): 363-364.

Shen L, Liu CC, An CY, Ji HF. 2016. How does curcumin work with poor bioavailability? Clues from experimental and theoretical studies. *Sci Rep*. 6: 20872.

Shoji M, Nakagawa K, Watanabe A, Tsuduki T, Yamada T, Kuwahara S *et al*. 2014. Comparison of the effects of curcumin and curcumin glucuronide in human hepatocellular carcinoma HepG2 cells. *Food Chem*. 151: 126-132.

Singh S, Aggarwal BB. 1995. Activation of transcription factor NF-kappa B is suppressed by curcumin (diferulolylmethane). *J Biol Chem*. 270(42): 24995-25000.

Sirijaroonwong S, Unchern S, Morales NP, Phisalaphong C. 2007. Free radical scavenging activity of curcumin and its derivatives. *Thai J Pharmacol*. 29(1): 60-63.

Somparn P, Phisalaphong C, Nakornchai S, Unchern S, Morales NP. 2007. Comparative antioxidant activities of curcumin and its demethoxy and hydrogenated derivatives. *Biol Pharm Bull*. 30(1): 74-78.

Vareed SK, Kakarala M, Ruffin MT, Crowell JA, Normolle DP, Djuric Z *et al*. 2008. Pharmacokinetics of curcumin conjugate metabolites in healthy human subjects. *Cancer Epidemiol Biomarkers Prev*. 17(6): 1411-1417.

Vogel H, Pelletier J. 1815. Examen chimique de la racine de curmuma. *J de Pharmacie*. I: 289-300.

Wang YJ, Pan MH, Cheng AL, Lin LI, Ho YS, Hsieh CY, Lin JK. 1997. Stability of curcumin in buffer solutions and characterization of its degradation products. *J Pharm Biomed Anal*. 15(12):1867-1876.

Wei-Xin P, Yang-De Z, Ke Y, Ye-Cheng X. 2007. Chemical constituents of *Zingiber officinale* (Zingiberaceae). *Acta Bot Yunnanica*. 29(1): 125-128.

Yu Q, Liu Y, Wu Y, Chen Y. 2018. Dihydrocurcumin ameliorates the lipid accumulation, oxidative stress and insulin resistance in oleic acid-induced L02 and HepG2 cells. *Biomed Pharmacother*. 103: 1327-1336.

Scope of the book

Considering the potential of metabolites, this book aims to bring out the pharmacological potential and the utility of the phase I metabolites of curcumin/curcuminoids especially the reductive metabolites, namely, Dihydrocurcumin, Tetrahydrocurcumin/Tetrahydrocurcuminoids, Hexahydrocurcumin and Octahydrocurcumin, their occurrence, chemical synthesis and biological significance with respect to curcumin.

Chapter 2

Dihydrocurcumin (DHC)
A Transient Metabolite With Tangible Benefits

Scope of this Review

The focus of this review is to further look into the sources of DHC and to understand the biological activities in comparison with curcumin.

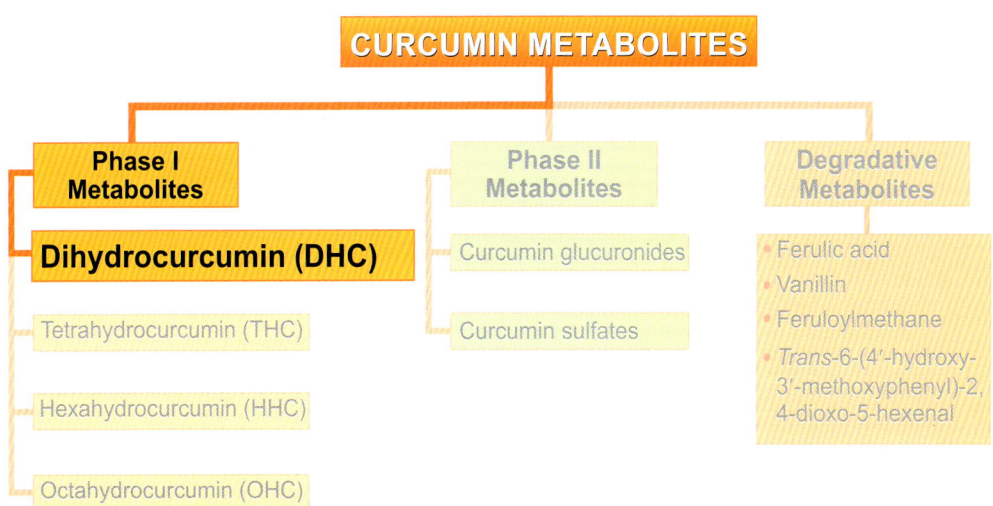

Chapter 2
DIHYDROCURCUMIN (DHC): A TRANSIENT METABOLITE WITH TANGIBLE BENEFITS

DIHYDROCURCUMIN (DHC): A TRANSIENT METABOLITE WITH TANGIBLE BENEFITS

Introduction

Curcumin, the naturally occurring polyphenolic compound which gives the yellow color to turmeric isolated from the rhizomes of *Curcuma longa* has shown multiple therapeutic activities (Govindarajan, 1980). While curcumin is identified as one of the major curcuminoids, with several pharmacological activities, dihydrocurcumin (DHC) **(6)** existing as keto-enol tautomer (Fig. 7), an intermediate reductive metabolite of curcumin formed in the body, is also found to have potential anti-inflammatory activities (Matsuda *et al.*, 2004).

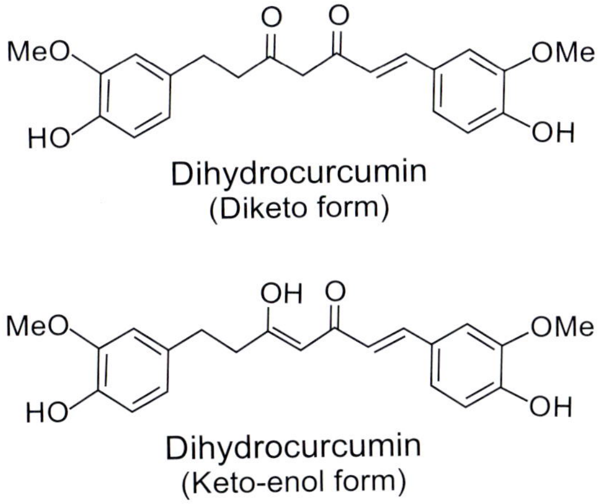

Fig. 7: Chemical structure of Dihydrocurcumin (DHC) **(6)**.

Natural Occurrence

Dihydrocurcumin (DHC) has been isolated from the rhizomes (Ravindranath and Satyanarayana, 1980), as well as from the root tuber (Wang et al., 2008) of *C. longa*. It occurs naturally in the African plant *Aframomum letestuianum* belonging to Zingiberaceae family, isolated and identified by Kamnaing et al. (2003) who named it as Letestuianin B. It has also been isolated and identified from the acetone extract of the rhizomes of *Curcuma zedoaria* cultivated in Thailand by Matsuda et al. (2004). It exists predominantly in keto-enol form (Fig. 7) in solution as deduced from its NMR in $CDCl_3$. In a recent study, Jia et al. identified DHC by characterizing curcuminoids in turmeric using ultra-high-performance liquid chromatography-quadrupole time of flight tandem mass spectrometry (UHPLC-QTOF-MS/MS) (Jia et al., 2017). Interestingly, an earlier study (Kita et al., 2009) reported that content of dihydrocurcuminoids (DHCs) was found to be more in the cell clumps, leaves and roots of *C. longa* than curcuminoids, whereas curcuminoids were found to be more abundant than DHCs in the rhizome (Table 1).

Table 1: The content of curcuminoids and DHCs in the rhizome, leaves and roots of *C. longa*. (Adapted from Kita et al., 2009)

	Contents (µg/g) dry weight			
	Cell clump	Cultured plant		
		Rhizome[a]	Leaf[b]	Root[b]
Total Curcuminoids	0.39	4785.99	0.23	0.04
Curcumin	0.07	1694.93	0.11	0.01
Demethoxycurcumin	0.31	1686.63	0.08	0.01
Bisdemethoxycurcumin	0.01	1404.43	0.04	0.02
Total Dihydrocurcuminoids	12.45	1893.15	8.23	3.45
Dihydrocurcumin	2.03	1252.58	6.82	1.02
Dihydrodemethoxycurcumin	10.11	394.36	1.26	2.17
Dihydrobisdemethoxycurcumin	0.31	246.21	0.15	0.26

[a] Average of six samples prepared from six plants and analyzed individually
[b] Samples from six plants were combined and analyzed

DIHYDROCURCUMIN (DHC): A TRANSIENT METABOLITE WITH TANGIBLE BENEFITS

Crystal Structure

Lozada *et al.* studied the crystal structure of DHC by X-ray crystallography. The molecule exists in its keto-enol form in the solid state. There is intramolecular hydrogen bonding between the enolic-OH and ketone carbonyl. The crystal structure is given in Fig. 8.

The molecule is nonplanar. The enone part of the molecule is essentially orthogonal to the rest of the structure. Dihydrocurcumin crystallizes into triclinic, *P1*. The unit cell dimensions at 293 K are $a=7.4733(6)$, $b=11.4315(9)$, $c=12.7458(10)$Å, $\alpha=113.272(2)$, $\beta=103.374(2)$, $\gamma=97.340(2)$°C, $V=943.46(13)$Å^3, $D_x=1.304$ g/cm^3, and $Z=2$. R value is $R=0.050$ for 3333 reflections. The packing of the molecules in the lattice is directed by O–H⋯O intermolecular hydrogen bonds, C–H⋯O contacts and van der Waals forces (Lozada *et al.*, 2005).

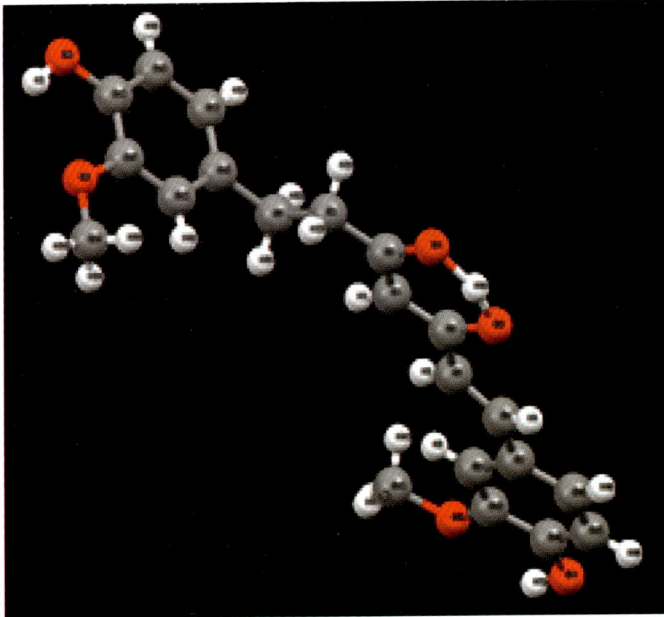

Fig. 8: Molecular structure of DHC with atom labeling.
(Adapted from Lozada *et al.*, 2005)

Metabolic Biotransformation - In vivo

Pan *et al.* examined the biotransformation of curcumin and characterized the structures of its metabolites in the plasma after oral or intraperitoneal administration of curcumin (0.1 g/kg) in mice. Based on the chemical structures of the metabolites determined by mass spectrometry/mass spectrometry (MS/MS) analysis, it was reported that curcumin was first biotransformed to DHC and THC and subsequently they were converted to monoglucuronide conjugates (Pan *et al.*, 1999).

Pharmacokinetics and Tissue Distribution - In vivo

Wang *et al.* investigated the pharmacokinetics and tissue distribution of curcumin and its metabolites in mice after intravenous administration of curcumin (20 mg/kg). It was shown that curcumin, DHC and THC were detected in plasma. Also, curcumin and THC were detected in liver while curcumin and DHC were detected in kidney whereas, only curcumin was detected in brain (Wang *et al.*, 2018).

A Metabolic Product of Gut Microbiota

Hassaninasab *et al.* reported for the first time that *Escherichia coli* (Strain K-12), a substrain of H10B isolated from human feces has the capacity to metabolize curcumin. The curcumin-converting enzyme, obtained from *E. coli* had a molecular mass of about 82-kDa and consisted of two identical subunits. This enzyme was named as "NADPH-dependent curcumin-dihydrocurcumin reductase" (CurA) and was reported to have a narrow substrate spectrum, preferentially acting on curcumin. The microbial metabolism of curcumin by the purified enzyme was found to be comprised of a two-step reduction in which curcumin being converted to NADPH-dependent-intermediate product DHC, and then into THC (Fig. 9) (Hassaninasab *et al.*, 2011).

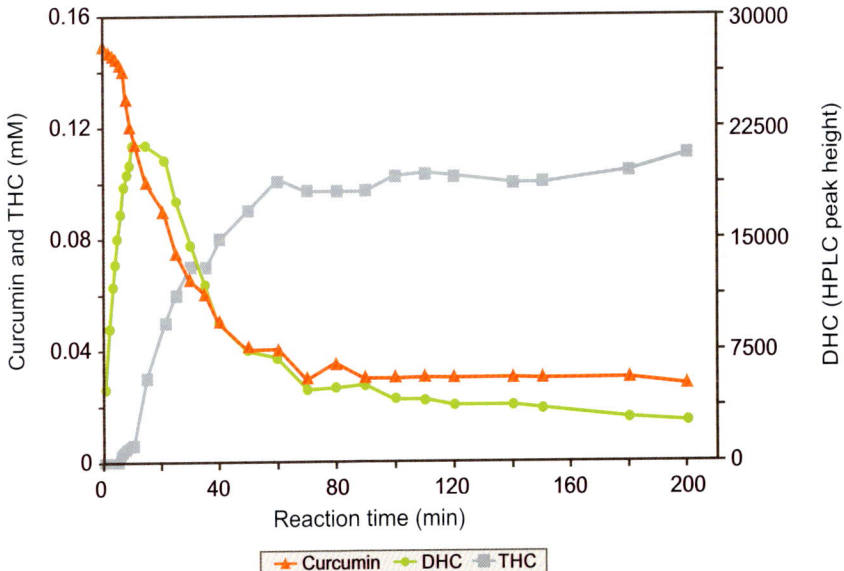

Fig. 9: Time course of curcumin conversion to DHC and THC.
(Adapted from Hassaninasab *et al.*, 2011)

Chapter 2
DIHYDROCURCUMIN (DHC): A TRANSIENT METABOLITE WITH TANGIBLE BENEFITS

Subsequently, Tan *et al.* studied the colonic bacteria mediated transformation of curcuminoids using *E. fergusonii* ATCC 35469 and *E. coli* ATCC 8739 from human fecal isolates, and *E. coli* DH10B in a modified medium for colonic bacteria (Tan *et al.*, 2014). *Escherichia coli* strain used in this study was also used by Hassaninasab *et al.* for the identification of the enzyme CurA. Interestingly, the metabolites of curcumin, DHC and THC, including ferulic acid were found in the fermentated cultures of all the three strains (Hassaninasab *et al.*, 2011).

Overall, the findings from the above two studies provide insights into the gut microbiota mediated metabolism of curcuminoids. In this process curcumin is converted to DHC and then to THC by the enzyme "CurA", through the reduction of the two C=C bonds one after the other on the heptadienone chain (Fig. 10).

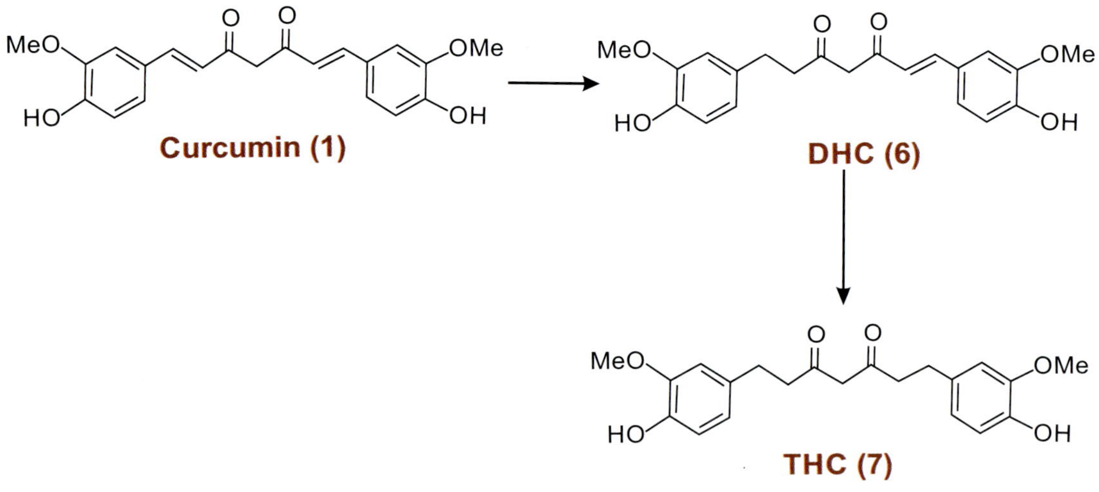

Fig. 10: Conversion of Curcumin (1) to DHC (6) and THC (7).

Pharmacological Significance

The effect of DHC on lipid accumulation, oxidative stress and insulin resistance were investigated *in vitro* using normal liver cells (L02) and hepatocarcinoma cells (HepG2) by Yu *et al.* (2018).

Cytotoxic Effects

Cell viability was investigated *in vitro* after pretreatment with oleic acid (OA) and a subsequent treatment with DHC at different concentrations in both HepG2 and L02 cells. Dihydrocurcumin concentrations at 0-20 µM in HepG2 and 0-50 µM in L02 did not compromise the cell viability *in vitro*. However, at higher concentrations (50 µM and 100 µM) a decrease in viability was observed in HepG2 cells, while 100 µM of DHC reduced the viability of L02 cells (Fig. 11) (Yu *et al.*, 2018).

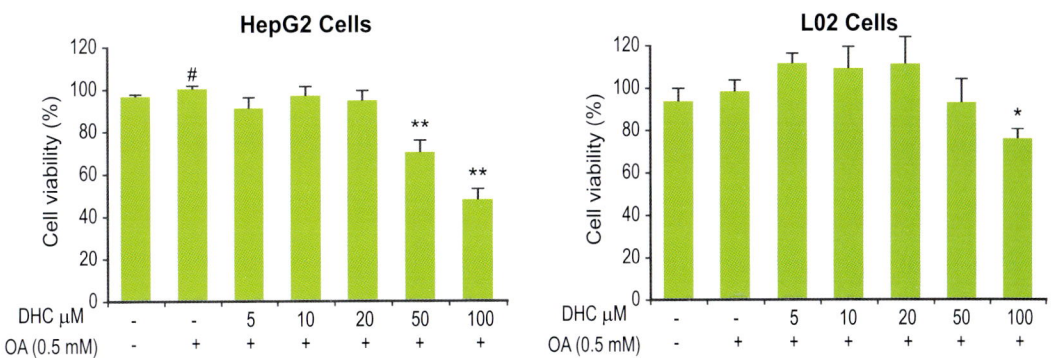

n=3; #$p<0.05$, Control vs. OA group; *$p<0.05$ and **$p<0.01$, DHC-treated vs. OA group. OA: Oleic Acid

Fig. 11: Effects of DHC on cell viability in HepG2 and L02 cells.
(Adapted from Yu *et al.*, 2018)

Antioxidant Potential

The effect of DHC was distinctly different in primary liver cells and cancerous liver cells. In HepG2 cells, OA-induced intracellular reactive oxygen species (ROS) content was further increased by DHC treatment in a dose-dependent manner ($p<0.05$), while in L02 cells DHC treatment significantly reduced the OA-induced ROS (Fig. 12). On the other hand, the OA-pretreatment for 24 h decreased the protein level of nuclear factor E2-related factor 2 (Nrf2) in both tested cells (HepG2) and normal liver cells (L02) as compared with the control group, whereas DHC treatment resulted in dose-dependent increase in protein level of Nrf2 in both the cells (Fig. 13). The transcription factor Nrf2 regulates the expression of a series of antioxidant related detoxifying genes against oxidative stress in the liver. Findings from the study suggest that DHC reduced the levels of cellular oxidative stress via activating the Nrf2 signaling pathways, and downregulated CYP4A protein and ROS levels in L02 cells, in contrast to the uniform increase in Nrf2, CYP4A and ROS in HepG2 cells (Yu *et al.*, 2018). Increase in ROS leading to apoptosis is a well-known anticancer mechanism of curcuminoids. Thus, the observed effects are likely to be a balanced result of DHC-induced antioxidant and antitumor activities.

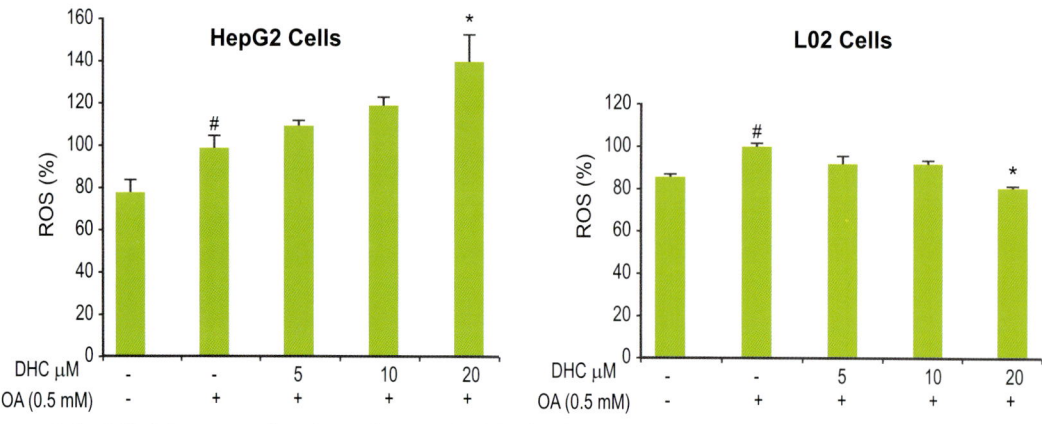

n=3, #$p<0.01$, OA-pretreated vs. Control group; *$p<0.05$, DHC-treated vs. OA-pretreated group.
OA: Oleic Acid; ROS: Reactive Oxygen Species

Fig. 12: Effects of DHC on ROS in HepG2 and L02 cells.
(Adapted from Yu *et al.*, 2018)

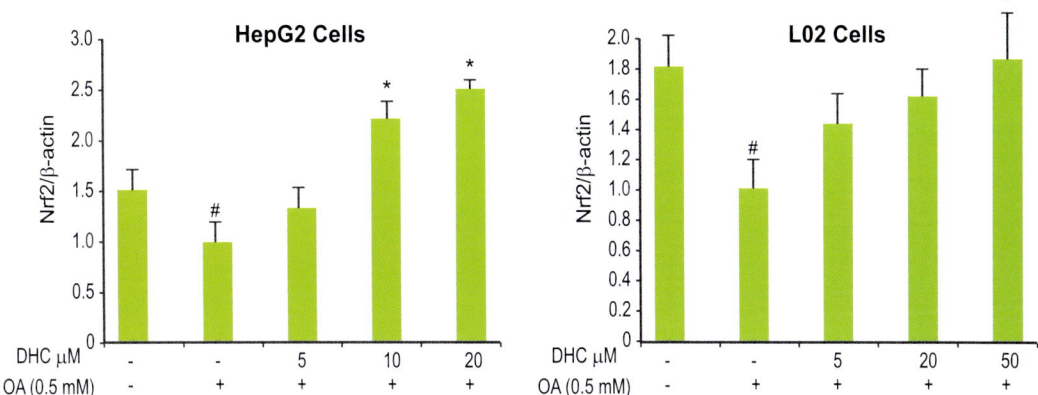

n=3, #p<0.05, OA-pretreated vs. Control group; *p<0.05, DHC-treated vs OA-pretreated group.
Nrf2: Nuclear Factor E2-Related Factor 2; OA: Oleic Acid

Fig. 13: Effects of DHC on the protein expression of Nrf2 in HepG2 and L02 cells.
(Adapted from Yu *et al.*, 2018)

Inhibition of oleic acid (OA)-induced Lipid Accumulation

Oleic acid pretreatment dramatically increased the intracellular triglyceride (TG) content compared with normal control. Dihydrocurcumin treatment was found to decrease TG content in a dose-dependent manner. Dihydrocurcumin treatment was shown to decrease lipid accumulation significantly, at 10 μM and 20 μM in HepG2 cells, and at 50 μM DHC in L02 cells (Fig. 14).

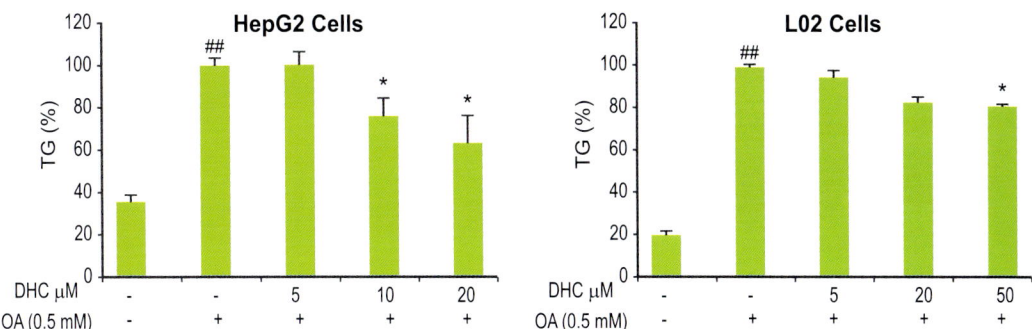

n=3, ##p<0.01, OA vs. Control group; *p<0.05, DHC-treated vs. OA-pretreated group.
OA: Oleic Acid; TG: Triglyceride

Fig. 14: Effects of DHC on TG in HepG2 and L02 cells.
(Adapted from Yu *et al.*, 2018)

Compared to the control group, OA-pretreatment increased the mRNA expression of patatin-like phospholipase domain containing protein 3 (PNPLA3) and the sterol regulatory element binding protein-1C (SREBP-1C), and decreased peroxisome proliferator-activated receptor α (PPARα) mRNA expression and the ratio of PPARα to SREBP-1C mRNA expression. While, treatment of cells with DHC in a dose-dependent manner decreased mRNA expression of PNPLA3 (Fig. 15A) and SREBP-1C (Fig. 15B), whereas it increased PPARα mRNA expression (Fig. 15C) and ratio of PPARα to SREBP-1C mRNA level (Fig. 15D). Dihydrocurcumin was shown to exert significant effects on expression levels of both the genes and proteins.

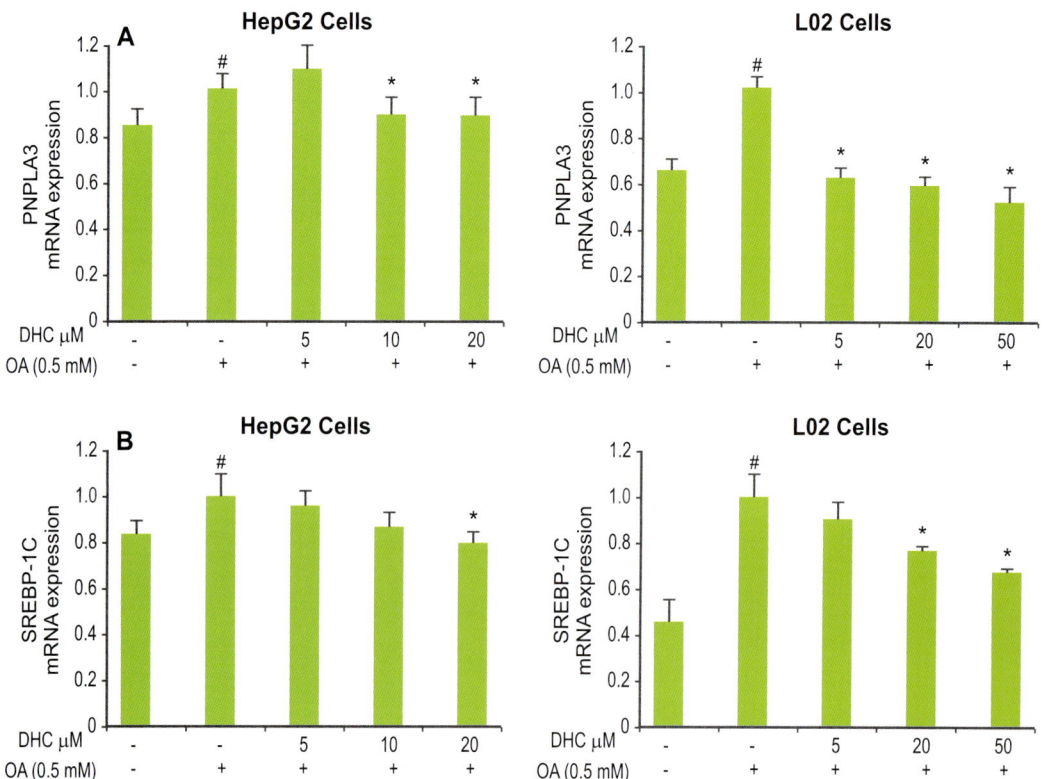

n=3, #p<0.01, OA-pretreated vs. Control group; *p<0.05, DHC-treated vs. OA-pretreated group. OA: Oleic Acid; PNPLA3: Patatin-like phospholipase domain containing protein 3; SREBP-1C: Sterol Regulatory Element Binding Protein-1C

Fig. 15A,B: Effects of DHC on PNPLA3 and SREBP-1C mRNA expression in HepG2 and L02 cells. (Adapted from Yu *et al.*, 2018)

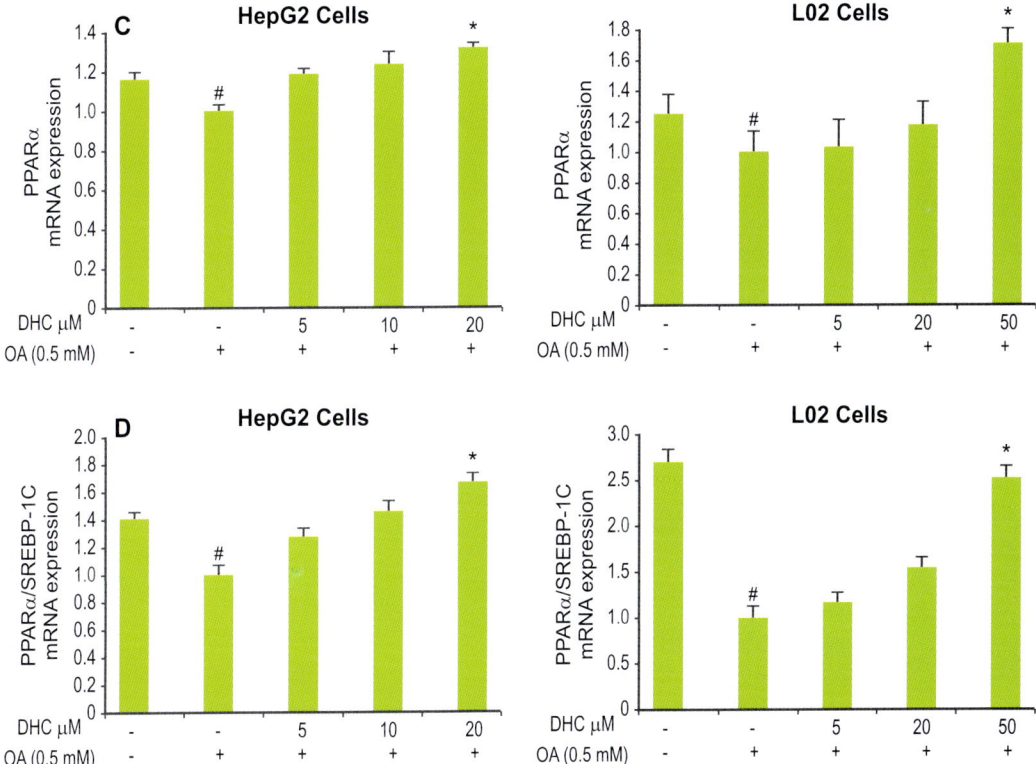

n=3, #p<0.01, OA-pretreated vs. Control group; *p<0.05, DHC-treated vs. OA-pretreated group. OA: Oleic Acid; PPARα: Peroxisome Proliferator Activated Receptor-α; SREBP-1C: Sterol Regulatory Element Binding Protein-1C

Fig. 15C,D: Effects of DHC on the PPARα mRNA expression and PPARα and SREBP-1C mRNA expression ratio in HepG2 and L02 cells. (Adapted from Yu *et al.*, 2018)

In summary, DHC decreased the levels of cellular triglycerides by regulating or modulating the mRNA and protein expression levels of SREBP-1C, PNPLA3 and PPARα (Yu *et al.*, 2018).

Insulin Resistance

Dihydrocurcumin improved the hepatocellular glucose uptake by increasing the protein expression levels of pAKT and PI3K. The results presented in the study by Yu *et al.* support the fact that DHC improved OA induced steatosis by normalizing the lipid metabolism, insulin resistance and oxidative stress in L02 and HepG2 cells. Although DHC and THC are the metabolites of curcumin, the pharmacological activity of DHC greatly contributes to overall total effect of curcumin against nonalcoholic fatty liver disease (Yu *et al.*, 2018).

Anti-allergic Activity

An aqueous-acetone extract of the *C. zedoaria* rhizomes was shown to suppress the release of β-hexosaminidase, which is a marker of mast cell degranulation in RBL-2H3. Among other components present in *C. zedoaria* extract, curcumin and DHC inhibited β-hexosaminidase activity. However, curcumin showed higher activity against β-hexosaminidase compared to DHC (Matsuda *et al.*, 2004).

Trypanocidal Activity

Dihydrocurcumin from *A. letestuianum* was tested for its growth inhibitory activity against bloodstream forms of *African trypanosomes*, *Trypanosoma b. brucei* and *Trypanosoma b. rhodesiense* isolates grown *in vitro*. Dihydrocurcumin showed greater inhibitory activity against *T. b. brucei* isolates (IC$_{50}$ value of 67 µg/mL) than *T. b. rhodesiense* (IC$_{50}$ value of 100 µg/mL), suggesting that DHC plays a potential role in trypanocidal activity (Kamnaing *et al.*, 2003).

Conclusion

Several preclinical and clinical studies have already shown that curcumin has many useful health-promoting properties. Its metabolite, DHC, augments these properties of curcumin especially the anticancer, antioxidant, lipid-lowering and anti-allergic activities as disclosed by the evidence reviewed in this chapter. The synergistic activities of the metabolite DHC, and others later to be discussed, with their parent molecule appear to explain the useful pleiotropic activities of curcumin.

Chapter 2
DIHYDROCURCUMIN (DHC): A TRANSIENT METABOLITE WITH TANGIBLE BENEFITS

References

Govindarajan VS. 1980. Turmeric—chemistry, technology, and quality. *Crit Rev Food Sci Nutr*. 12(3): 199-301.

Hassaninasab A, Hashimoto Y, Tomita-Yokotani K, Kobayashi M. 2011. Discovery of the curcumin metabolic pathway involving a unique enzyme in an intestinal microorganism. *Proc Natl Acad Sci USA*. 108(16): 6615-6620.

Jia S, Du Z, Song C, Jin S, Zhang Y, Feng Y et al. 2017. Identification and characterization of curcuminoids in turmeric using ultra-high performance liquid chromatography-quadrupole time of flight tandem mass spectrometry. *J Chromatogr A*. 1521: 110-122.

Kamnaing P, Tsopmo A, Tanifum EA, Tchuendem MH, Tane P, Ayafor JF et al. 2003. Trypanocidal diarylheptanoids from *Aframomum letestuianum*. *J Nat Prod*. 66(3): 364-367.

Kita T, Imai S, Sawada H, Seto H. 2009. Isolation of dihydrocurcuminoids from cell clumps and their distribution in various parts of turmeric (*Curcuma longa*). *Biosci Biotechnol Biochem*. 73(5): 1113-1117.

Lozada MC, Lobato CE, Enriquez RG, Ortiz B, Gnecco D, Reynolds WF et al. 2005. Crystal structures and synthesis of 5-hydroxy-1,7-bis (4-hydroxy-3-methoxyphenyl)-hept-4,6-dien-3-one. *Analytical Sciences: X-ray Structure Analysis Online*. 21: x59-x60.

Matsuda H, Tewtrakul S, Morikawa T, Nakamura A, Yoshikawa M. 2004. Anti-allergic principles from Thai zedoary: structural requirements of curcuminoids for inhibition of degranulation and effect on the release of TNF-α and IL-4 in RBL-2H3 cells. *Bioorg Med Chem*. 12(22): 5891-5898.

Pan MH, Huang TM, Lin JK. 1999. Biotransformation of curcumin through reduction and glucuronidation in mice. *Drug Metab Dispos*. 27(4): 486-494.

Ravindranath V, Satyanarayana M. 1980. An unsymmetrical diarylheptanoid from *Curcuma longa*. *Phytochemistry*. 19(9): 2031-2032.

Tan S, Rupasinghe TW, Tull DL, Boughton B, Oliver C, McSweeny C et al. 2014. Degradation of curcuminoids by *in vitro* pure culture fermentation. *J Agric Food Chem*. 62(45): 11005-11015.

Wang J, Yu X, Zhang L, Wang L, Peng Z, Chen Y. 2018. The pharmacokinetics and tissue distribution of curcumin and its metabolites in mice. *Biomed Chromatogr*. e4267.

Wang LY, Zhang M, Zhang CF, Wang ZT. 2008. Diaryl derivatives from the root tuber of *Curcuma longa*. *Biochem Syst Ecol*. 36(5): 476-480.

Yu Q, Liu Y, Wu Y, Chen Y. 2018. Dihydrocurcumin ameliorates the lipid accumulation, oxidative stress and insulin resistance in oleic acid-induced L02 and HepG2 cells. *Biomed Pharmacother*. 103: 1327-1336.

Chapter 3

Tetrahydrocurcumin (THC)
The Major Metabolite With Major Benefits

Scope of this Review

This review addresses the significance of THC, a major metabolite of curcumin, which include its natural occurrence in plants, chemical synthesis, its excellent safety margin, microbial biotransformation and absorption across the intestinal tissues. This review also focuses on the understanding of the dazzling array of pharmacological properties of THC, including slowing down the aging process and its use in oral and skin care products because of its colorless nature, a problem usually associated with curcumin.

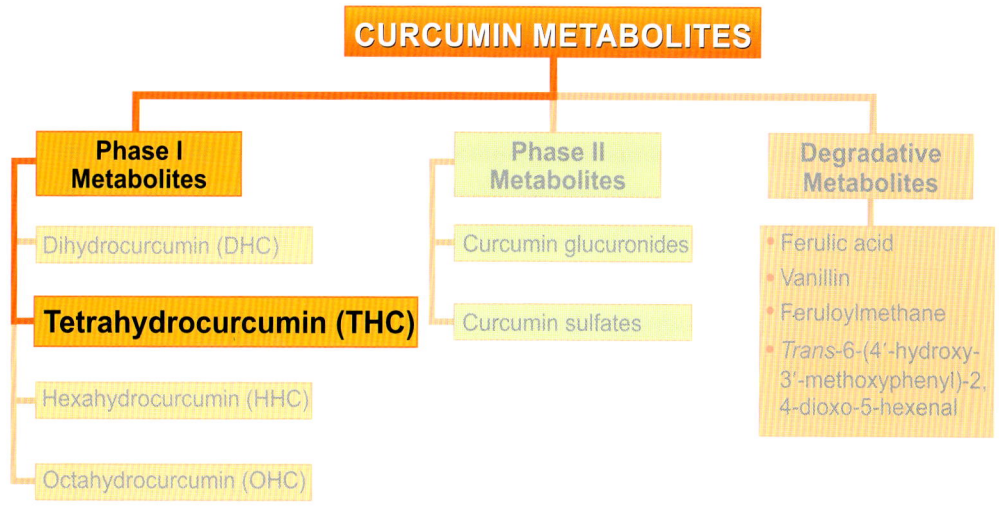

Chapter 3
TETRAHYDROCURCUMIN (THC): THE MAJOR METABOLITE WITH MAJOR BENEFITS

Chapter 3
TETRAHYDROCURCUMIN (THC): THE MAJOR METABOLITE WITH MAJOR BENEFITS

Introduction

Turmeric (*Curcuma longa L.*) is an important tropical spice commercially traded for its aroma and coloring properties. Active compounds in turmeric are typically classified as either volatile or non-volatile compounds (Surwase *et al.*, 2011).

1. Major non-volatile compounds are curcuminoids, which includes curcumin, demethoxycurcumin (DMC) and bisdemethoxycurcumin (BDMC) (Fig. 1)

2. Major volatile compounds identified in turmeric oil are *ar*-turmerone, α-turmerone, β-turmerone (curlone), *ar*-curcumene, zingiberene, α-phellandrene, 1,8-cineol and some other sesquiterpenes. Turmerones are sesquiterpenoid cyclic ketones, accounts for 40-50% of the volatile oil

The rhizomes of turmeric abound in phenolic compounds known as curcuminoids (1–6%) which are responsible for the characteristic yellow color. Sabinsa has developed a proprietary curcuminoids composition that comprises curcumin (75–81%), DMC (15–19%) and BDMC (2.5–6.5%) [US Patent Number 5,861,415]. Curcumin (1,7-bis (4'-hydroxy-3'-methoxyphenyl)-1,6-heptadiene-3,5-dione) is the most important compound in turmeric and was first isolated in 1815 (Vogel and Pelletier, 1815). It is a yellowish crystalline, odorless powder (melting point 184–186 °C), poorly soluble in water, petroleum ether and benzene; soluble in ethyl alcohol, glacial acetic acid, and in propylene

Chapter 3
TETRAHYDROCURCUMIN (THC): THE MAJOR METABOLITE WITH MAJOR BENEFITS

glycol; very soluble in acetone and diethyl ether. Absorption spectra of curcumin and curcuminoids are very similar, with their maximum absorption (λ_{Max}) at 429 nm and 424 nm, respectively (Sharma *et al.*, 2005). In addition, curcumin is considered as a non-toxic chemical to mammals even at very high doses (5-10%) by weight of diet (Samaha *et al.*, 1997; Weber *et al.*, 2005). Most of the commercial curcuminoids sold as "curcumin", are mixtures of the three curcuminoids. Curcumin C3 Complex®, the branded composition of natural curcuminoids, pioneered and patented by Sabinsa, is a well characterized and clinically documented composition. The Curcumin C3 Complex® is standardized to contain not less than 95% curcuminoids by HPLC analysis and is currently being used by several clinical researchers with Investigational New Drug (IND) approval from the US FDA and other regulatory organizations overseas.

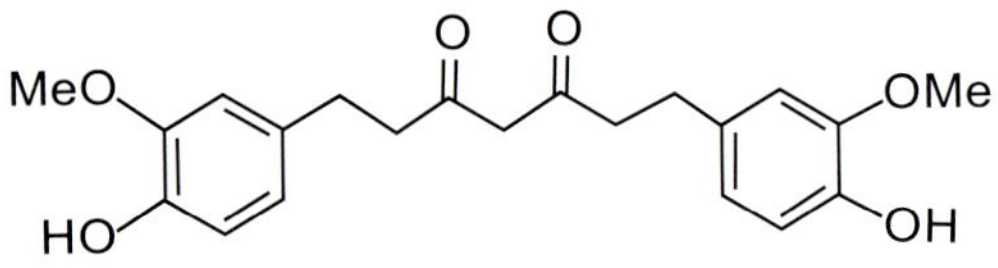

Tetrahydrocurcumin (THC) (7)

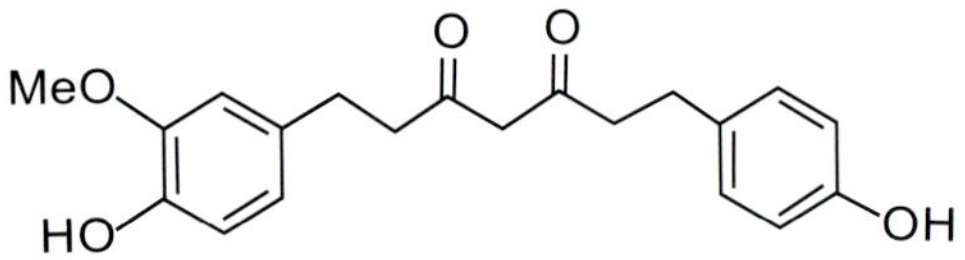

Tetrahydrodemethoxycurcumin (THDMC) (17)

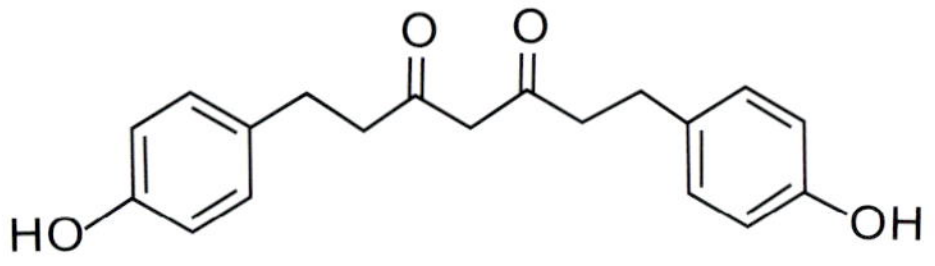

Tetrahydrobisdemethoxycurcumin (THBDMC) (18)

Fig. 16: Structures of Tetrahydrocurcuminoids (THCs).

The hydrogenated colorless derivatives of curcuminoids, namely Tetrahydrocurcuminoids (THCs) (Fig. 16) include Tetrahydrocurcumin (THC) **(7)**, Tetrahydrodemethoxycurcumin (THDMC) **(17)** and Tetrahydrobisdemethoxycurcumin (THBDMC) **(18)**. Curcumin and THC are the major constituents (≥ 75% of the total content) of the turmeric and reduced (hydrogenated) turmeric preparations, respectively. Tetrahydrocurcumin has higher physiological and pharmacological activities than its parent compound. The therapeutic interest for THC lies in their low toxicity and their beneficial biological activities (Maheshwari *et al.*, 2006). Several independent studies reported the significant antioxidant effects of THC (Portes *et al.*, 2007).

Chapter 3
TETRAHYDROCURCUMIN (THC): THE MAJOR METABOLITE WITH MAJOR BENEFITS

Tetrahydrocurcuminoids appear to be the "major active metabolites" formed when curcuminoids are intraperitoneally administered to mice. Structurally, THC and curcumin have identical β-diketone structures and phenolic groups. However, THC lacks the double bonds of curcumin (Okada *et al.*, 2001).

Characteristics of Tetrahydrocurcumin

Chemical Name : 1,7-Bis(4'-hydroxy-3'-methoxyphenyl)-3,5-heptanedione

CAS Number : 36062-04-1

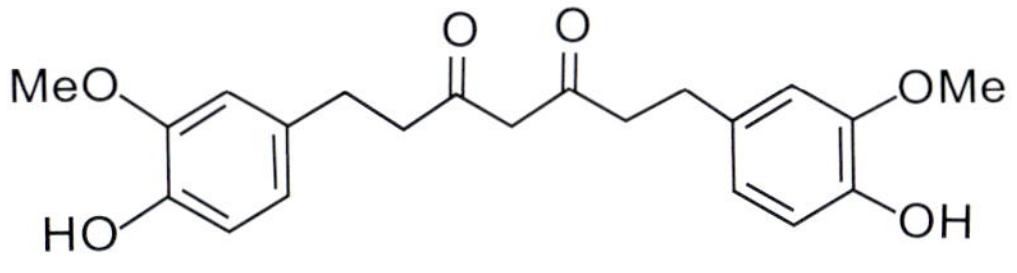

Tetrahydrocurcumin (7)

Molecular Formula : $C_{21}H_{24}O_6$

General Properties

    Molecular Weight : 372.41

    Melting Range : 97–99 °C

    Appearance : Off white to white powder

    Solubility : Insoluble in water and soluble in organic solvents like acetone, ethyl acetate, chloroform and isopropanol

Chapter 3
TETRAHYDROCURCUMIN (THC): THE MAJOR METABOLITE WITH MAJOR BENEFITS

Natural Occurrence

Tetrahydrocurcumin has been isolated as a natural product from *Zingiber* and *Curcuma* species of the family Zingiberaceae. Tetrahydrocurcumin (3,5-dione-1,7-bis (4'-hydroxy-3'-methoxyphenyl) heptane) from the rhizomes of *Z. officinale* Rosc (Ginger) was isolated along with other compounds (Peng *et al.*, 2007). Subsequently, Li *et al.* (2012) isolated THC from the rhizomes of *Z. officinale*, along with other diarylheptanoids. Han *et al.* (2015) characterized the metabolites from above ground and root parts of *Z. mioga* and *Z. officinale* by UHPLC-Q-TOF-MS/MS and gas chromatography time-of-flight mass spectrometry (GC-TOF-MS). Tetrahydrocurcumin, [8]-gingerol, and [8]-paradol were the distinguishing metabolites between *Z. mioga* and *Z. officinale* that were present in different quantities. The roots of *Z. officinale* had relatively high contents of THC, diarylheptanoid, and galanganol C and showed high antioxidant activities. More recently, several compounds were isolated from the chloroform extract of *Z. officinale* rhizome and characterized as [6]-dehydrogingerol, *N*-methyl-2-pyrolidinone, [6]-gingerol, [8]-gingerol, [6]-shogaol, THC, HHC and *meso*-3, 5-diacetoxy-1,7-bis (4'-hydroxy-3'-methoxyphenyl) heptane. The structures were elucidated by analysing their spectroscopic data (Sharma and Sahai, 2018).

The minor constituents, THDMC and THBDMC, also occur naturally in the *Curcuma* species. Both THDMC and THBDMC are found in the rhizome of Thai Zeodary (*Curcuma zedoaria*), an anti-inflammatory material in Thai traditional medicine system (Matsuda *et al.*, 2004). Additionally, analysis at Sami Labs, the R&D and manufacturing arm of Sabinsa, also showed the presence of THC in *C. zedoaria* as identified by TLC and confirmed by Mass Spectral fragmentation studies. Thus, all the three constituents of THCs, namely THC, THDMC and THBDMC are found to occur naturally in plants that have been consumed either as part of the food or traditional medicine. Recent studies also identified THCs during characterization of curcuminoids in turmeric using UHPLC-Q-TOF- MS/MS (Jia *et al.*, 2017) and by NMR (Friesen *et al.*, 2019).

Biotransformation of Curcumin to THC

Curcumin is first biotransformed to DHC and THC, and these compounds are subsequently converted to monoglucuronide conjugates including curcumin-glucuronide, dihydrocurcumin-glucuronide and tetrahydrocurcumin-glucuronide in mouse (Lin *et al.*, 2000). In human and rat hepatocytes, curcumin is metabolized into curcumin glucuronide, curcumin sulfate, THC, HHC and OHC (Ireson *et al.*, 2002). In a recent study, *Marchantia polymorpha* cells have been shown to convert curcumin into THC with 90% yield in one day (Shimoda *et al.*, 2012).

In commercial preparations of THCs, the curcuminoids are converted to THCs under low pressure hydrogenation with palladium carbon (Pd/C) (Majeed *et al.*, 2007; Patent #EP1171144) or Raney Nickel (Ni) as the catalyst.

Identification & Quantification

Recently Novaes *et al.* (2017) analyzed THC by using ultra-high performance liquid chromatography (UHPLC). The HPLC analysis was performed in a Shimadzu Nexera UHPLC system coupled with Shimadzu LCMS 8040 triple quadrupole mass spectrometer (Shimadzu, Kyoto, Japan). Waters Acquity UPLC BEH C18 column under isocratic conditions with 45% aqueous acetonitrile in 0.1% formic acid and a flow rate of 0.4 mL/min was used for the chromatography. Under the chromatographic conditions, the tautomers of THC were resolved into the keto and enol forms with the retention times at 1.4 and 2.7 min respectively. The analysis was nearly identical with the earlier reports of Liu *et al.* (2006). The

Chapter 3
TETRAHYDROCURCUMIN (THC): THE MAJOR METABOLITE WITH MAJOR BENEFITS

presence of THC in keto-enol forms was determined by multiple reaction monitoring (MRM) in positive mode using curcumin as a reference standard and found to be almost with 1:1 ratio (Fig. 17). The concentration of THC was quantified by summation of both (keto and enol) the peak areas.

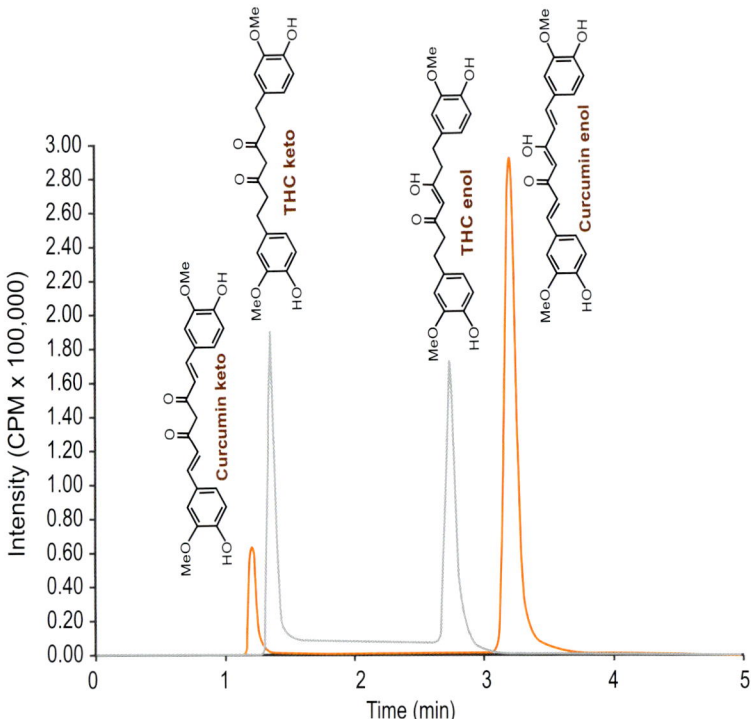

Fig. 17: Chromatograms of THC and curcumin as enol and keto forms determined by UHPLC/LC–MS/MS assay (Concentration: 1 µg/mL in acetonitrile).
(Adapted from Novaes *et al*. 2017)

A typical HPLC method was adopted for quantification of THCs.

The HPLC analysis was performed in a Shimadzu LC-20AD HPLC system with BDS Hypersil C18 (Thermo) (250 x 4.6 cm, 5 µM) column, Ultra-violet/Photo-diode array (UV/PDA) detector and detection at 280 nm.

The HPLC analysis was performed by isocratic elution with mobile phase acetonitrile and 0.1% formic acid in water in the ratio of 50:50 and a flow rate at 1 mL/min. The eluent was filtered through 0.45 µm millipore filter paper and degassed in an ultrasonic bath before use. A 20 µL of sample solution was injected for the analysis.

The sample solution was prepared by dissolving 50 mg of THCs with 50 mL of methanol in a 100 mL of volumetric flask. After sonication for 15 min, the volume was adjusted up to 100 mL with methanol.

The HPLC patterns of THCs showed three peaks and the order of elution was observed based on the relative retention time (RRT) values for enol forms.

    Tetrahydrobisdemethoxycurcumin   : RRT - 1.112

    Tetrahydrodemethoxycurcumin   : RRT - 1.053

    Tetrahydrocurcumin   : RRT - 1.000

Preparation of THC by Hydrogenation

Tetrahydrocurcumin is prepared by hydrogenation (Fig. 18) of curcumin in an inert solvent in the presence of a metallic catalyst like Pd/C or Raney Ni (Mimura *et al.*, 1993). Subsequent studies also derived THC from curcumin by hydrogenation (Matsuda *et al.*, 2004) by following previously established protocols (Sui *et al.*, 1993).

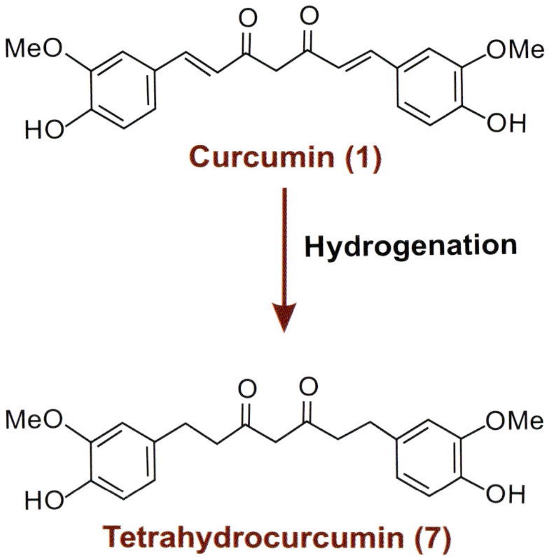

Fig. 18: Preparation of THC

Chapter 3
TETRAHYDROCURCUMIN (THC): THE MAJOR METABOLITE WITH MAJOR BENEFITS

Crystal Structure

The three-dimensional crystal structure of THC has been studied by X-ray crystallography (Girija *et al.*, 2004). The molecule is non-planar, and the benzene rings positioned at the ends of the heptane chain are orthogonally placed with a dihedral angle of 84.09°, which is very close to 90°. This means that the benzene rings are almost perpendicular to each other. The crystal structure of THC is given below (Fig. 19):

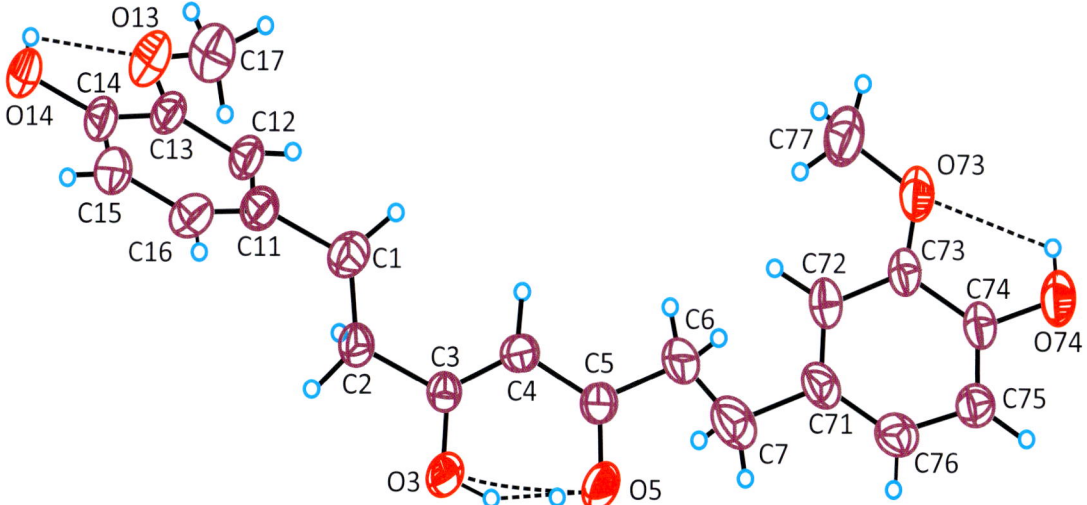

Fig. 19: Crystal structure of THC.
(Adapted from Girija *et al.*, 2004)

The molecular geometry and H-atom locations reveal that the 'heptane-3,5-dione' moiety exists in the keto-enol form, with the enolic hydroxyl H-atom equally disordered between the O-3 and O-5 dione moiety. Of the possible tautomeric forms, in the crystal phase, β-diketones prefer the *cis*-enol arrangement stabilized by a strong intramolecular hydrogen bond.

X-ray diffraction study confirms the existence of tautomeric form. The tautomerism is given in Fig. 20.

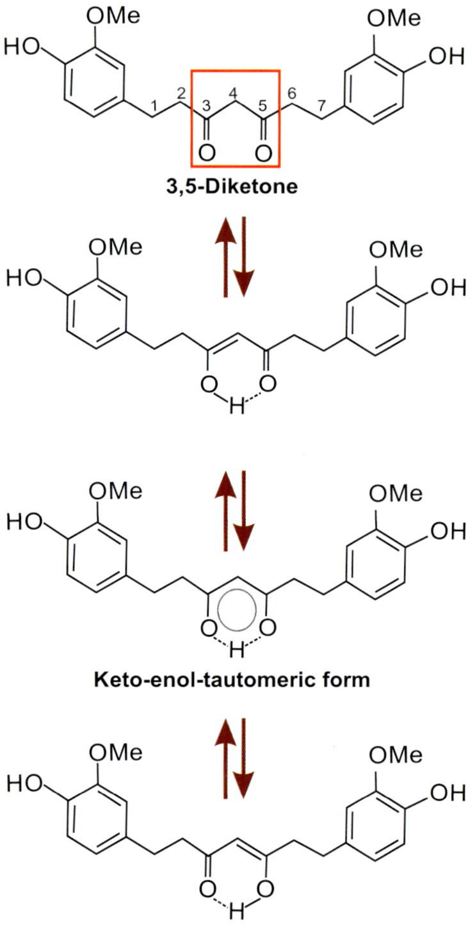

Fig. 20: Tautomeric forms of THC.

Chapter 3
TETRAHYDROCURCUMIN (THC): THE MAJOR METABOLITE WITH MAJOR BENEFITS

Microbial Transformation

Tetrahydrocurcumin, a partially reduced derivative of curcumin found in turmeric, appears to be the major active metabolite formed when curcumin is administered intraperitoneally to the mice (Anand et al., 2008).

A recent and very interesting finding demonstrated that curcumin in the human intestine is converted into THC by *E. coli* and that the resulting THC may be responsible for curcuminoids-mediated biological activities in the human body (Fig. 21) (Hassaninasab et al., 2011). The study found that purified "NADPH-dependent Curcumin/Dihydrocurcumin reductase" (CurA) enzyme from *E. coli* strain K-12, sub strain DH10B catalyzed two reaction steps wherein curcumin was first reduced to DHC followed by the latter's sequential reduction to THC. Thus, the study led to the discovery of two-step curcumin metabolic pathway catalyzed by CurA. The products DHC and THC were generated from curcumin through reductive destruction of the chromatic diarylheptatrienone chain. The lack of production of further reduced reaction products suggested that CurA catalyzes reduction of only compounds with C-C double bonds. The CurA was found to be substrate-specific, NADPH dependent, metal independent and stable at wide pH range (4.5–12.0). All these evidences show that CurA could be a potent catalyst for the production of large amount of value-added product *in vitro*.

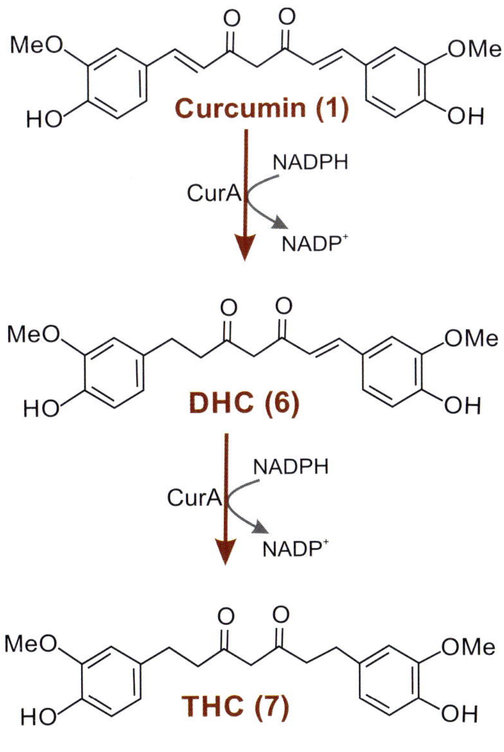

Fig. 21: Metabolic pathway of curcumin in intestine. (Adapted from Hassaninasab et al., 2011)

The study provides immense support for the understanding that THC represents the predominant, more biologically active metabolite of curcumin.

Subsequently, Tan *et al.* (2014) elucidated the metabolism of curcuminoids using pure culture of *E. fergusonii* (ATCC 35469) and two other *E. coli* strains (ATCC 8739 and DH10B), which also contain the YncB gene that encodes for CurA, cultured in modified medium for colon bacteria (mMCB) with or without pig cecal fluid. The authors have demonstrated that the metabolism of curcuminoids (curcumin, DMC and BDMC) by three different *Escherichia* bacterial cultures resulted in the metabolism of curcumin to DHC, THC and ferulic acid (FA). This study provided further supporting evidence on the breakdown products of curcumin and the relative abundance of different curcumin metabolites.

In this context, Tan *et al.* (2015) used an *in vitro* model containing human starters and showed that after 24 h of human fecal fermentation, the three curcuminoids, curcumin, DMC and BDMC were degraded resulting in the formation of THC, dihydroferulic acid (DFA) and an unidentified molecule as a major metabolite of curcuminoids. It was concluded that ingested curcuminoids have potential beneficial effects, which might be attributed to their colonic metabolites, such as THC, which is common with other polyphenolic dietary sources.

Curcumin has also been converted to THC by microbial transformation with the yeast *Debaryomyces hansenii* (Kamiya et al., 1999; Sakai and Kamiya, 2003). Maehara *et al.* (2011) investigated the microbial conversion of curcumin by an endophytic fungus *Diaporthe* sp (CLO-13), isolated from the rhizome of *C. longa*. Findings from this study revealed the existence of four colorless derivatives, namely (3R,5R)-THC **(19)**, (3R,5S)-HHC named neohexahydrocurcumin **(20)**, (3S,5S)-OHC **(21)** and *meso*-OHC **(22)** (Fig. 22). It was reported that THC and the other three derivatives inhibited the peroxidation of microsomal and mitochondrial lipids prepared from rat liver.

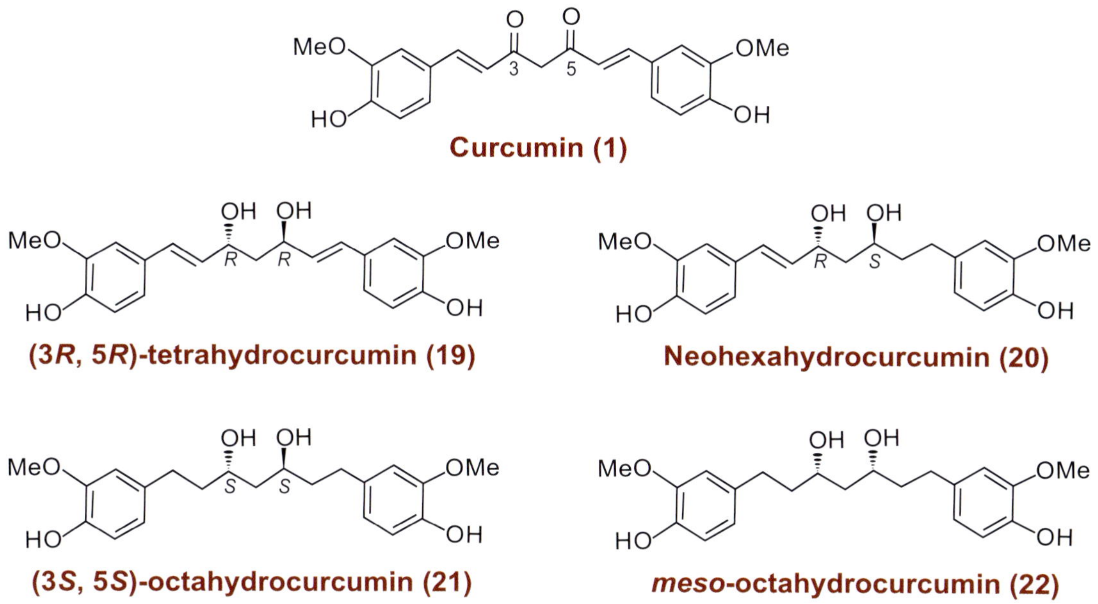

Chapter 3
TETRAHYDROCURCUMIN (THC): THE MAJOR METABOLITE WITH MAJOR BENEFITS

Curcumin (1)

(3R, 5R)-tetrahydrocurcumin (19)

Neohexahydrocurcumin (20)

(3S, 5S)-octahydrocurcumin (21)

***meso*-octahydrocurcumin (22)**

Fig. 22: Chemical structures of curcumin and its microbial conversion products.

Among the four reduction products, THC and HHC as major products, and DHC and OHC as minor ones were detected in humans and animals, whereas only DHC and THC were identified in microorganism using purified enzymes. It is suggested that THC converted from curcumin in the human intestine is responsible for various activities in the human body. It has been reported that THC is more potent than curcumin with respect to anti-inflammatory (Mukhopadhyay *et al.*, 1982), antidiabetic and anti-hyperlipidemic (Pari and Murugan, 2007a) activity, and has equally potent antioxidant activity (Osawa *et al.*, 1995; Sugiyama *et al.*, 1996).

Absorption Characteristics: Curcumin vs. THC

Distribution of Curcumin vs. THC in Serum and Liver *(Okada et al., 2001)*

In an animal study on the amelioration of oxidative stress induced renal injury, two separate groups of mice (n=6) were fed with diet containing 0.5% of curcumin and 0.5% of THC for one month. The distribution of curcumin and THC was determined in serum and liver tissue at the end of the study.

The concentration of THC in liver and serum was higher than curcumin in both groups (Tables 2 & 3), thus providing proof that orally ingested curcumin is converted to THC which is more easily absorbed from the GI tract.

Table 2: Distribution of curcuminoids in liver and serum of mice fed with curcumin.

	Liver		Blood Serum
	Free (nmol/mg)	Conjugate (nmol/mg)	Free + Conjugate (nmol/mL)
Curcumin	Not Detected	Not Detected	0.6 ± 0.1
THC	Not Detected	3.5 ± 0.4	14.4 ± 3.9

Table 3: Distribution of curcuminoids in liver and serum of mice fed with THC.

	Liver		Blood Serum
	Free (nmol/mg)	Conjugate (nmol/mg)	Free + Conjugate (nmol/mL)
Curcumin	Not Detected	Not Detected	Not Detected
THC	2.5 ± 0.6	7.9 ± 1.6	43.4 ± 15.5

Chapter 3
TETRAHYDROCURCUMIN (THC): THE MAJOR METABOLITE WITH MAJOR BENEFITS

Pharmacokinetics and Tissue Distribution of Curcumin and THC

Nano formulation of curcumin has been extensively used to improve its limited bioavailability and prolong its presence in the plasma, following oral administration and thereby optimizing its therapeutic potential. Lipocurc™ (liposomal curcumin) is a nano formulation that was developed for parenteral administration. The pharmacokinetics and safety of intravenously administered Lipocurc™ have been extensively studied in animal models and in Phase I clinical study in human.

The safety, pharmacokinetics, excretion and tissue distribution of curcumin and its metabolite, THC were studied in Beagle dogs following intravenous infusion of Lipocurc™ at a dose of 10 mg/kg over a 2 h and 8 h infusion times (Helson *et al.*, 2012; Matabudul *et al.*, 2012). Infusion of Lipocurc™ in dogs at two different time periods resulted in higher plasma levels of curcumin and THC with a 2 h infusion compared to an 8 h infusion. **Tetrahydrocurcuin levels in the plasma were 6.3–9.6 fold higher than curcumin during both infusion rates**, indicating the putative existence of a faster curcumin reducing enzyme in blood or tissues and comparatively slow rate of blood THC clearance. The plasma half-lives of both compounds following 2 h infusion was observed to be in the range of 0.4–0.7 h resulting from both hepatic and renal clearance.

Interestingly, Matabudul *et al.* (2012) reported that both curcumin and THC were extensively distributed in tissues, with the lung and liver having the highest levels. Tissue partition coefficients for curcumin and THC were also higher for the 8 h infusion than the 2 h infusion. The tissue THC/curcumin ratio varied in a tissue specific manner and was lower for the 8 h compared to the 2 h infusion. Tissue levels of curcumin were considerably higher following the 8 h infusion of curcumin, despite much lower plasma curcumin concentrations. Pharmacokinetic and distribution data of curcumin and THC in plasma and tissues reflect their net contribution to therapeutic effects.

Chapter 3
TETRAHYDROCURCUMIN (THC): THE MAJOR METABOLITE WITH MAJOR BENEFITS

Tan *et al.* (2016) used LC–MS/MS method with a basic mobile phase for the quantification of THC in human plasma over the concentration range of 5–2500 ng/mL and suggested that a mobile phase could be selected based mainly on its merits to facilitate LC separation and/or MS detection.

Storka *et al.* (2015) conducted a Phase I clinical study to address the safety and tolerability of liposomal curcumin in humans. A single intravenous dose of liposomal curcumin in healthy humans showed dose-dependent increase in the plasma concentrations of curcumin and its metabolite, THC in the first 15 minutes, which remained stable during the infusion time. The authors observed that the plasma exposure to THC post-infusion compared to during infusion was not decreased as much as for curcumin, suggesting that curcumin cleared rapidly from the plasma into tissues is still being metabolized to THC post-infusion. It was concluded that a single intravenous dose of liposomal curcumin is considered safe up to a dose of 120 mg/m^2 when infused over a period of 2 h.

Zhongfa *et al.* (2012) used a nano-emulsion preparation containing 20% curcumin (w/w) to examine the pharmacokinetics of curcuminoids and curcumin metabolites in mice. A 10-fold increase in the area under the curve ($AUC_{(0 \to 24h)}$) and >40 fold increase in the C_{max} was seen after the oral dose of nano-emulsion in comparison to curcumin suspension in 1% methylcellulose. The plasma pharmacokinetics was studied for the two natural congeners, DMC and BDMC, and three metabolites, THC, curcumin-*O*-glucuronide, and curcumin-*O*-sulfate in mice after an oral dose of NEC. Tetrahydrocurcumin could be detected in mouse plasma 30 minutes after oral administration and the terminal elimination half-life of the metabolites were found to be in the following order: Curcumin-*O*-glucuronide > Curcumin > DMC > THC > BDMC > Curcumin-*O*-sulfate. The ratio of AUC/dose was higher for BDMC followed by DMC and curcumin, in mice after an oral dose of 1 g/kg NEC, hence the bioavailability of both BDMC and DMC are more than that of curcumin.

A recent study investigated the absorption of solubilized THC (provided by Sabinsa) released from the self- microemulsifying drug delivery system (SMEDDS) floating tablets using Caco-2 cell monolayers. The SMEDDS consists of colloidal silicon dioxide, HPMC

Chapter 3
TETRAHYDROCURCUMIN (THC): THE MAJOR METABOLITE WITH MAJOR BENEFITS

K4M, sodium bicarbonate, tartaric acid, lactose and silicified-microcrystalline cellulose. The results of the Caco-2 permeation studies showed that both liquid and solid SMEDDS formulations showed a comparatively higher (three to five fold) transport of THC than the unformulated drug. The findings suggested that the oral bioavailability of THC could be improved by a self-microemulsifying tablet (Sermkaew *et al.*, 2013).

Plyduang *et al.* (2014) investigated the drug loading and release of THC conjugated with a hydrophilic polymer, carboxymethylcellulose (CMC) to the colon of rats. SabiWhite® (Tetrahydrocurcumin Ultra-Pure) was provided by Sabinsa. The active molecule, 4-amino-THC, was readily released from the conjugates in the colon within 24 h, and with only very small amounts released in the upper GI tract over 12 h. The cytotoxic activity of the 4-amino-THC was compared to curcumin and THC with normal and colon cancer cell lines. The results of this study confirmed that THC and curcumin were potent inhibitors of cell growth, and their effects occurred in a dose-dependent manner on HT-29 cells. The cytotoxic activity of 4-amino-THC was less than THC and curcumin in cancer cell lines. Only least cytotoxicity was observed in normal colon cells.

Jager *et al.* (2014) compared the levels of curcuminoids (curcumin, DMC, BDMC) and the metabolite THC after oral administration of three different curcumin formulations: curcumin phytosome formulation, cellulosic derivatives and natural antioxidants (CHC) in comparison to a standardized curcumin mixture. Based on the AUC, it was observed that the plasma concentration of THC, was increased significantly with the CHC formulation of curcumin.

In a recent study, Bolger *et al.* (2017) investigated the distribution of curcumin in Beagle dog and human blood cells and hepatocytes using a concentration of 2 µM curcumin (as Lipocurc™), this dose was found to be constant in intravenous infusion studies with Lipocurc™ carried out earlier. It has been reported that Lipocurc™ was distributed in red blood cells and peripheral blood mononuclear cells (PBMCs). Compared to red blood cells, a higher concentration was observed in PBMCs, particularly when expressed on a per cell basis. Although curcumin metabolism to THC was observed across all blood cell types, there was a significant species difference on the disposition and metabolism of curcumin between dog and human blood cells. The disposition of curcumin in blood cells is, therefore, species-dependent and of pharmacokinetic relevance. The same group in a recent study, investigated the distribution of liposomal curcumin and its metabolism to THC in human PBMCs obtained from healthy individuals (PBMC$_{HI}$) and chronic lymphocytic leukemia (CLL) patients (PBMC$_{CLL}$) *in vitro*. Peripheral blood mononuclear cells from CLL patients displayed a 2.2–2.6 fold higher distribution of curcumin compared to PBMC$_{HI}$ but the metabolism of curcumin to THC was not markedly different in the two samples. The study concluded that the distribution of curcumin into PBMCs from CLL patients was higher compared to PBMCs from healthy individuals leading to its therapeutic benefit (Bolger *et al.*, 2018).

Recently, the pharmacokinetics and tissue distribution of curcumin and its metabolites in mice were investigated (Wang *et al.*, 2018) after intravenous administration of curcumin (20 mg/kg). It has been reported that AUC for curcumin was high (107.0 ± 18.3 mg/L min) in the plasma. In the case of curcumin metabolites, the plasma absorption value for THC was higher (12.0 ± 4.0 mg/L min) than DHC (6.0 ± 1.2 mg/L min). The findings also show that curcumin and THC were detected in liver, while curcumin and DHC, and not THC were detected in kidney. Interestingly, only curcumin was detected in the brain. Overall findings indicated that THC was the major metabolite of curcumin detected in the plasma. The exposure of curcumin in plasma was 6-fold greater than that in liver, kidney and brain.

Pharmacological Significance

Antioxidant Potential

Free radicals play a major role in the pathogenesis and progression of various diseases, including neurodegenerative diseases, myocardial ischemia/reperfusion (I/R) injury and cancer as well as deteriorating changes associated with aging. The antioxidant potential of curcumin comparable to α-tocopherol has been well established in many *in vitro* models. The therapeutic benefits of curcumin have been demonstrated in several animal models of oxidative stress such as Alzheimer's disease, ethanol-induced injury in brain, liver, kidney and myocardial ischemic damage, despite the claim about its poor bioavailability. It is suggested that THC, the metabolite of curcumin may be the mediator of major antioxidant activity *in vivo* (Somparn *et al.*, 2007).

Mechanisms of Action

Tetrahydrocurcuminoids counteract free radicals in 2 ways

- **PREVENTION** of free radical formation
- **INTERVENTION** whereby already preformed radicals are quenched

Tetrahydrocurcuminoids have been recognized as **BIOPROTECTANT**® composition.

A set of studies performed by Sabinsa (Figs. 23 & 24) revealed that THCs were found to be more potent antioxidants than the commonly used antioxidant, vitamin C.

Chapter 3
TETRAHYDROCURCUMIN (THC): THE MAJOR METABOLITE WITH MAJOR BENEFITS

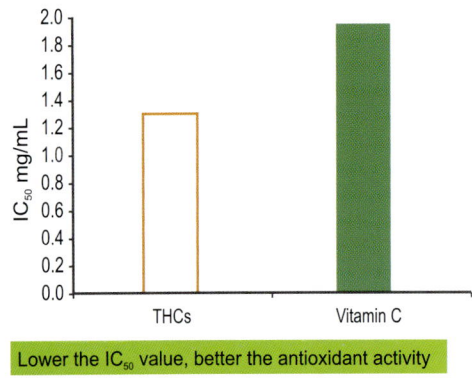

Fig. 23: Comparison of antioxidant activity of THCs with vitamin C by DPPH method.

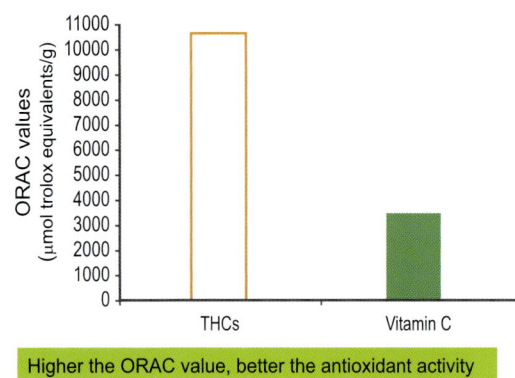

Fig. 24: Comparison of antioxidant activity of THCs with vitamin C by ORAC method.

In the 1,1 diphenyl-2-picrylhydrazyl (DPPH) radical scavenging method, the ability of an antioxidant to bind with and quench the DPPH radical (a very stable free radical species) is measured, using various concentrations of the selected antioxidants.

A compound with high antioxidant potential effectively traps this radical, thereby, preventing propagation and the resultant chain reaction.

Recently, attention has been focused on THC, because this compound appears to exert a greater antioxidant activity than curcumin in both *in vitro* and *in vivo* systems (Okada *et al.*, 2001; Pari and Murugan, 2004). Sugiyama *et al.* demonstrated that THC exhibited similar physiological and pharmacological properties as the active form of curcumin *in vivo* (Sugiyama *et al.*, 1996), while Naito *et al.* showed an involvement of THC in biochemical and molecular actions at the cellular level in ameliorating oxidative stress in cholesterol-fed rabbits (Naito *et al.*, 2002). Tetrahydrocurcumin has been reported to have more potent antioxidant activity than curcumin (Okada *et al.*, 2001). In a series of studies conducted by Sabinsa (Majeed *et al.*, 1995), the free radical scavenging ability of curcumin, BDMC and THC were evaluated by using DPPH assay. As shown in Fig. 25, all the compounds tested significantly neutralized free radicals in a dose-dependent manner. Among compounds tested, THC was found to be the most effective, followed by curcumin and BDMC.

Chapter 3
TETRAHYDROCURCUMIN (THC): THE MAJOR METABOLITE WITH MAJOR BENEFITS

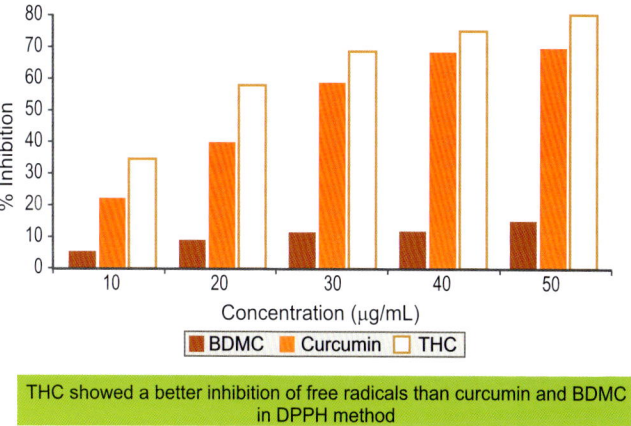

Fig. 25: Effects of THC, Curcumin and BDMC on free radical scavenging activity.
(Adapted from Majeed *et al.*, 1995)

Studies performed for understanding the molecular mechanism revealed that the phenolic hydroxy groups rather than the β-diketone moiety of THC are accountable for the enhanced antioxidant activity of THC compared to that of curcumin (Fig. 26) (Portes *et al.*, 2007).

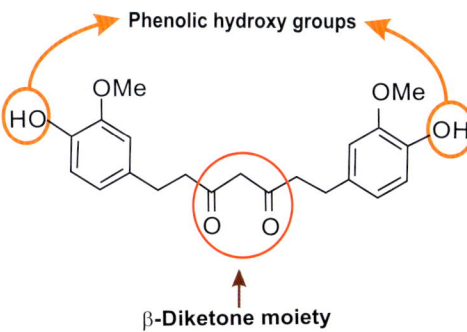

Fig. 26: Structure of THC.

Inhibition of AAPH-induced Linoleic Acid Oxidation by Curcuminoids (Somparn et al., 2007)

The 2,2'-azobis (2-amidinopropane) dihydrochloride (AAPH) is a water-soluble azo compound, which is used extensively as a free radical generator often in the study of lipid peroxidation and the characterization of antioxidants. A comparative study to identify antioxidant activity of curcumin, DMC, BDMC, and the hydrogenated derivatives (THC, HHC and OHC) was carried out using DPPH radical, AAPH-induced linoleic oxidation and AAPH-induced red blood cell hemolysis assays. The DPPH scavenging activity was significantly higher in hydrogenated derivatives of curcumin than a reference antioxidant, trolox (Fig. 27).

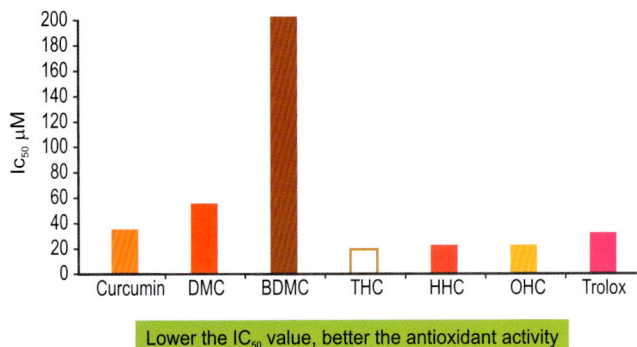

Fig. 27: DPPH radical scavenging activity of curcumin, its derivatives and trolox.
(Adapted from Somparn et al., 2007)

It was revealed that the hydrogenated derivatives had stronger antioxidant activity on lipid peroxidation (Fig. 28) and red blood cell hemolysis (Fig. 29). By using AAPH-induced linoleic acid oxidation model, the stoichiometric number of peroxyl radicals trapped per molecule of hydrogenated derivatives were found to be 3.4, 3.8 and 3.1 for THC, HHC and OHC, respectively. For curcumin and DMC, the values observed were 2.7 and 2.0, respectively, that are similar to trolox, whereas the value was 1.4 for BDMC.

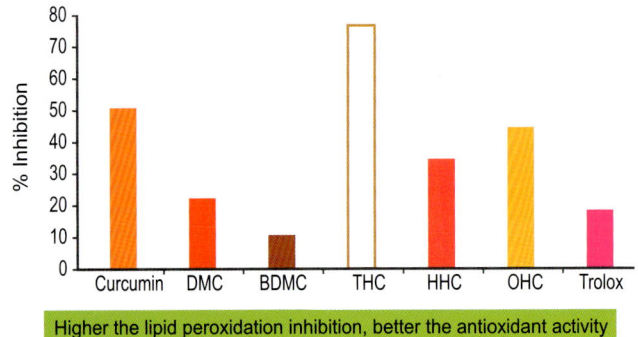

Fig. 28: Lipid peroxidation inhibition by curcumin, its derivatives and trolox.
(Adapted from Somparn et al., 2007)

TETRAHYDROCURCUMIN (THC): THE MAJOR METABOLITE WITH MAJOR BENEFITS

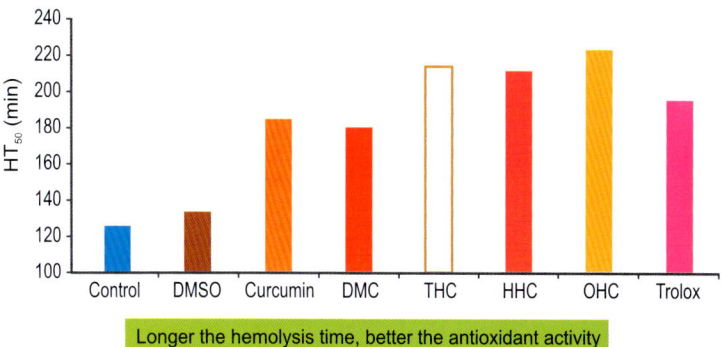

Fig. 29: Hemolysis (HT_{50}) activity (50% maximal time) of curcumin and its derivatives, and trolox at 30 µM. (Adapted from Somparn et al., 2007)

Inhibition of AAPH-induced hemolysis in red blood cells decreased in the order of OHC >THC = HHC > Trolox > Curcumin = DMC. Lower antioxidant activity was observed in dimethoxy derivatives of curcumin, indicating the role of the *ortho*-methoxy phenolic groups in antioxidant activity. However, hydrogenation at conjugated double bonds of the central seven carbon chain and β-diketone of curcumin to THC, HHC and OHC improved the antioxidant activity significantly.

Antioxidant activity of curcumin and its derivatives

1. DPPH Scavenging Activity (Fig. 27)
   THC > HHC = OHC > Trolox > Curcumin > DMC >>> BDMC

2. AAPH-induced Linoleic Acid Oxidation (Fig. 28)
   THC > Curcumin ≥ OHC ≥ HHC > DMC ≥ Trolox > BDMC

3. AAPH-induced RBC Hemolysis (Fig. 29)
   OHC > THC = HHC > Trolox > Curcumin = DMC

Tetrahydrocurcumin was found to inhibit the peroxidation of microsomal and mitochondrial lipids prepared from rat liver (Maehara et al., 2011). Recently, Morales et al. (2015)

evaluated the free radical scavenging capacity of curcumin, its demethoxy derivatives and hydrogenated derivatives THC, HHC and OHC towards DPPH, nitric oxide radical (NO), hydroxyl radical (HO) and superoxide anion radical (O_2^-). Corroborating with the earlier results, the study demonstrated that THC showed higher or comparable scavenging potency as curcumin towards all of the tested free radicals. Curcumin and its derivatives showed better scavenging of DPPH and NO but were not effective hydroxyl radical or superoxide anion radical scavengers. Based on these results, the authors suggest that curcumin and its derivatives principally act as chain breaking antioxidants rather than as direct free radical scavengers.

The antioxidant activity of two *Zingiber* species, namely *Z. mioga* and *Z. officinale*, and their different structural parts, namely *Z. mioga* root (ZMR), *Z. mioga* aboveground (ZMA), *Z. officinale* root (ZOR), and *Z. officinale* aboveground (ZOA) were compared using the ABTS (2,2'-azino-bis(3-ethylbenzothiazoline-6-sulphonic acid)), DPPH, and FRAP (Fluorescence recovery after photobleaching) assay methods by Han *et al.* (2015). The highest antioxidant activity corresponded to the root parts of *Z. officinale*, followed by the aboveground parts of *Z. officinale*. The results of the antioxidant activity assays ABTS, DPPH, and FRAP were consistent in the following order: ZOR > ZOA > ZMA > ZMR. The highest antioxidant activity was observed, particularly, in the below ground part (root) of *Z. officinale*, which was attributed to the presence of the secondary metabolite, such as THC, having high antioxidant activity (Figs. 30A & 30B).

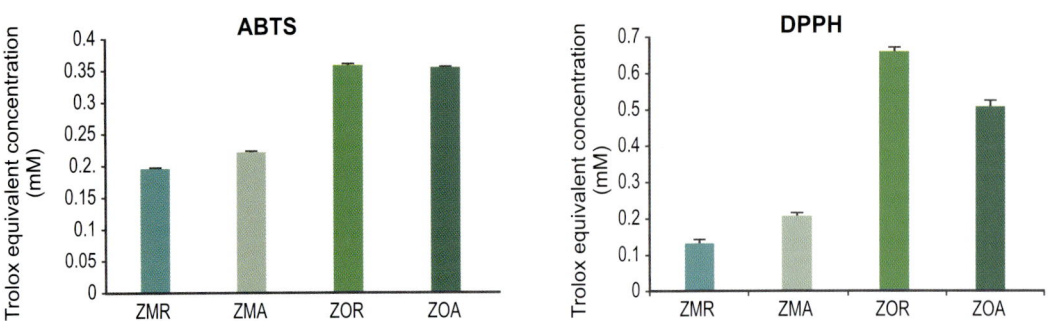

ZMR: *Z. mioga* Root; ZMA: *Z. mioga* Aboveground; ZOR: *Z. officinale* Root; ZOA: *Z. officinale* Aboveground.

Fig. 30A: Antioxidant activity assay, ABTS and DPPH of *Z. officinale* and *Z. mioga* with the two different structural parts. (Adapted from Han *et al.*, 2015)

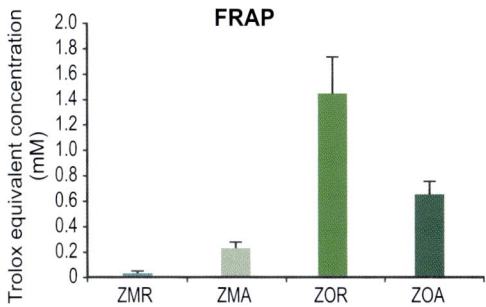

ZMR: *Z. mioga* Root; ZMA: *Z. mioga* Aboveground; ZOR: *Z. officinale* Root; ZOA: *Z. officinale* Aboveground.

Fig. 30B: Antioxidant activity assay, FRAP of *Z. officinale* and *Z. mioga* with the two different structural parts. (Adapted from Han *et al.*, 2015)

Prabhu *et al.* (2011) investigated the scavenging response of THCs (provided by Sabinsa) using series of *in vitro* models compared with standard antioxidant trolox and curcumin. It was shown that THCs exhibited its radical scavenging effect in concentration-dependent manner on super oxide, hydroxyl radicals, ferric ions, DPPH and ABTS. This study shows that THCs are good antioxidants compared to the standard antioxidant, trolox.

More recently, Novaes *et al.* (2017) measured the antioxidant activity of THC and other curcuminoids. The total antioxidant activity of THC and curcumin was calculated with respect to trolox as a measure of antioxidant capacity. It was shown that both THC and curcumin showed their greatest antioxidant effect at 100 µg/mL (Fig. 31)

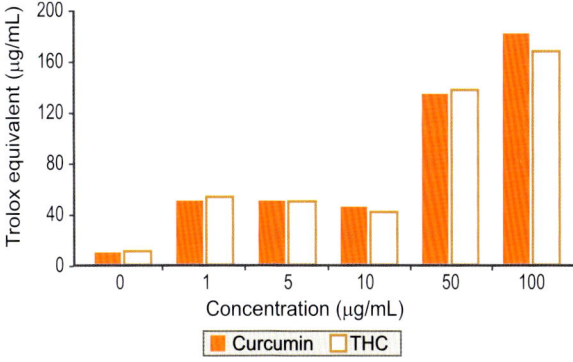

Fig. 31: The antioxidant activity of THC and curcumin. (Adapted from Novaes *et al.*, 2017)

Comparative Antioxidant Activity of THCs and THCs-Phosphatidylcholine Liposome *(Arunothayanun et al., 2005)*

Decoloration reaction of ABTS radicals was used to compare the antioxidant capacity of THCs as well as THCs encapsulated in phosphatidylcholine liposomes (see page 148 for additional details).

Fig. 32 shows the % ABTS radical cation remaining after 1 h incubation of THCs, curcuminoids, curcumin and vitamin E, prepared as alcoholic solutions in various concentrations, to the solution containing ABTS free radicals.

It has been shown that curcuminoids exhibit higher antioxidant capacity than pure curcumin, but THCs supersede curcuminoids easily in their antioxidant potential.

The comparative antioxidant potential of THCs, curcuminoids and curcumin is shown in the Table 4.

These results suggest that the lower concentration of THCs can be used instead of curcuminoids or vitamin E to achieve the same antioxidant effect.

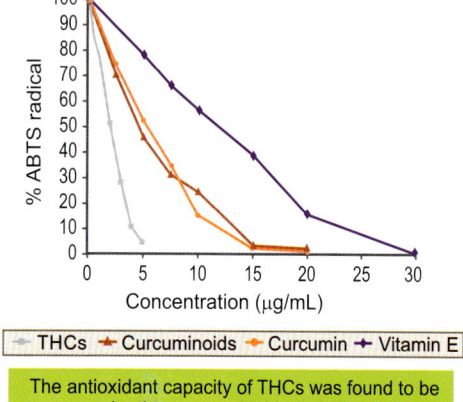

The antioxidant capacity of THCs was found to be superior than curcuminoids and vitamin E

Fig. 32: % ABTS radical cation remaining after 1 h incubation of THCs, curcuminoids, curcumin and vitamin E. (Adapted from Arunothayanun *et al.*, 2005)

Table 4: Comparative antioxidant potential.

Antioxidants	Antioxidant Potential (IC$_{50}$ µg/mL)
THCs	2.0 ± 0.1
Curcuminoids	4.6 ± 0.3
Curcumin	5.3 ± 0.4
Vitamin E	11.6 ± 1.7

Lower the IC$_{50}$ value, better the antioxidant activity

Fig. 33 shows that THCs could enhance the reduction of free radicals when used in combination with vitamin E.

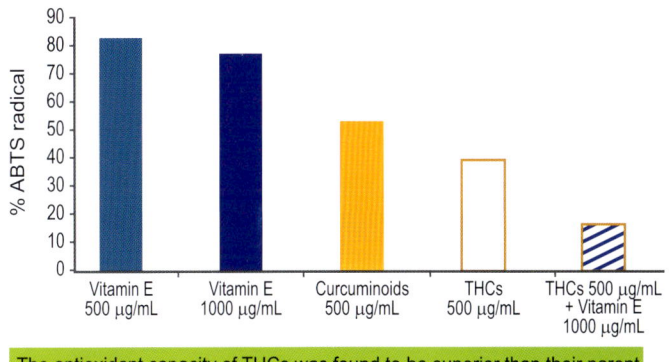

Fig. 33: ABTS (%) radical cation remaining after 1 h incubation of alcoholic solutions of vitamin E, curcuminoids, THCs or mixture of THCs and vitamin E.
(Adapted from Arunothayanun *et al.*, 2005)

Reactive oxygen species (ROS) is known to induce endothelial nitric oxide synthase (eNOS) and activate matrix metalloproteinase (MMPs) (Xu and Touyz, 2006). **Sangartit *et al.* (2014)** examined whether THC with its strong antioxidant potential can improve NO bioavailability, inhibit MMP activation and thereby attenuate vascular oxidative stress in mice during cadmium (Cd) exposure. Cadmium profoundly suppressed eNOS but enhanced inducible nitric oxide synthase (iNOS) expression in mice aortas, revealing the alteration of the eNOS/iNOS pathway in Cd exposure. In addition, a marked increase in urinary nitrate/nitrite was found in Cd exposed mice. On the other hand, it was shown that THC upregulated eNOS and downregulated iNOS protein expressions in the aortic tissue (Figs. 34A & 34B), as well as decreased urinary nitrate/nitrite level in Cd exposed mice. It was suggested that THC restored the NO bioavailability in the vascular system, suppressed MMP-induced vascular remodeling (Figs. 34C & 34D), reduced oxidant formation and maintained antioxidant, glutathione (GSH).

Chapter 3
TETRAHYDROCURCUMIN (THC): THE MAJOR METABOLITE WITH MAJOR BENEFITS

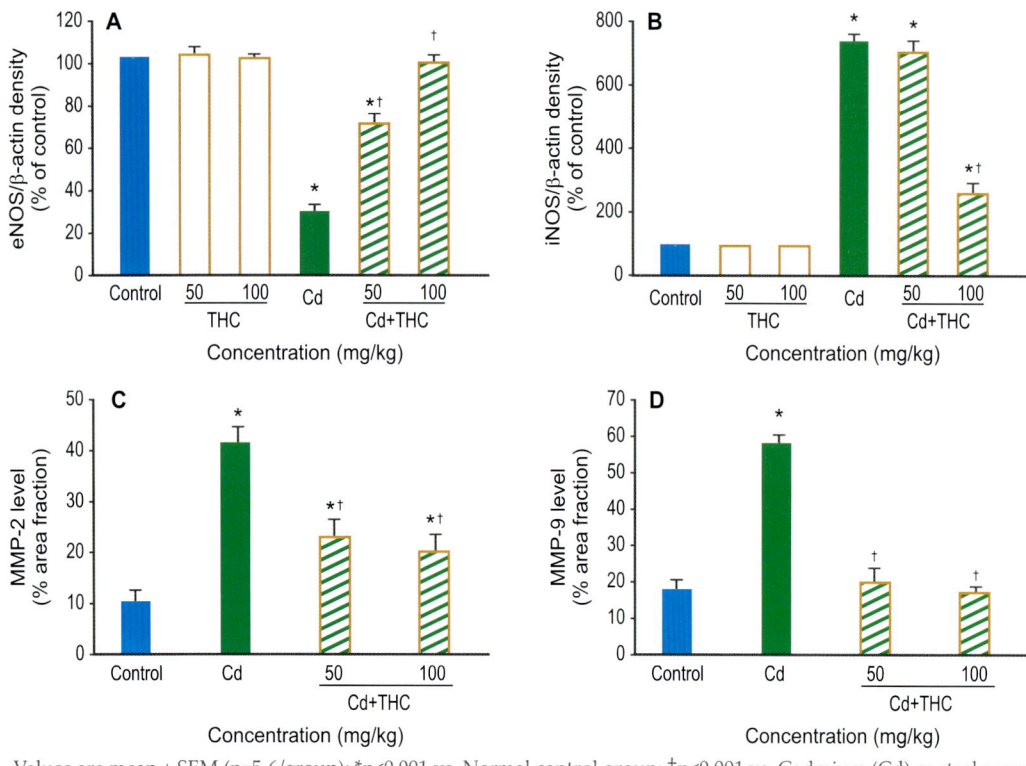

Fig. 34: Antioxidant potential of THC on eNOS (A), iNOS (B), MMP-2 (C) and MMP-9 (D) protein expressions in the aortas of mice.
(Adapted from Sangartit et al., 2014)

Deferiprone, an oral iron chelator, is widely used in patients with β-thalassemia major (an inherited blood disorder resulting in excessive destruction of red blood cells, leading to anemia) to prevent the deleterious effects of iron accumulation by decreasing body iron and non-transferrin bound iron (NTBI) (Sajid et al., 2009). However, deferiprone may exert adverse effects, especially agranulocytosis and thrombocytopenia, a condition is characterized by severe reduction in blood platelet counts (Ricchi et al., 2010). In a subsequent study, the same group (Sangartit et al., 2016) investigated whether combined therapy with antioxidant THC and deferiprone could reduce the adverse effects of iron chelator and mitigate iron toxicity. Hemodynamics, vascular reactivity, baroreflex sensitivity, and the levels of antioxidant status were examined with or without supplementation of THC, deferiprone, or combination of THC and deferiprone using a model of iron sucrose-induced iron overload in experimental animals.

The authors have demonstrated that a combination of deferiprone and THC exerts iron chelating and antioxidant properties by restoring blood pressure, hemodynamics, vascular function, and baroreflex sensitivity following iron overload. It was also shown that THC restored endothelial protective effects by increasing eNOS, thereby restoring vascular responses and blood pressure. In addition, THC also increased antioxidant GSH and restored redox status in iron-overloaded mice, suggesting THC enhanced GSH levels by scavenging ROS intermediates (Fig. 35).

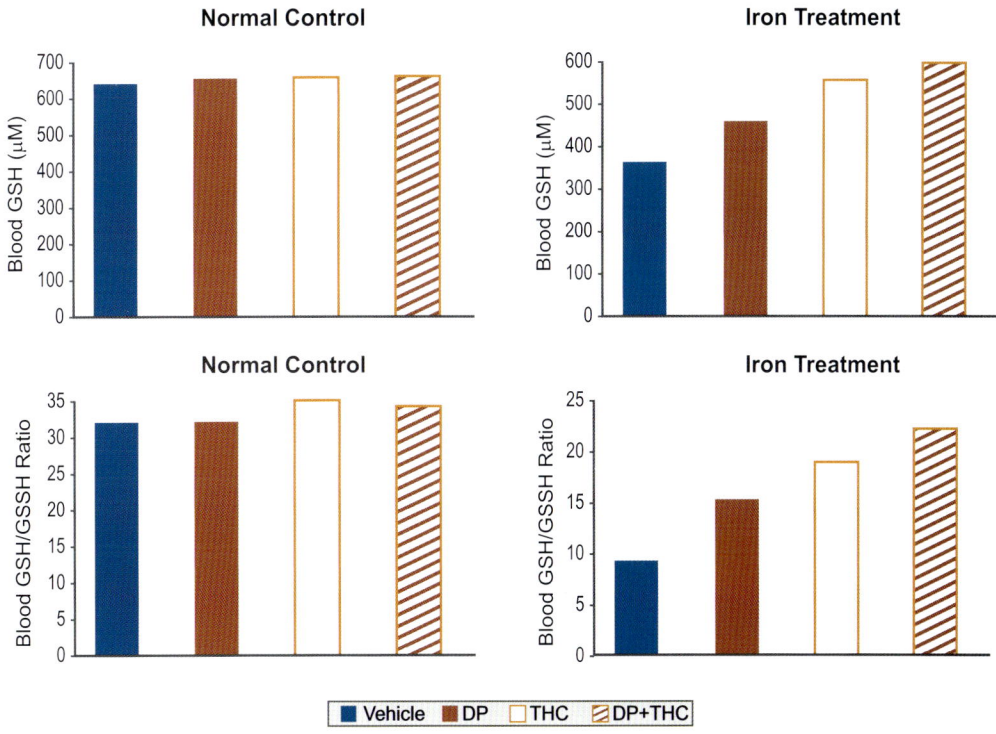

Fig. 35: Effect of deferiprone (DP) and/or THC on antioxidant status.
(Adapted from Sangartit et al., 2016)

In summary, several studies have clearly demonstrated that THC is a potent antioxidant (Arunothayanun *et al.*, 2005; Naito *et al.*, 2002; Somparn *et al.*, 2007; Sugiyama *et al.*, 1996) **and recent studies are in agreement with the earlier findings** (Han *et al.*, 2015; Maehara *et al.*, 2011; Morales *et al.*, 2015; Novaes *et al.*, 2017; Sangartit *et al.*, 2014 & 2016).

Anti-inflammatory Potential

Curcuminoids are potent anti-inflammatory agents. The anti-inflammatory potency of curcumin, curcumin analogs and phenylbutazone were compared in carrageenan-induced foot paw edema and cotton pellet granuloma models of inflammation in rats (Itokawa *et al.*, 2008). The inflammatory potency was found to follow the order: Sodium curcuminate (NaC) > THC > Curcumin > phenylbutazone (PB). Tetrahydrocurcumin was effective at almost half the dose of the parent compound, curcumin. The study revealed that curcumin analogs are more active in alleviating acute inflammation (Fig. 36). The presence of the β-diketone moiety as a link between the two phenyl groups is deemed important for the anti-inflammatory activity (Itokawa *et al.*, 2008).

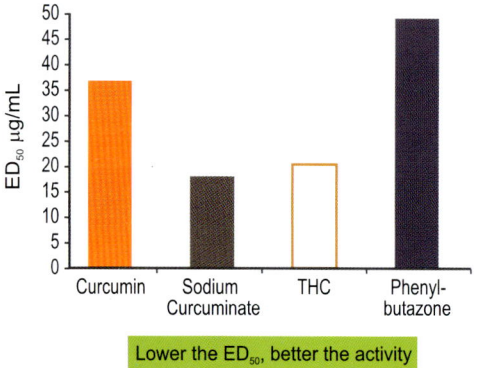

Fig. 36: Effect of curcumin derivatives and phenylbutazone on carrageenan-induced paw edema in rats. (Adapted from Itokawa *et al.*, 2008)

TETRAHYDROCURCUMIN (THC): THE MAJOR METABOLITE WITH MAJOR BENEFITS

In a neuroinflammation animal study (chronic and acute) using THCs (provided by Sabinsa), Begum *et al.* (2008) first reported measurable amounts of the unconjugated THC metabolite in both the plasma and brain in mice continually fed with curcumin for a long duration and THCs showed efficacy in preventing the oxidative damage of central nervous system (CNS). It was shown in both acute and chronic inflammation models that the brain inflammatory markers iNOS and IL-1β were inhibited more effectively by THC than curcumin with lower IC_{50} concentration (0.186 and 0.701 μM for iNOS and 1.286 vs. 1.722 μM for IL-1β). The brain lipid peroxidation products, F2 isoprostanes, were significantly lowered with THC treatment at the EC_{50} value of 0.501 μM compared to that of 1.067 μM for curcumin. Tetrahydrocurcuminoids also reduced the soluble β-amyloid peptide (Aβ) without impacting on insoluble form (Begum *et al.*, 2008).

In a recent study, Novaes *et al.* (2017) investigated the anti-inflammatory properties of curcumin and THC in rats after oral administration. Both curcumin and THC inhibited lipoxygenase activity at concentrations as low as 1 μg/mL compared to the untreated control (Novaes *et al.*, 2017). The above findings collectively suggest the anti-inflammatory potential of THC *in vivo* (Fig. 37).

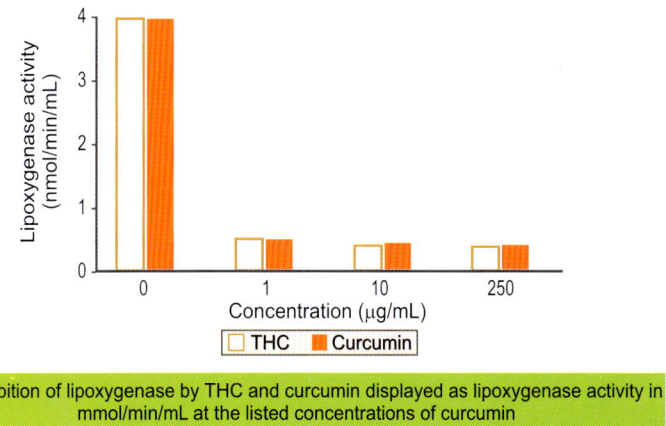

The inhibition of lipoxygenase by THC and curcumin displayed as lipoxygenase activity in mmol/min/mL at the listed concentrations of curcumin

Fig. 37: The anti-inflammatory activity of THC and curcumin. (Adapted from Novaes *et al.*, 2017)

TETRAHYDROCURCUMIN (THC): THE MAJOR METABOLITE WITH MAJOR BENEFITS

Zhao *et al*. (2015) evaluated curcumin and its three major metabolites, THC, HHC, and OHC for their anti-inflammatory properties using lipopolysaccharide (LPS)-stimulated macrophage cells (RAW 264.7 cells). Tetrahydrocurcumin at a concentration of 100 μM significantly inhibited the release of proinflammatory cytokines TNF-α and IL-6 compared to HHC and OHC (Fig. 38).

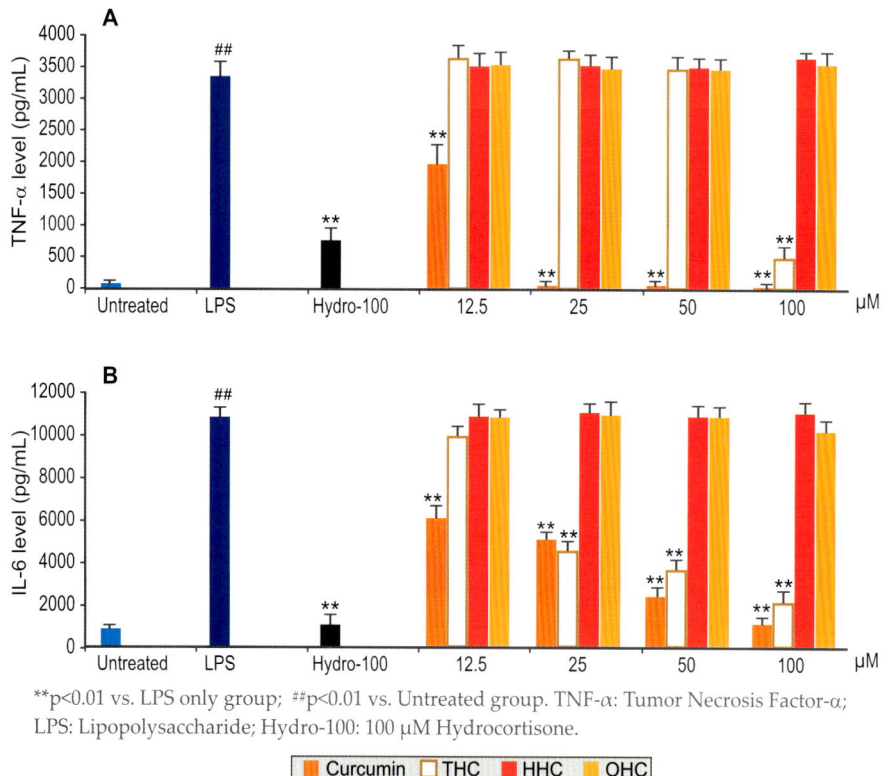

**p<0.01 vs. LPS only group; ##p<0.01 vs. Untreated group. TNF-α: Tumor Necrosis Factor-α; LPS: Lipopolysaccharide; Hydro-100: 100 μM Hydrocortisone.

Fig. 38: Effects of curcumin and its metabolites on TNF-α and IL-6 in RAW 264.7 cells. TNF-α (A) and IL-6 (B). (Adapted from Zhao *et al*., 2015)

The authors also provide evidence that THC at a concentration of 50 μM, exhibited a more potent effect on iNOS expression compared to that of the other metabolites at similar concentrations (Fig. 39). In addition, it was also shown that curcumin and its metabolites at 50 μM concentrations inhibited IκB-α degradation and thereby, prevented the translocation of NF-κB to the nucleus (Fig. 40). Overall, THC was found to be the most pharmacologically active metabolite of curcumin.

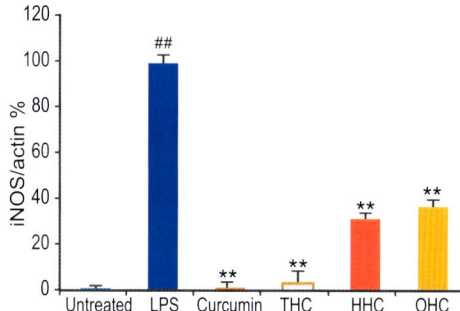

**p<0.01 vs. LPS only group; ##p<0.01 vs. Untreated group;
iNOS: Inducible nitric oxide synthase; LPS: Lipopolysaccharide.

Fig. 39: THC inhibits LPS-induced overexpression of iNOS in RAW 264.7 cells. Densitometric analysis of iNOS protein expression. (Adapted from Zhao *et al*., 2015)

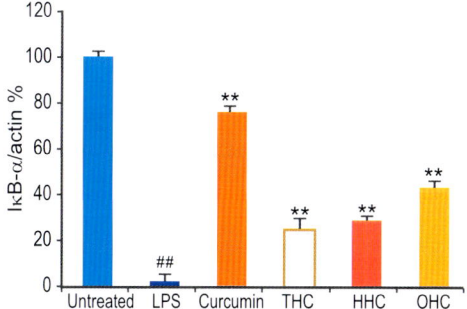

**p<0.01 vs. LPS only group; ##p<0.01 vs. Untreated group;
LPS: Lipopolysaccharide.

Fig. 40: THC inhibits the LPS-induced degradation of IκB-α in RAW 264.7 cells. Densitometric analysis of IκB-α protein expression. (Adapted from Zhao *et al*., 2015)

Recently, Zhang *et al*. (2018a) compared the *in vivo* anti-inflammatory effects of THC and curcumin using three common inflammatory animal models, namely

    a) Xylene-induced ear edema in mice
    b) The vascular permeability assay using acetic acid-induced murine model
    c) Carrageen-induced paw edema, a non-immune and an acute inflammatory model

The results indicated that THC in a dose-dependent manner suppressed the formation of ear edema induced by xylene (Fig. 41A), paw edema provoked by carrageenan (Fig. 41B) and inhibited the Evans blue dye leakage in peritoneal cavity elicited by acetic acid (Fig. 41C).

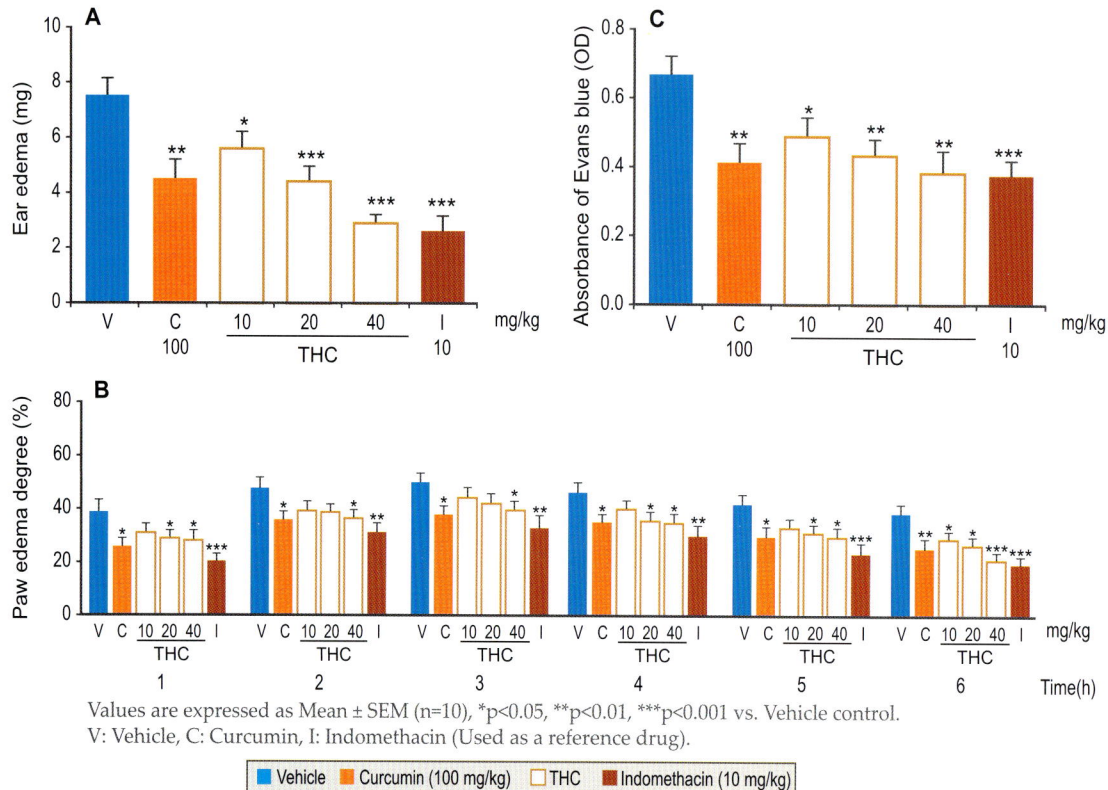

Fig. 41: Effect of THC on xylene-induced ear edema (A) carrageenan-induced paw edema (B) and acetic-acid-induced vascular permeability (C) in mice. (Adapted from Zhang et al., 2018a)

The authors also describe that THC possessed a better safety profile than curcumin with an LD_{50} value greater than 10,000 mg/kg. It was shown that THC alleviated acute inflammation by reducing the production of pro-inflammatory mediators, IL-1β, IL-6, TNF-α and PGE2, at the tissue levels. In addition, THC drastically suppressed COX-2 expression without affecting the expression of COX-1. Furthermore, THC exhibited superior inhibitory effects on pro-inflammatory mediators, including COX-2, when compared with curcumin. The results suggest that THC might possess a better effect than curcumin in selectively inhibiting the COX-2 activity.

The authors (Zhang *et al.*, 2018a) suggested that the structural differences between curcumin and THC may be the reason for the differential anti-inflammatory effects *in vivo*. Hydrogenation of the conjugated double bonds of the heptadiene backbone of curcumin and its transformation to THC could possibly increase the anti-inflammatory activity which enabled the inhibition of carrageenan-induced paw edema in mice significantly. It was also shown that THC treatment exhibited potent anti-inflammatory effects, by inhibition of NF-κB pathways through the inactivation of TAK1 and suppression of COX-2 and other inflammatory mediators. In conclusion, it was reported that THC showed more marked anti-inflammatory activity than curcumin, demonstrating that THC could be an important bioactive anti-inflammatory form of curcumin *in vivo*, suggesting THC as a promising new chemical entity for further development of potent anti-inflammatory therapeutics. Overall these findings demonstrate that the combination of THC with curcumin could have a potential synergistic effect on total anti-inflammatory activities.

Anti-glycation Potential

Glycation is a non-enzymatic chemical process in which human DNA, lipids and proteins are damaged by the attachment of reducing sugars such as glucose, ultimately leading to the formation of highly reactive Advanced Glycation End products (AGEs). This process has been associated with deleterious health effects. An anti-glycation agent inhibits the glycation process and prevents the formation of AGEs (e.g. free radicals, α-dicarbonyl species, protein cross-links etc). Administration of THCs to diabetic rats (streptozotocin-nicotinamide-induced) has been shown to decrease the AGEs and collagen cross-linking (Table 5). The antiperoxidative properties of THC were suggested for its antiglycation activity (Pari and Murugan, 2007b).

Table 5: Anti-glycation activity of THCs measured in the tail tendon in normal and experimental rats.
(Adapted from Pari and Murugan, 2007b)

Groups	Hydroxyproline (mg/100 mg tissue)	Total collagen (mg/100 mg tissue)	Extent of glycation (µg of glucose/ mg collagen)	Fluorescence (AU/µmol hydroxyproline)
Normal	8.97 ± 0.61	65.53 ± 4.46	11.09 ± 0.76	28.23 ± 1.92
Diabetic control	15.98 ± 0.94	121.02 ± 7.14	23.19 ± 1.37	55.47 ± 3.27
Diabetic + THCs (80 mg/kg)	9.76 ± 0.71	73.46 ± 5.36	12.88 ± 0.94	32.20 ± 2.35
Diabetic + Curcumin (80 mg/kg)	10.52 ± 0.59	81.16 ± 4.61	14.90 ± 1.03	39.08 ± 2.22

Values are mean ± SD from six rats in each group; AU: Arbitrary Units

In another study, Pari and Karthikesan (2009) demonstrated that THCs (80 mg/kg) provided significant protection of glycation of membrane proteins against STZ-NA-induced diabetic rats. Interestingly, it was observed that THCs and chlorogenic acid (CGA) synergistically exerted significant protective effect over glycation of membrane proteins against STZ-NA-induced diabetic rats.

Chapter 3
TETRAHYDROCURCUMIN (THC): THE MAJOR METABOLITE WITH MAJOR BENEFITS

Cardioprotective Potential

Cardiovascular disease includes atherosclerosis, hypertension and other related illnesses, and thus making it one of the leading causes of death worldwide. Atherosclerosis, a disease state, occurs because of thickening of artery wall, mainly due to the accumulation of fats, such as cholesterol. The chronic inflammatory response causes hardening or furring of the arterial walls, known as an arteriosclerotic vascular disease (ASVD), triggered by low-density lipoproteins (LDL).

It is reported that when rabbits were fed with diets containing 1% cholesterol with THC, a reduction in the atherosclerotic lesions area compared to control was observed (Naito *et al.*, 2002).

Tetrahydrocurcuminoids (provided by Sabinsa) and rutin were evaluated for cardioprotective effect in experimentally induced myocardial infarction (MI) in rats. The I/R injury model of MI in male rats developed cardiac necrosis, increase in lipid peroxidation, aspartate transaminase (AST), alanine transferase (ALT) and a decrease in antioxidant status with reduced glutathione and catalase. Treatment with THC and rutin considerably decreased the infarct size in rats induced by MI-I/R compared to the control group. Similarly, THC and rutin also decreased MI-I/R induced lipid peroxidation. Thus, it was suggested that one of the potential modes of action of cardio-protection by THC and rutin could possibly by suppressing the MI-I/R induced oxidative stress in rats. These findings were further confirmed by histopathological examination (Ali *et al.*, 2009).

Trans-Fatty acids (TFAs) are well-recognized risk factors for coronary heart disease. The TFAs can not only originate from exogenous food sources but could also generate endogenously from tissues in the body. Oxidative radicals could stress cell membranes to release TFAs. Three possible free radicals including thiyl radicals, sulfhydryl radicals and nitrogen dioxide have been recognized as the free radical paths for the generation of TFA. Hung *et al.*, using cell culture models, tested several antioxidants for their efficacy to block the production of *trans*-isomers of arachidonic acid (thiyl induced isomerism). It was reported that among the antioxidants tested THC, curcumin and resveratrol excelled as preventive agents (Table 6) (Hung et al., 2011).

Table 6: Inhibitory effects of antioxidants on thiyl radical-induced TAA (*trans* arachidonic acid) formation. (Adapted from Hung et al., 2011)

Antioxidants	all-*cis*	mono-*trans*	di-*trans*	tri-*trans*	all-*trans*	Inhibition (%)
Control	24.43 ± 0.99	30.49 ± 2.35	25.31 ± 1.17	14.64 ± 1.70	5.13 ± 0.99	0.00 ± 0.00
Curcumin	57.34 ± 1.42	24.08 ± 0.94	11.41 ± 0.50	5.46 ± 0.18	1.71 ± 0.14	43.53 ± 2.38
THC	56.11 ± 4.71	25.70 ± 5.59	11.51 ± 1.65	4.55 ± 1.73	2.12 ± 0.94	41.86 ± 6.87
Resveratrol	54.88 ± 3.02	25.97 ± 1.86	12.59 ± 1.04	5.19 ± 0.64	1.37 ± 0.29	40.32 ± 3.20
α-Tocopherol	43.25 ± 1.51	29.53 ± 1.53	16.56 ± 0.41	7.81 ± 0.48	2.85 ± 0.52	24.90 ± 1.36
Retinol acetate	42.78 ± 3.38	30.57 ± 2.67	16.34 ± 1.13	7.30 ± 0.08	3.01 ± 1.16	24.31 ± 3.50
Vitamin C	40.23 ± 4.13	30.02 ± 3.51	18.55 ± 1.73	8.21 ± 0.81	3.00 ± 1.15	20.90 ± 5.57
Gallic acid	37.56 ± 4.51	27.81 ± 4.47	21.20 ± 1.75	10.09 ± 1.11	3.34 ± 1.80	17.31 ± 7.00
Sesamol	37.03 ± 4.53	31.12 ± 1.72	19.56 ± 1.51	8.62 ± 1.91	3.68 ± 1.46	16.63 ± 6.56

In the above study, the authors produced thiyl radicals utilizing UV irradiation of 2-mercaptoethanol to induce *cis-trans* isomerization of arachidonic acid. The time of UV irradiation was 30 min and the concentration of antioxidants used was 500 μM.

Wongeakin *et al.* (2009) compared the effect of curcumin vs. THC on the diabetes-induced endothelial dysfunction in a streptozotocin-induced Wistar Furth diabetic rat model. It was characterized by the impairment of acetylcholine-activated vasorelaxation and increased leukocyte-endothelial cell interaction. Results of this study showed that curcumin and THC are effective in protecting the function of endothelial cells against diabetes-induced dysfunction, and may be used as therapeutic agents for protecting diabetes-induced endothelial cell dysfunction which is a major underlining cause for diabetic cardiovascular complications.

Nakmareong *et al.* (2011 & 2012) investigated the effect of THC on hemodynamic status, aortic elasticity and oxidative stress in rats with *N*-nitro-*L*-arginine methyl ester

(L-NAME)-induced hypertension. It has been reported that THC significantly reversed L-NAME-induced deleterious effects by reducing aortic wall thickness and stiffness. These effects of THC were associated with increased aortic eNOS expression, elevated plasma nitrate/nitrite, decreased oxidative stress with reduced superoxide production and enhanced blood glutathione level. Based on the results, the authors claim that THC attenuates the detrimental effect of L-NAME by improving the hemodynamic status and aortic elasticity concomitant with reduction of oxidative stress.

The effect of THC on alleviating hypertension, vascular dysfunction and vascular remodeling in mice exposed to Cd was investigated by Sangartit *et al.* (2014). Exposure to Cd for 8 weeks markedly increased its concentration in blood and tissues, including heart, aorta, liver and kidney of mice, whereas supplementation with THC significantly decreased Cd

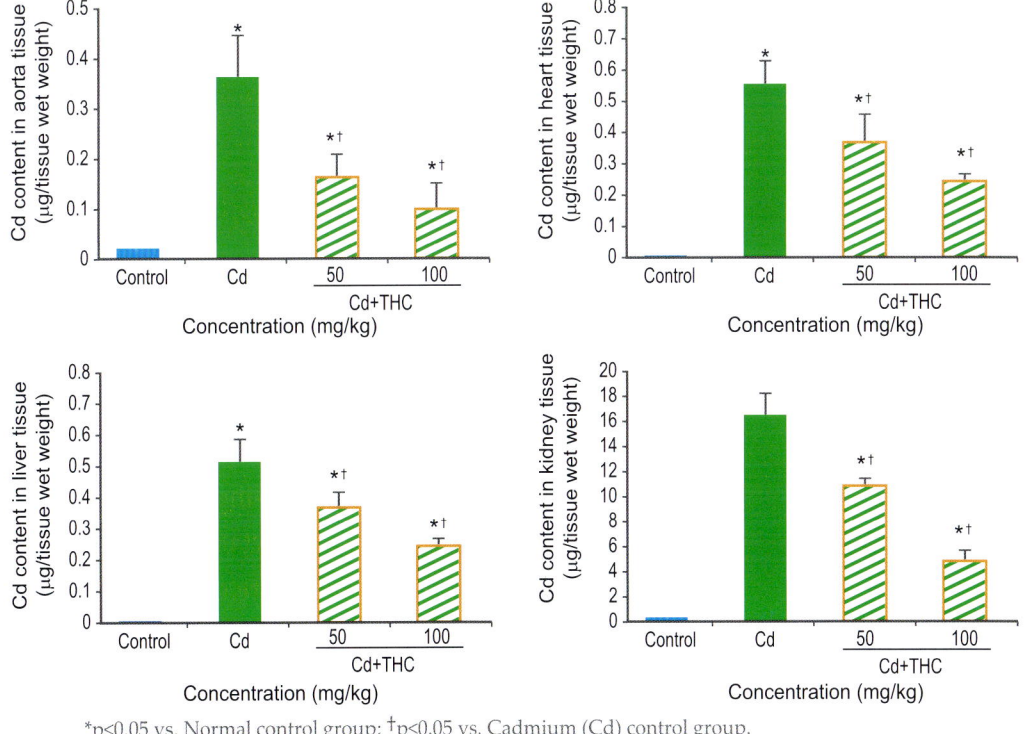

*p<0.05 vs. Normal control group; †p<0.05 vs. Cadmium (Cd) control group.

Fig. 42A: Effect of THC on Cd accumulation in the tissues of mice exposed to Cd.
(Adapted from Sangartit *et al.*, 2014)

accumulations in blood and tissues in a dose-dependent manner, thereby reducing oxidative stress, decreasing vascular superoxide production and the levels of MDA in plasma and tissues (Figs. 42A & 42B).

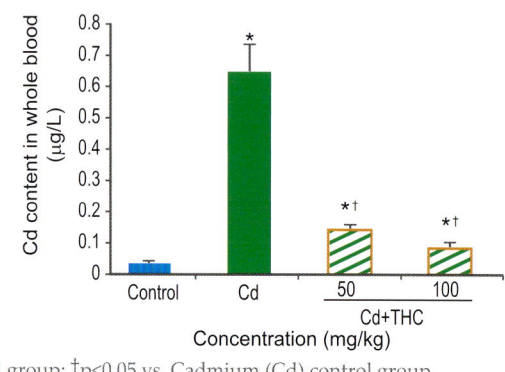

*$p<0.05$ vs. Normal control group; †$p<0.05$ vs. Cadmium (Cd) control group.

Fig. 42B: Effect of THC on Cd accumulation in the blood of mice exposed to Cd.
(Adapted from Sangartit *et al.*, 2014)

In a subsequent study, Sangartit *et al.* (2016) evaluated the effect of THC in combination with deferiprone that possess both chelating and free radical scavenging properties, respectively, against cardiovascular dysfunction in iron-overloaded experimental animals. Results from this study show that long-term administration of iron sucrose induced hypertension, which was associated with marked increase in arterial blood pressure (systolic blood pressure, diastolic blood pressure, and mean arterial pressure) in iron-overloaded mice compared with those of normal controls. Although deferiprone or THC as a single agent was able to reduce excess iron in the iron-loaded condition, THC has lesser effect on iron chelation than deferiprone. However, THC in combination with deferiprone exerted synergic beneficial effects acting as antioxidant and iron chelator, respectively, in alleviating hypertension, vascular dysfunction, and baroreflex sensitivity in mice.

More recently, Lau *et al.* (2018) investigated beneficial cardiac effects of dietary 1% THC in the subtotal 5/6 nephrectomized female Sprague-Dawley rats (Charles River, Wilmington,

MA). Female rats develop more proteinuria and renal fibrosis when subjected to 5/6 nephrectomy, as compared to male rats (Fleck et al., 2006). In this model, one kidney is removed first, and approximately 50% of the remaining kidney is removed by polar excision in 1-2 weeks. Subtotal nephrectomy, so-called 5/6 nephrectomy, is probably the most established method to mimic chronic kidney disease (CKD) and cardiac-renal syndrome in humans (Zhang and Kompa, 2014). Chronic kidney disease animals showed increased proteinuria, decreased creatinine clearance, hypertension, and cardiac hypertrophy and dietary THC improved all of these parameters (Table 7 and Fig. 43).

Table 7: Body weights, normalized heart weights, and blood and urine biochemical data in control and dietary THC treatment groups. (Adapted from Lau et al., 2018)

	Control (n=6)	CKD (n=6)	CKD+THC (n=9)
Body weight (g)	282 ± 18	260 ± 13	257 ± 11
Heart weight/body weight (g/kg)[a]	3.5 ± 0.3	4.6 ± 0.5[#]	4.3 ± 0.8
Hemoglobin (g/dL)	14.1 ± 0.5	13.7 ± 1.1	12.3 ± 1.5
BUN at start of special diet (mg/dL)	N/A	63 ± 10	69 ± 15
Terminal BUN (mg/dL)[a]	20.6 ± 3.4	87.1 ± 32.9[#]	61.3 ± 25.5[#]
Plasma creatinine (mg/dL)[a]	0.4 ± 0.1	1.4 ± 0.5[#]	1.1 ± 0.2[#]
Creatinine clearance (mL/min*kg)	5.2 ± 1.2	1.8 ± 1.1[#]	2.8 ± 0.7[#]
24 h Total urine protein (mg)[a]	18 ± 17	663 ± 252[#]	528 ± 119
Plasma C-reactive protein (mg/mL)	1.9 ± 1.1	2.8 ± 1.2	2.7 ± 0.9
Plasma galectin-3 (ng/mL)	444 ± 148	475 ± 162	400 ± 208

Values are mean ± SD; [#]$p<0.05$ vs. Control; BUN: Blood Urea Nitrogen; CKD: Chronic Kidney Disease.
[a]Data with unequal variances by Bartlett's test, analyzed using Kruskal-Wallis test.

Chapter 3
TETRAHYDROCURCUMIN (THC): THE MAJOR METABOLITE WITH MAJOR BENEFITS

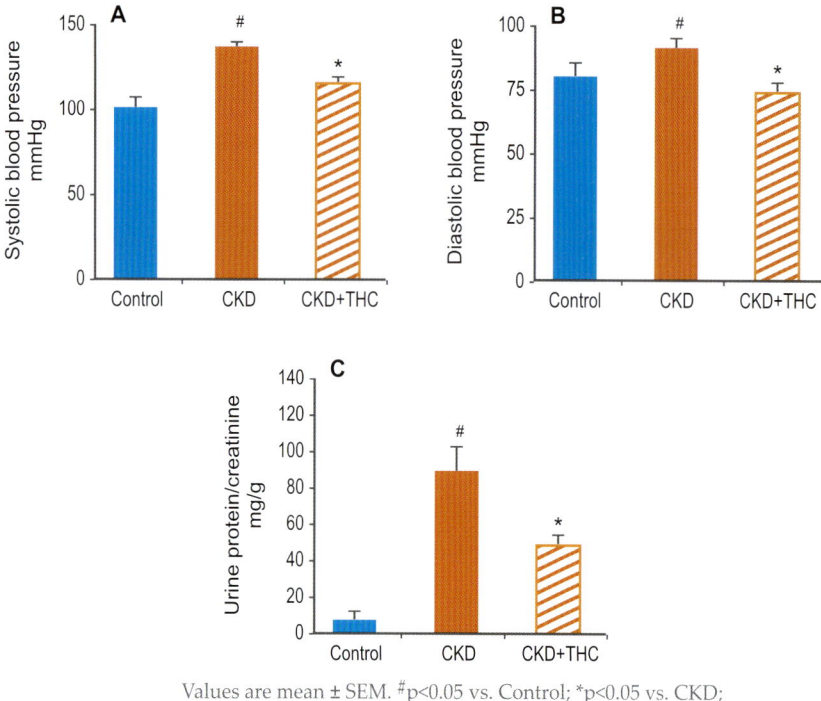

Values are mean ± SEM. #$p<0.05$ vs. Control; *$p<0.05$ vs. CKD; CKD: Chronic Kidney Disease.

Fig. 43: Effect of THC on blood pressure and proteinuria in 5/6 nephrectomized CKD rats. Systolic and diastolic blood pressure (A, B); Proteinuria determined by urine protein/creatinine ratio (C). (Adapted from Lau *et al.*, 2018)

In summary, it was shown that 1% THC diet ameliorated proteinuria, hypertension, and cardiac hypertrophy in 5/6 nephrectomized rats, suggesting the cardioprotective outcomes (normalized blood pressure, decreased cardiac hypertrophy) reflecting direct myocardial benefits of THC.

Nephroprotective Potential

Kidneys play key roles in body function such as filtering the blood, removal of waste products like urea, uric acid etc., maintaining a balance in the levels of electrolyte in the body and controlling blood pressure. They are also the source of hormone erythropoietin that stimulates bone marrow to make red blood cells.

Tetrahydrocurcumin ameliorated the oxidative stress induced renal injury in mice (Okada et al., 2001). The renal protective effect of curcumin and THC were studied in male ddY mice against ferric nitrilotriacetate (Fe-NTA)-induced oxidative renal damage. An enhanced quantity of free radical-related lipid peroxidation products, aldehyde modified proteins and modified DNA bases such as 8-hydroxy-2'-deoxyguanosine (8-OHdG) were observed after treatment of Fe-NTA for 3 h. Therefore, to evaluate the oxidative suppression, the formation of thiobarbituric acid-like reactive substance (TBARS), as well as 8-OHdG and 4-hydroxy-2-nonenal (HNE) were measured in the kidney.

Mice were fed with a diet containing 0.5 g/100 g per kg bw curcumin or THC for 4 weeks. Tetrahydrocurcumin significantly inhibited 2-thiobarbituric acid reactive substances and HNE-modified proteins and 8-hydroxy-29-deoxyguanosine formation in the kidney; whereas curcumin inhibited only HNE-modified protein formation. The HPLC and electron spin resonance spin trapping with 5,5-dimethyl-1-pyrroline-*N*-oxide were used to evaluate the pharmacokinetics and radical scavenging capacities of curcumin and THC. The amounts of THC and its conjugates (as sulfates and glucuronides) in the liver and serum were larger in THC group than in the curcumin group. Also, the absorbance of THC from the GI tract was more than curcumin. When compared to curcumin, THC pronouncedly induced several antioxidant enzymes, such as glutathione peroxidase, glutathione *S*-transferase and NADPH: QR, and scavenged Fe-NTA-induced free radicals *in vitro* better than curcumin. The results suggested that curcumin was converted to THC *in vivo* and found to be more promising chemopreventive agent (Okada et al., 2001).

In an earlier study, Murugan and Pari (2005) have reported the nephroprotective effect of THCs against erythromycin estolate reduced toxicity. Subsequently, the authors investigated the possible role of THCs (80 mg/kg) in the protection against chloroquine (CQ)-induced peroxidative damage in renal tissue of female Wistar rats (Pari and Murugan, 2006). In this study, increased serum urea, creatinine and decreased levels of creatinine clearance were observed in CQ-treated rats reflecting the renal damage. Administration of THCs was shown to protect the kidney function from CQ by decreasing serum urea and creatinine levels and significantly increasing the levels of creatinine clearance (Table 8).

Table 8: Effect of THCs on the levels of kidney function markers of rats with chloroquine-induced peroxidative damage. (Adapted from Pari and Murugan, 2006)

Groups	Urea (mg/dL)	Creatinine (mg/dL)	Creatinine clearance (mg/min.)
Normal	25.03 ± 1.38^a	0.36 ± 0.02^a	0.44 ± 0.03^a
Normal + Curcumin (80 mg/kg)	23.00 ± 1.41^b	0.34 ± 0.02^e	0.48 ± 0.02^b
Normal + THCs (80 mg/kg)	20.45 ± 1.14^c	0.33 ± 0.01^b	0.47 ± 0.02^b
Normal + CQ (970 mg/kg)	51.40 ± 2.57^d	0.70 ± 0.04^c	0.25 ± 0.05^c
CQ (970 mg/kg) + Curcumin (80 mg/kg)	29.00 ± 1.73^e	0.40 ± 0.24^d	0.35 ± 0.06^d
CQ (970 mg/kg) + THCs (80 mg/kg)	27.05 ± 1.85^f	0.38 ± 0.18^a	0.39 ± 0.04^e

Values are mean ± SD for six rats in each group. Values not sharing a common superscript letter differ significantly at p<0.05 (DMRT). CQ: Chloroquine.

Chloroquine caused oxidative stress leading to the formation of free radicals and enhanced lipid peroxidation resulting in renal injury. Tetrahydrocurcuminoids treatment was shown to protect the cells through attenuation of lipid peroxidation and to reduce the production of free radical derivatives by decreasing the levels of kidney TBARs and hydroperoxides.

Murugan and Pari (2007a & 2007b) also studied the effect of THCs on renal functional markers and protein levels in STZ-NA-induced diabetic rats. It was shown that diabetic rats have decreased levels of kidney function markers, such as urea, uric acid, creatinine and increased levels of albumin. Treatment with THCs and curcumin reversed these parameters to near normal levels (Table 9).

Chapter 3
TETRAHYDROCURCUMIN (THC): THE MAJOR METABOLITE WITH MAJOR BENEFITS

Table 9: Effect of THCs on renal functional markers in STZ-NA-induced diabetes rats.
(Adapted from Murugan and Pari, 2007a)

Groups	Urea in urine (mg/dL)	Uric acid (mg/dL)	Creatinine (mg/dL)	Albumin (μg/dL)	Urine volume (mL/day)
Control rats	146.78 ± 8.72*	7.97 ± 4.74*	2.85 ± 0.17*	149.31 ± 7.26*	9.38 ± 0.56*
Diabetic control	108.65 ± 7.46⁺	5.75 ± 0.39⁺	1.73 ± 0.12⁺	314.88 ± 15.62⁺	21.69 ± 1.49⁺
Diabetic + THCs (80 mg/kg)	136.15 ± 8.65#	7.53 ± 0.39#	2.60 ± 0.16#	164.38 ± 9.35*#	11.19 ± 0.71#
Diabetic + Curcumin (80 mg/kg)	112.43 ± 7.05$	7.03 ± 0.12$	2.38 ± 0.13$	180.03 ± 9.81#	12.51 ± 0.68$

Values are mean ± S.D. for six rats in each group.
Values not sharing a common superscript symbol differ significantly at p< 0.05 (Duncan's multiple range test).

Moreover, Song *et al.* (2015) investigated the molecular mechanisms associated with the effects of THC on cisplatin-induced nephrotoxicity using *in vitro* cell culture and *in vivo* animal models. The authors used renal tubular cells (LLC-PK1) to determine the protective effect of THC against cisplatin-induced oxidative damage. Cisplatin treatment significantly decreased cell viability to about 50% compared to that of untreated control cells, whereas pretreatment with THC markedly restored cell viability in a dose-dependent manner. No cytotoxic effects of THC were observed at the treatment doses and these doses effectively protected cisplatin-induced cell damage (Fig. 44).

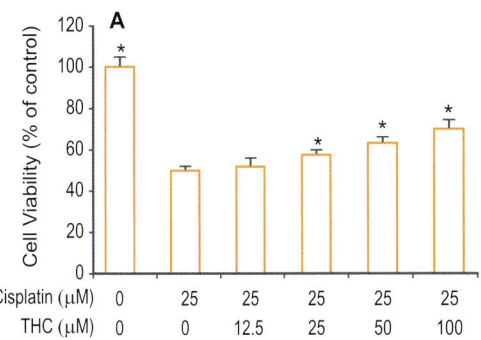
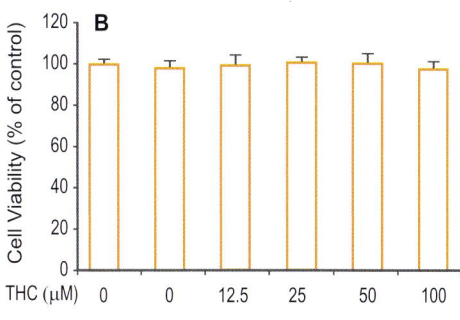

*p<0.05 vs. Cisplatin-treated control value.

Fig. 44: Effect of THC on cisplatin-induced nephrotoxicity in LLC-PK1 cells.
(A) Dose-dependent protective effect of THC against cisplatin-induced nephrotoxicity in cells.
(B) No cytotoxic effects of THC were observed at the treatment doses and these doses effectively protected cisplatin-induced cell damage.
(Adapted from Song *et al.*, 2015)

Chapter 3
TETRAHYDROCURCUMIN (THC): THE MAJOR METABOLITE WITH MAJOR BENEFITS

Next, the effect of THC on cisplatin-induced oxidative renal damage was examined in rats. Tetrahydrocurcumin treatment did not ameliorate cisplatin-induced body weight reduction and kidney weight increase. However, co-treatment with THC recovered the renal functional parameters, decreased creatinine clearance in cisplatin-treated rats (Fig. 45). It was concluded that kidney cell damage induced by cisplatin was significantly inhibited by THC treatment. In addition, the renal dysfunction of cisplatin-treated rats was markedly ameliorated by THC administration. The renoprotective effect of THC was associated with the caspase-dependent anti-inflammatory pathway. Taken together, these results demonstrate the renoprotective effect of THC in cisplatin-treated rats and, therefore, its use can be considered to prevent kidney damage during or after chemotherapy.

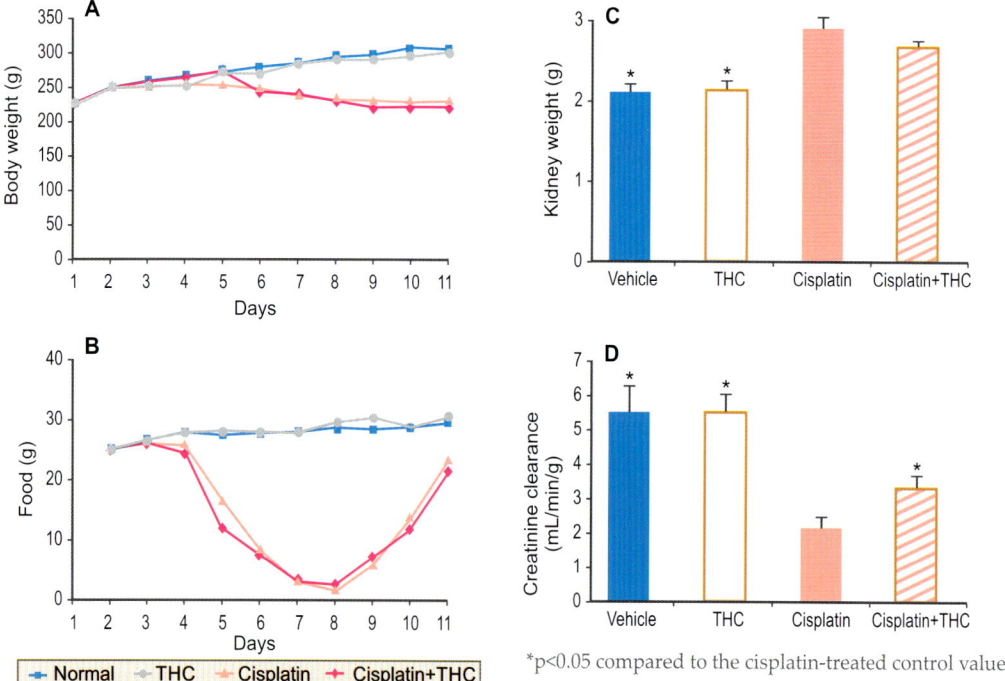

Fig. 45: Effect of THC on body weight, kidney weight, food intake, and the renal function parameter in the cisplatin-induced renal damage rat model.
(A) Changes in body weight; (B) Changes in food intake; (C) Changes in kidney weight and (D) Creatinine clearance. (Adapted from Song *et al.*, 2015)

Chapter 3
TETRAHYDROCURCUMIN (THC): THE MAJOR METABOLITE WITH MAJOR BENEFITS

In a recent study Park *et al.* (2018) used LLC-PK1 cells to determine the protective effect and mechanism of THC against FK506-induced renal damage. It was reported that FK506 treatment (50 μM) reduced the cell viability by 55% compared to that of the control. The reduction in cell viability was ameliorated by THC co-treatment in a dose-dependent manner and observed upto 88% cell viability restoration after co-treatment with THC at a dose of 12 μM (Fig. 46A). In addition, THC showed antioxidant effect by restoration of GSH (Fig. 46B) and anti-apoptotic effect by inhibiting the activation of caspase-3 and caspase-9. Thus, THC may act as an adjuvant therapy to reduce adverse effects of FK506 in the kidney.

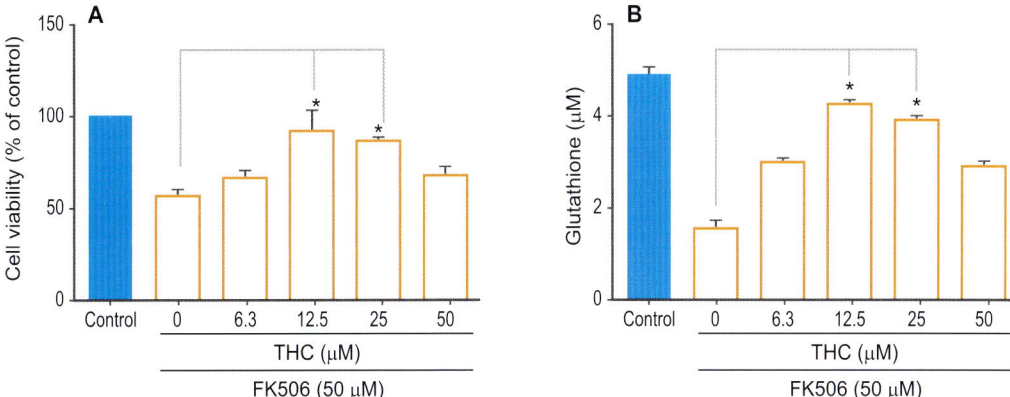

Results were expressed as the percentile of absorbance of treated samples compared to that of the control. Values are expressed as mean (SD) (*p<0.05, THC vs. FK506-treated cells).

Fig. 46: Effect of THC on FK506-induced cytotoxicity in LLC-PK1 cells.
(A) Cell viability measured by MTT assay; (B) Antioxidant effect measured by Glutathione assay.
(Adapted from Park *et al.*, 2018)

More recently, to investigate the beneficial renal effect of dietary THC, Lau *et al.* (2018) administered 1% THC to a well-established 5/6 nephrectomized CKD rats, which exhibit mass reduction of nephron. The effect of THC on proteinuria, fibrosis, and inflammation was evaluated. It was reported that dietary THC treatment restored the levels of metalloenzyme copper-zinc superoxide dismutase (CuZn SOD), the antioxidant (scavenging) enzymes and glutathione peroxidase (GPX-1) in the remnant kidney of the CKD rats. In addition, apoptosis and fibrosis were also shown to increase remnant kidney of the CKD rats whereas caspase-3 and α-smooth muscle actin (αSM-actin) were decreased by THC diet. Further, the increased iNOS level was downregulated by THC treatment.

Chapter 3
TETRAHYDROCURCUMIN (THC): THE MAJOR METABOLITE WITH MAJOR BENEFITS

Tetrahydrocurcumin treatment-associated improvements on the markers of oxidative stress, apoptosis, and fibrosis in kidney lysates are illustrated in Fig. 47.

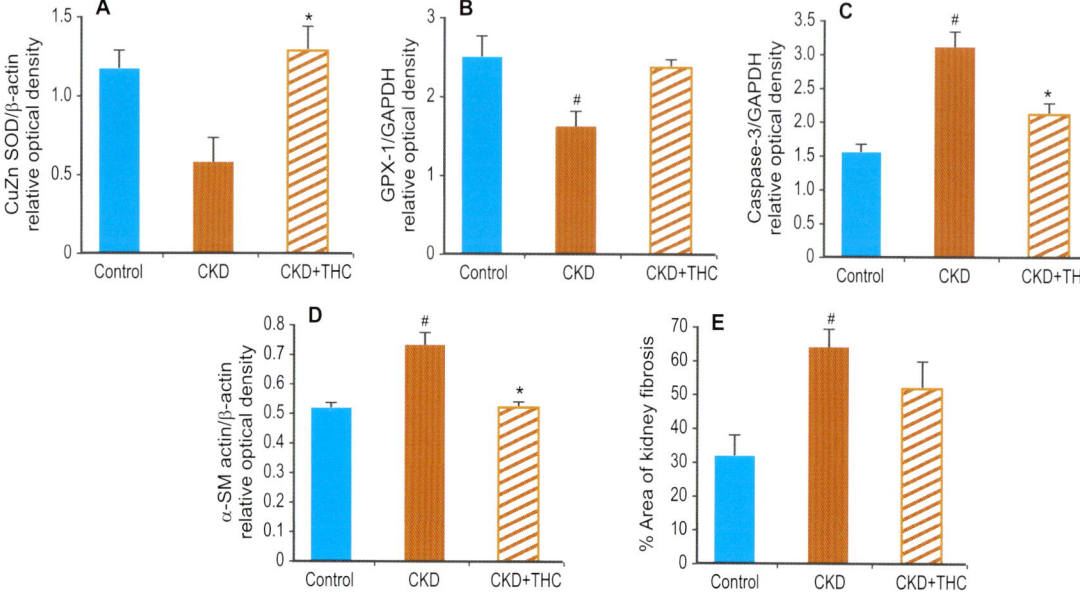

#$p<0.05$ vs. Control; *$p<0.05$ vs. CKD (Chronic Kidney Disease).

Fig. 47: THC diet improved the protein markers of oxidative stress and kidney fibrosis.
The antioxidant (scavenging) proteins:
(A) Copper-zinc superoxide dismutase (CuZn SOD)
(B) Glutathione peroxidase (GPX-1) was decreased in CKD and levels were restored with dietary THC therapy-the apoptosis marker
(C) Caspase-3 and the fibrosis marker
(D) α-Smooth muscle actin (α-SM-actin) was increased in the remnant kidney from CKD rats and were decreased with THC therapy
(E) Kidney fibrosis was decreased ~20% with THC therapy

(Adapted from Lau *et al.*, 2018)

In summary, 1% THC diet improved expression of antioxidant enzymes in the remnant kidney, decreased renal apoptosis and fibrosis in 5/6 nephrectomized rats. It has been reported that the renoprotective effects, decreased production of ROS, with subsequent downregulation of the caspase-3 apoptosis pathway, observed in this study are consistent with reports from other rodent models (Okada *et al.*, 2001; Pari and Murugan, 2005 & 2006). Similarly, THCs also have been shown to decrease albuminuria and blunt rise in serum creatinine in rats with diabetic nephropathy (Murugan and Pari, 2005, 2006 & 2007c; Pari and Murugan, 2007b).

… Chapter 3
TETRAHYDROCURCUMIN (THC): THE MAJOR METABOLITE WITH MAJOR BENEFITS

Hepatoprotective Potential

Liver is a vital organ which aids in digestion, removal of toxic and waste products from the body etc. It plays a major role in metabolism with wide range of functions such as protein synthesis, glycogen storage, hormone production, detoxification etc. It secretes bile, which helps in the intestinal absorption of fats and the fat-soluble vitamins.

Injuries and other damages to the liver are known to cause jaundice, hepatitis, cirrhosis, haemochromatosis, Wilson's disease, non-alcoholic fatty liver disease, and cancer. Several factors have been shown to be involved either in the induction or progression of hepatic injury, including chemicals or drugs, oxidative stress, viral infections, excessive consumption of alcohol, bile acid build-up, over activation of hepatocytes, Kupfer cells, fat-storing stellate cells and leukocytes. Alterations of ALT, AST, alkaline phosphatase (ALP), albumin, gamma-glutamyl transpeptidase, bilirubin, extracellular matrix proteins and transforming growth factor (TGF)-β1, the common biochemical markers, are being used often as indicators of liver damage.

Protection afforded by THCs and curcumin (both THCs and curcumin were provided by Sabinsa) on CQ-induced hepatotoxicity was evaluated in female Wistar rats. Animals were pretreated with THCs and curcumin at 80 mg/kg for 8 days orally before the single oral administration of CQ to induce hepatotoxicity. Treatment was followed for another 7 days. Control animals received only CQ treatment. In the CQ-treated rats, THC significantly reduced the activities of AST, ALP, ALT, bilirubin levels and lipid peroxidation products by increasing the activity of plasma and liver vitamin C and E, glutathione, superoxide dismutase, catalase and glutathione peroxidase. Histopathology (Fig. 48) indicated the almost normal appearance of the liver with THC treatment in contrast to feathery degeneration and microvesicular type of fatty regeneration, sinusoidal dilation and focal necrosis in the control rats. Thus, the findings revealed that THCs were found to have more significant hepatoprotective effect than curcumin (Pari and Amali, 2005) in CQ-induced hepatotoxicity model.

Chapter 3
TETRAHYDROCURCUMIN (THC): THE MAJOR METABOLITE WITH MAJOR BENEFITS

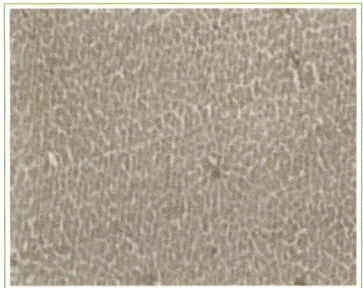
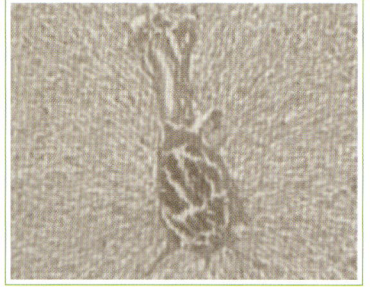

Hepatocytes show feathery degeneration and microvesicular type of fatty generation in Chloroquine treated liver

Sinusoidal dilation and focal necrosis

A. Control –Normal rat liver

B. Normal + Chloroquine treated rat liver

C. Normal + Chloroquine toxicity in treated rat liver

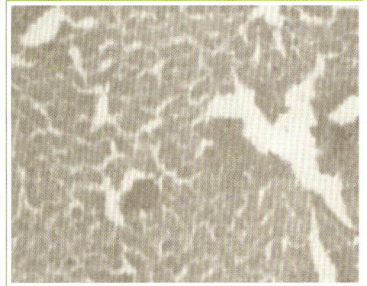
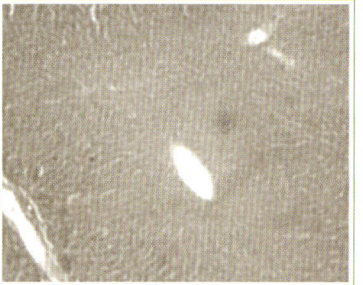
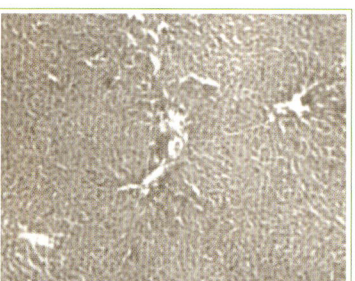

Normal hepatocytes with focal necrosis

Normal appearance of liver

Normal hepatocytes with mild portal inflammation and normal hepatocytes

D. Chloroquine + Curcumin treated rat liver

E. Normal + THCs

F. Chloroquine + THCs treated rat liver

Fig. 48: Histopathology of CQ-treated rat liver.
(Adapted from Pari and Amali, 2005)

In addition, THC treatment altered the pathology of the liver by changing into mild inflammation and cell infiltration in CQ-treated rats (Pari and Amali, 2005).

In another study, THCs (provided by Sabinsa) showed significant hepatoprotective effect against erythromycin estolate-induced hepatotoxicity in rats. The level of serum enzymes such as AST, ALT, ALP, bilirubin, cholesterol, triglycerides, phospholipids, free fatty acids and plasma TBARS and hydroperoxides in rats treated with erythromycin estolate were significantly reduced by THCs. Histopathological examination of liver section showed that

TETRAHYDROCURCUMIN (THC): THE MAJOR METABOLITE WITH MAJOR BENEFITS

THCs could prevent hepatocyte damage and degeneration induced by erythromycin estolate. The effects of THCs were comparable or better than silymarin, a known hepatoprotective molecule (Pari and Murugan, 2004).

Muthumani and Miltonprabu (2015) investigated the hepatoprotective effect of THCs (provided by Sabinsa) over arsenic (a potent hepatotoxin) induced toxicity in rat liver. Hepatotoxicity was measured by the increased activities of serum hepato-specific enzymes, namely ALT, ALP, AST and bilirubin along with increased elevation of lipid peroxidative markers, TBARS. The results indicated that THCs reduced the levels of liver enzymes including transaminases, ALP, LDH and bilirubin in rats. Treatment with THCs also reduced the oxidative stress, dyslipidemia, mitochondrial damage and improved mitochondrial structure and function in arsenic exposed rat liver (Fig. 49).

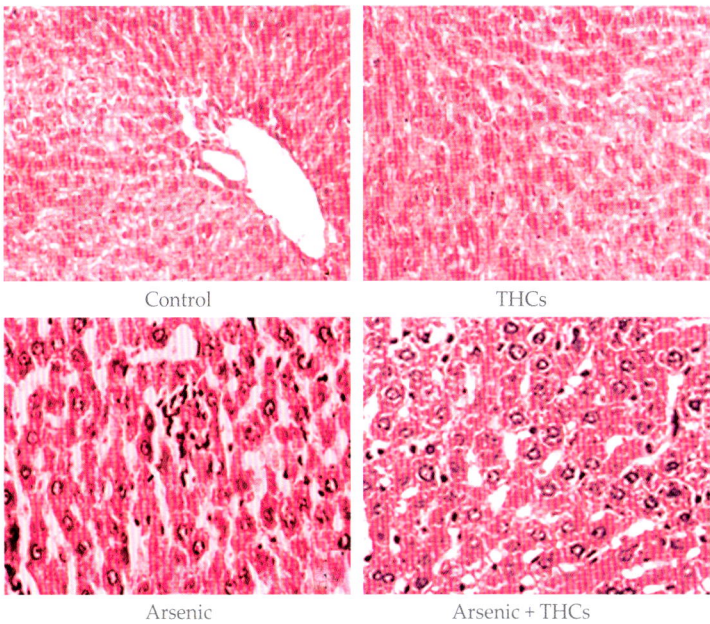

Control group showing normal hepatic architecture; Arsenic treated group without THCs treatment showing loss of hepatic architecture and many fatty droplets, vacuolated cytoplasm, pyknotic nuclei, focal necrotic areas accompanied with inflammatory cell infiltrations; Arsenic + THCs (80 mg/kg/bw) group displaying marked improvement in the hepatic architecture which is comparable to that of the arsenic treated group; and THCs (80 mg/kg/bw) alone group showing normal histological architecture of the liver tissue.

Fig. 49: Photomicrographs (40x) of rat liver (H & E) sections from control and arsenic treated groups with or without THCs treatment. (Adapted from Muthumani and Miltonprabu, 2015)

Chapter 3
TETRAHYDROCURCUMIN (THC): THE MAJOR METABOLITE WITH MAJOR BENEFITS

Most recently, Ramakrishnan *et al.* (2017) studied the protective role of THCs (provided by Sabinsa) on Cd-induced oxidative damage in rats. Tetrahydrocurcuminoids (20, 40 and 80 mg/kg/bw) were orally administered followed by Cd for 4 weeks. Histopathological changes observed in Cd-intoxicated hepatic tissues were minimized on treatment with THCs. The authors concluded that THCs at the dose of 80 mg/kg/bw effectively subdue the Cd-induced toxicity and control the free radical-induced liver damage in rats (Fig. 50).

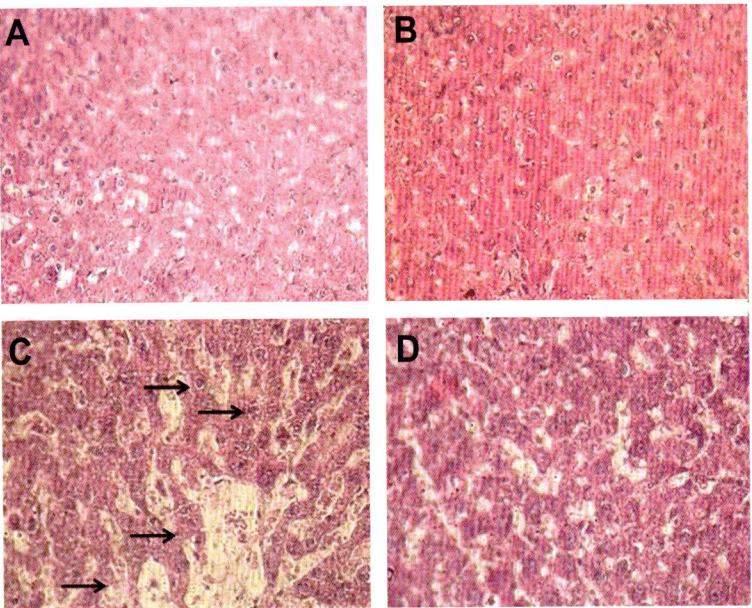

Fig. 50: Representative photomicrographs (40x) of liver section (H & E) from control, Cd and Cd + THCs treated rats.

(A) Liver section of a control rat displaying normal architecture of hepatocytes
(B) Liver section of THCs-alone-treated rats showing the normal histological architectural pattern of hepatocytes
(C) Section of Cd-treated rat liver exhibits marked disturbances of the normal architecture of the hepatocytes, with parenchymal necrosis, lymphatic infiltration and notable pyknotic nuclei
(D) Liver section of Cd + THCs-treated rats showing significant improvement of histological architecture with normal architectural pattern of hepatocytes

(Adapted from Ramakrishnan *et al.*, 2017)

Earlier studies have provided evidence that repeated and prolonged carbon tetrachloride (CCl_4) treatment induces liver fibrosis and cirrhosis (Liedtke *et al.*, 2013). In a recent study, Tsai *et al.* (2017) investigated the efficacy of THC against CCl_4-induced hepatic fibrogenesis in comparison with curcumin in rats. It was reported that CCl_4-induced advanced hepatic fibrosis was accompanied by high expressions of the fibrosis marker α-SMA, collagen I and TGF-β. Administration of THC at doses of 10 and 50 mg/kg improved hepatic histology caused by CCl_4 and significantly eliminated hepatic fibrogenesis, as evidenced by the diminished bridging collagen (Fig. 51) and fibrosis markers (Fig. 52). Tetrahydrocurcumin mediated anti-fibrogenic effect through the inhibition of Hepatic Stellate Cell (HSC) activation by interfering TGF-β signaling. Tetrahydrocurcumin also ameliorated CCl_4-induced hepatic apoptosis in rats by downregulating the activation of caspase-3, suggesting a cytoprotective effect of THC. Reduction of hepatocyte apoptosis by THC also represents a possible mechanism that contributes to the blockage of HSC activation in CCl_4-mediated fibrogenesis. Tetrahydrocurcumin administration also reduced hepatic collagen accumulation along with the activation of HSCs via down-regulation of TGF-β1 signaling and autophagy. Thus, the authors demonstrated that THC was more effective than curcumin in the abolishment of CCl_4-induced hepatic injury and fibrogenesis in rats.

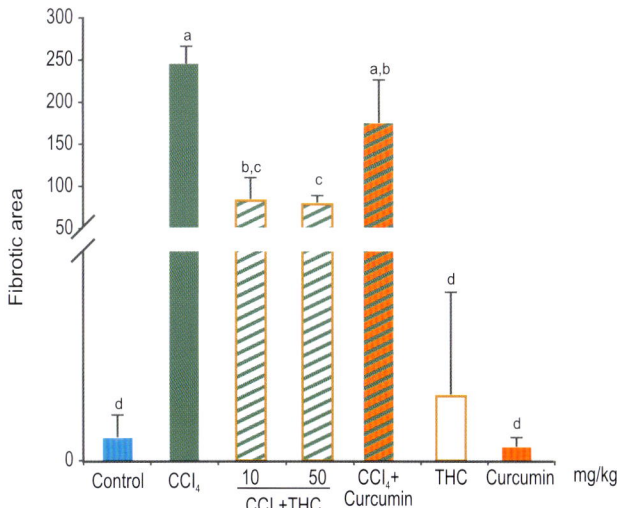

Values not sharing a common superscript letter differ significantly at p<0.05 (DMRT)

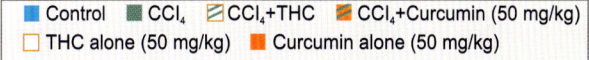

Fig. 51: Effect of THC on collagen deposition in CCl_4-treated SD rats.
Bar graph shows the quantification of representative images of sirius red from each group.
(Adapted from Tsai *et al.*, 2017)

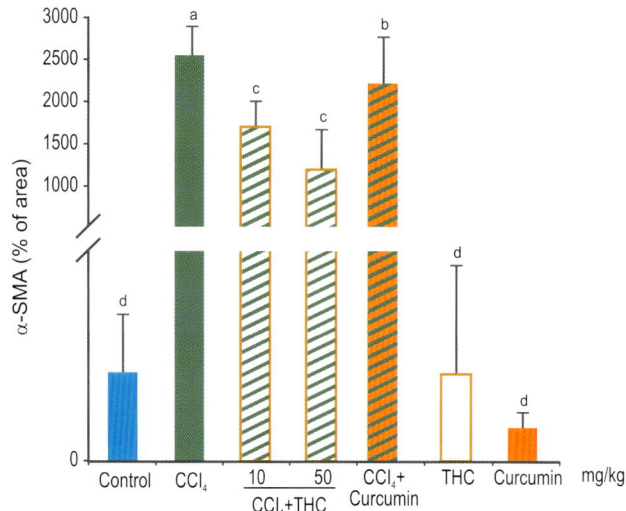

Values not sharing a common superscript letter differ significantly at p<0.05 (DMRT)

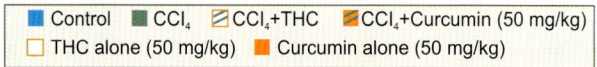

Fig. 52: Effect of THC on CCl_4-induced hepatic α-SMA expression
Bar graph showing quantification of the liver sections of experimental rats were stained with α-SMA positive cells for HSCs activation by immunohistochemical analysis.
(Adapted from Tsai *et al.*, 2017)

Acetaminophen (APAP) overdose is a leading cause of drug-induced hepatotoxicity that accounts for more than 40% of acute liver failure in the United States, Great Britain and Europe (Lee, 2017). Hepatotoxicity due to APAP overdose is associated with oxidative stress. In a recent study, Luo *et al.* (2019) investigated the potential mechanisms of THC against APAP-induced hepatotoxicity in comparison with curcumin using male Kunming mice. Findings of this study showed that pretreatment of mice with THC (100 mg/kg bw) substantially attenuated liver histopathological changes (Fig. 53) and enhanced liver function by decreasing the serum levels of ALT and AST in a dose-dependent manner (Figs. 54A & 54B).

Chapter 3
TETRAHYDROCURCUMIN (THC): THE MAJOR METABOLITE WITH MAJOR BENEFITS

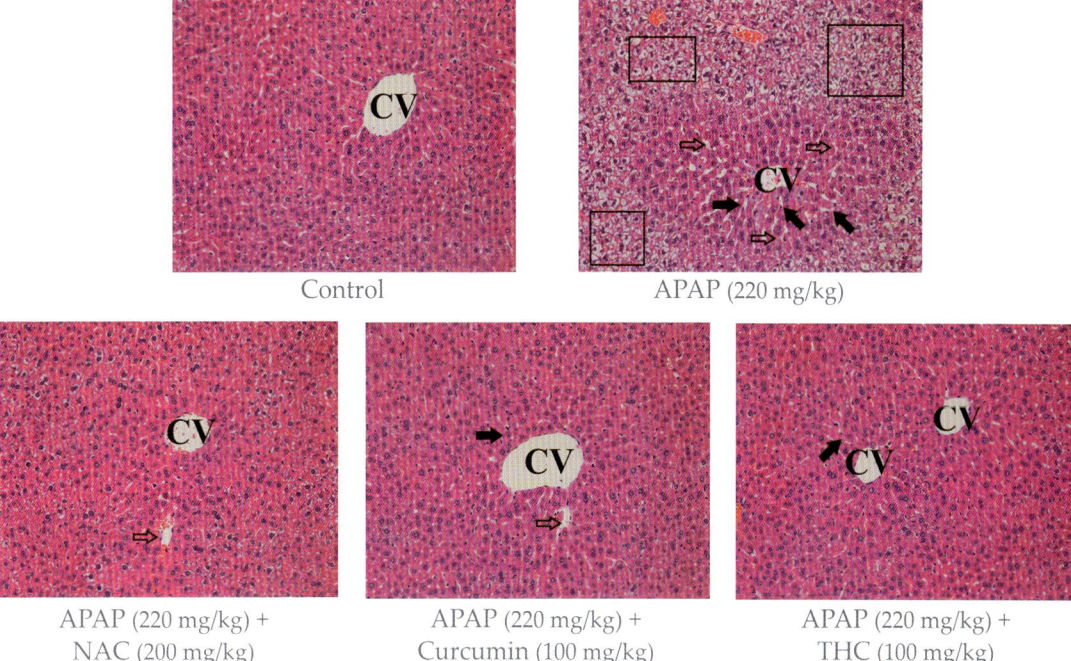

CV: Central Vessel; Solid arrows: Inflammatory cell infiltration; Open arrow: Sinusoidal dilation; Rectangle: Vacuolation; The scale indicates 50 μm.
APAP: Acetaminophen; NAC: N-acetyl cysteine.

Fig. 53: Effects of THC and curcumin on the liver histological alternations (original magnification × 100). (Adapted from Luo *et al.*, 2019)

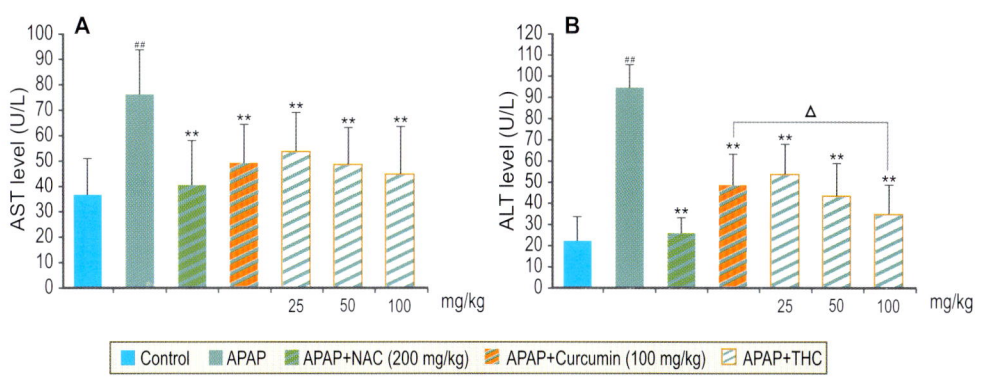

Values are expressed as the mean ± SD (n = 10); $^{\#\#}p<0.01$ vs. Control group. $^{**}p<0.01$ vs. APAP-treated group. $^{\Delta}p<0.05$ vs. Curcumin group.
NAC: N-acetyl cysteine; APAP: Acetaminophen; AST: Aspartate transaminase; ALT: Alanine transaminase.

Fig. 54: Effects of THC and curcumin on the levels of AST (A) and ALT (B) in serum.
(Adapted from Luo *et al.*, 2019)

Besides, THC significantly restored the hepatic antioxidant status by reducing the level of malondialdehyde (MDA) and ROS. Furthermore, THC as an antioxidant increased the levels of GSH, SOD, CAT and T-AOC (total antioxidant capacity). In addition, THC markedly suppressed the activity and expressions of CYP2E1 at the mRNA level by 2-fold. Moreover, THC activated the Keap1-Nrf2 pathway and enormously enhanced the translational activation of Nrf2-targeted genes against oxidative stress, via inhibiting the expression of Keap1 and blocking the interaction between Keap1 and Nrf2. Particularly, THC exerted superior hepatoprotective and antioxidant activities compared to curcumin.

Anti-hyperlipidemic Potential

The underlying cause of hyperlipidemia is associated with increased levels of lipids and/or lipoproteins in the blood, and a genetic mutation in hyperlipidemia-associated protein receptors, including diabetes. Changes in the concentration of lipids including cholesterol and triglycerides are complications observed frequently in case of diabetes mellitus and certainly contribute to the development of vascular disease (Howard *et al.*, 1978; Nikkila and Kekki, 1973).

Tetrahydrocurcuminoids were shown to have anti-hyperlipidemic effects in experimental diabetic rats (Murugan and Pari, 2006). It was reported that THC caused a significant reduction in lipid peroxidation (TBARs and hydroperoxides) and lipids (cholesterol, triglycerides, free fatty acids and phospholipids) than curcumin in serum and tissues of diabetic rats, suggesting its role in protection against lipid peroxidation and its anti-hyperlipidemic effect.

In a subsequent study, Pari and Murugan (2007a) demonstrated the anti-hyperlipidemic actions of THCs (provided by Sabinsa) in diabetic rats. The changes such as increased levels of serum total lipids (Fig. 55), low density lipids (LDL) (Fig. 56), very low-density lipids (VLDL) (Fig. 57) and decreased levels of high density lipids (HDL) (Fig. 58) in diabetic rats were reversed after administration of THCs. The treatment with THCs significantly reduced the levels of HMG CoA reductase (Fig. 59), cholesterol, triglycerides, free fatty acids and phospholipids (Figs. 60 & 61) to near-normal levels.

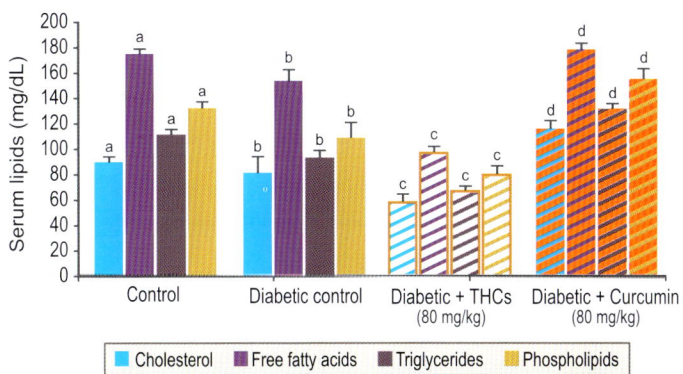

Values are mean ± SD for six rats in each group.
Values not sharing a common superscript letter differ significantly at p<0.05 (DMRT).

THCs were found to have better activity than curcumin in lowering serum lipids

Fig. 55: Influence of THCs and curcumin on serum cholesterol, free fatty acid, triglyceride and phospholipids in control and experimental rats.
(Adapted from Pari and Murugan, 2007a)

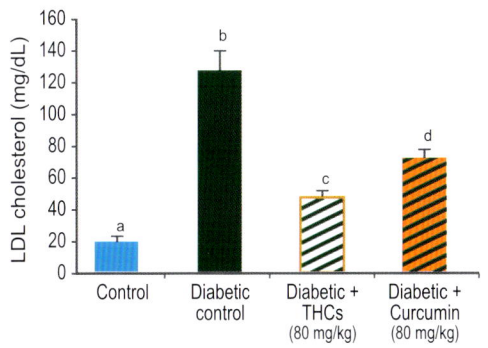
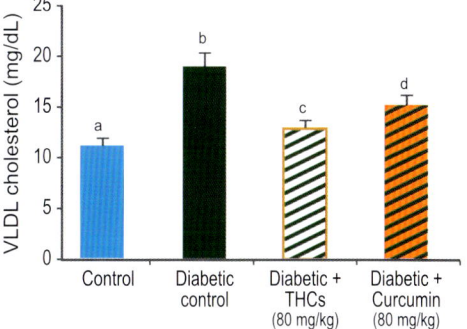

Values are mean ± SD for six rats in each group.
Values not sharing a common superscript letter differ significantly at p<0.05 (DMRT).

THCs were found to have better activity than curcumin in lowering LDL level

THCs were found to have better activity than curcumin in lowering VLDL level

Fig. 56: Influence of THCs and curcumin on the levels of LDL cholesterol in control and experimental rats.
(Adapted from Pari and Murugan, 2007a)

Fig. 57: Influence of THCs and curcumin on the levels of VLDL cholesterol in control and experimental rats.
(Adapted from Pari and Murugan, 2007a)

Chapter 3
TETRAHYDROCURCUMIN (THC): THE MAJOR METABOLITE WITH MAJOR BENEFITS

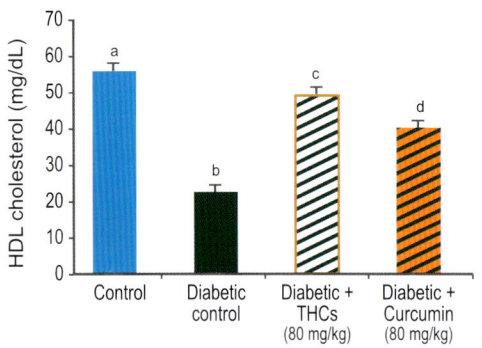

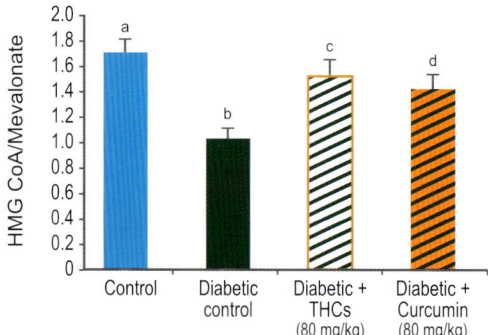

Values are mean ± SD for six rats in each group.
Values not sharing a common superscript letter differ significantly at p<0.05 (DMRT).

THCs were found to have better activity than curcumin in increasing HDL level

Higher the HMG CoA/Mevalonate ratio lower the enzyme activity

Fig. 58: Influence of THCs and curcumin on HDL cholesterol levels in control and experimental rats.
(Adapted from Pari and Murugan, 2007a)

Fig. 59: Influence of THCs and curcumin on hepatic HMG CoA reductase levels in control and experimental rats.
(Adapted from Pari and Murugan, 2007a)

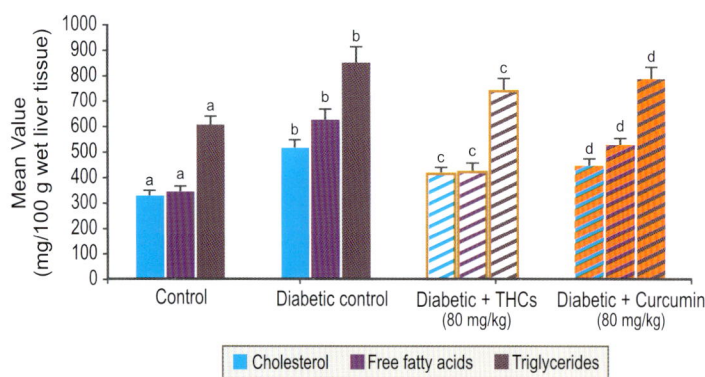

Values are mean ± SD for six rats in each group.
Values not sharing a common superscript letter differ significantly at p<0.05 (DMRT).

THCs were found to have better activity than curcumin in lowering cholesterol, free fatty acids and triglyceride levels

Fig. 60: Influence of THCs and curcumin on liver cholesterol, free fatty acids and triglyceride levels in control and experimental rats.
(Adapted from Pari and Murugan, 2007a)

TETRAHYDROCURCUMIN (THC): THE MAJOR METABOLITE WITH MAJOR BENEFITS

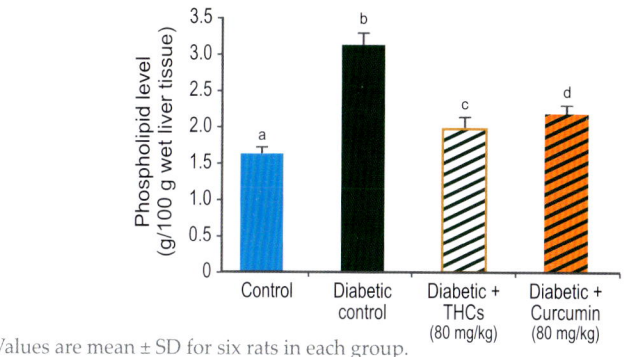

Values are mean ± SD for six rats in each group.
Values not sharing a common superscript letter differ significantly at p<0.05 (DMRT).

THCs were found to have better activity than curcumin in lowering phospholipid levels

Fig. 61: Influence of THCs and curcumin on liver phospholipid levels in control and experimental rats. (Adapted from Pari and Murugan, 2007a)

Wongeakin *et al.* (2009) reported that curcumin and THC changed the lipid profile (serum cholesterol, TG, HDL-C and LDL-C) significantly in STZ-induced diabetic rats, suggesting that curcumin and THC may have hypoglycemic and antilipidemic effects.

Karthikesan *et al.* (2010a) evaluated the anti-hyperlipidemic effect of THCs (provided by Sabinsa) and chlorogenic acid (CGA) alone and in combination on alterations in lipids, lipoproteins and enzymes involved in lipid metabolism in STZ-NA-induced type 2 diabetic rats. It was reported that administration of THCs ameliorated lipid abnormalities in experimental type 2 diabetes. In addition, CGA and THCs remarkably reduced the STZ-induced changes in lipid profile compared to the effects of CGA or THCs alone in diabetic rats.

Anticancer Activity

Cancer is defined as uncontrollable cell proliferation that invades and causes destruction to adjacent normal tissues or spread via lymph or blood to other organs sites in the body. When cancer cells at the originating site become clinically detectable, it is called the primary tumor. The infiltration of cancer cells into the surrounding normal tissues lead to a metastatic state. Metastasis is a complex cascade of events involving the migration of cancer cells from the site of origin to other parts of the body, namely lungs, liver, brain and bones through the bloodstream or lymphatic system. To migrate, malignant cells break away from the primary tumor, attach to and degrade proteins that make up the surrounding extra cellular matrix (ECM), which separates the tumor from adjoining tissue. Key proteases involved in the degradation of ECM are serine proteases (plasmins), urokinase plasminogen activator (uPA), cysteine proteases such as cathepsin B and L, and MMP.

Tumor angiogenesis, one of the critical steps associated with cancer metastasis, which is primarily involved in the formation of new capillary blood vessels from pre-existing vessels that promotes further tumor growth. It is a normal and vital process essential for growth and development, wound healing and granulation of tissue. However, it is also considered to be a fundamental step in transition of tumors from dormant to malignant state. Several growth factors namely, basic fibroblast growth factor (bFGF), and vascular endothelial growth factor (VEGF) secreted by tumor cells promote angiogenesis. In addition, cancerous cells do not produce anti-VEGF enzyme protein kinase G (PKG). Furthermore, PKG limits β-catenin in normal cells which promotes angiogenesis (Browning, 2008).

Since angiogenesis is also required for the spread of a tumor or metastasis, anti-angiogenic therapy is one of the most promising strategies for cancer treatment.

It is reported that curcumin and THC induce both anti-proliferation and anti-angiogenic effect. More potent anti-angiogenic effect was observed for THC, and it might be due to its higher antioxidant activity than curcumin (Aggarwal *et al.*, 2014; Yoysungnoen *et al.*, 2008).

Hepatocellular Carcinoma

Hepatocellular carcinoma (HCC), a highly malignant tumor, is characterized by active neovascularization that promotes tumor growth. One of the approaches for HCC treatment is the use of an anti-angiogenic agent. Sugiyama *et al.* provided evidence that THC exhibits strong antioxidant action; especially, THC has more potent physiological and pharmacological properties than curcuminoids including curcumin, DMC and BDMC (Sugiyama *et al.*, 1996).

Subsequently, Yoysungnoen *et al.* (2008) studied the *in vitro* effect of THC on HepG2 cells (an immortalized human liver carcinoma cells) and in male BALB/c nude mice to show the inhibitory effect of THC on tumor microvasculature. To evaluate the antiproliferative activities of THC *in vitro*, a standard 3-(4,5-dimethylthiazol-2- yl)-2,5-diphenyl-tetrazolium bromide (MTT) assay was employed. HepG2 cells (2×10^6 cells) were inoculated onto a dorsal skin-fold chamber in male BALB/c nude mice that were orally administered with curcumin or THC (300 mg/kg or 3000 mg/kg) daily to assess tumor growth inhibition. On the days of 7, 14 and 21, the tumor microvasculature was observed using fluorescence video microscopy (Fig. 62).

Results from this study showed that there was a substantial increase in the capillary vascularity in the HepG2-group on day 7 (52.43%), 14 (69.17%), and 21 (74.08%), as compared to control (33.04%, $p<0.001$). Interestingly, curcumin and THC significantly decreased in the capillary vascularity and this anti-angiogenic effect of curcumin and THC was found to be dose-dependent. However, THC treatment had more significant effect than curcumin, in particular, from the 21-day capillary vascularity (44.96% and 52.86%, $p<0.05$).

TETRAHYDROCURCUMIN (THC): THE MAJOR METABOLITE WITH MAJOR BENEFITS

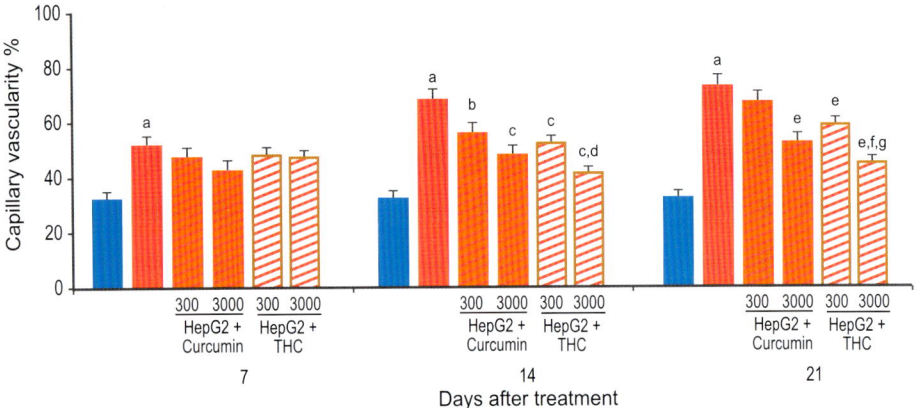

$^a p<0.001$, Control (normal) vs. HepG2 group with vehicle (vehicle control);
$^b p<0.005$, Curcumin (300 mg/kg/bw) vs. 14 d HepG2 group with vehicle;
$^c p<0.001$, Curcumin (3000 mg/kg/bw) and THC (300 & 3000 mg/kg/bw) vs. 14 d HepG2 group with vehicle;
$^d p<0.01$, THC (3000 mg/kg/bw) vs. 14 d HepG2-THC 300 group;
$^e p<0.001$, Curcumin (3000 mg/kg/bw) and THC (300 & 3000 mg/kg/bw) vs. 21 d HepG2 group with vehicle;
$^f p<0.001$, THC (3000 mg/kg/bw) vs. 21 d HepG2-THC 300 group;
$^g p<0.05$, THC (3000 mg/kg/bw) vs. 21 d HepG2-Curcumin 3000 group.

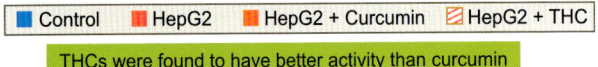

Fig. 62: Time course treatment effect (7-14 days) of curcumin or THC (300 and 3000 mg/kg/bw) on capillary vascularity (mean ± SE).
(Adapted from Yoysungnoen *et al.*, 2008)

From the above study, it was concluded that THC exerts its anti-angiogenic potential without any cytotoxic activities to HepG2 cells even at the highest dose studied. It is suggested that anti-angiogenic properties of curcumin and THC represent a common potential mechanism for their anticancer actions.

Liu *et al.* (2017) investigated the efficacy and associated mechanism of action of THC and curcumin against HCC in ascites tumor-bearing model in mice using hepatoma cell line (H22). Tetrahydrocurcumin treatment increased the survival rates of tumor bearing mice significantly and was more effective than curcumin in inhibiting tumor growth. Tetrahydrocurcumin induced the apoptosis of H22 cells by increasing the level of p53 and decreasing the level of mouse double minute 2 homolog (MDM2). Tetrahydrocurcumin also decreased the expression of Bcl-2 significantly and increased the expression of pro-apoptotic Bcl2-associated X protein (BAX), resulting in the release of cytochrome c.

Tetrahydrocurcumin significantly activated caspase-9 and induced cleavage of caspase-3 leading to apoptosis in H22 cells (Fig. 63). The results of this study indicate that THC was more effective than curcumin in inducing apoptosis of H22-induced ascites in tumor cells by activating the mitochondrial apoptosis pathway, suggesting THC could be a potentially effective agent for HCC treatment.

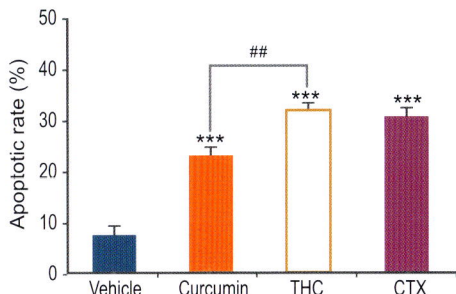

***$p<0.001$ vs. Vehicle control group; ##$p<0.01$ vs. Curcumin group.
CTX: Cyclophosphamide.

Fig. 63: Effects of THC on the apoptosis rate in a H22-induced ascites tumor model in mice.
(Adapted from Liu *et al.*, 2017)

Colon Cancer

A recent study found that THC was more effective in inhibiting the development of preneoplastic aberrant crypt foci (ACF) induced by 1, 2- dimethylhydrazine in colons of mice and cell proliferation than curcumin (Kim *et al.*, 1998). In a subsequent study, it was demonstrated that dietary administration of THC (provided by Sabinsa) disrupted the intercellular communication of crypt cells and also reduced the protein level of connexin-43 (Cx-43) (Fig. 64) an important molecule of gap junction and found

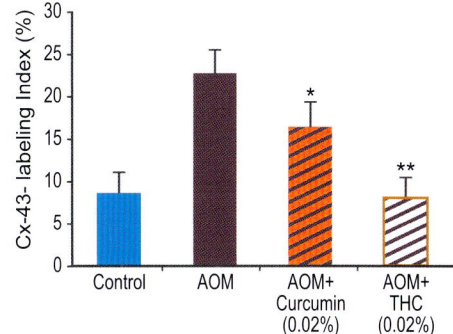

*$p<0.05$, **$p<0.01$ vs. Control group.
AOM: Azoxymethane.

Fig. 64: Inhibitory effects of curcumin and THC on AOM-induced Cx-43 protein expression in colorectal tissue.
(Adapted from Lai *et al.*, 2011)

to be more effective than curcumin in preventing azoxymethane-induced colon carcinogenesis (Lai *et al.*, 2011).

Breast Cancer

Human lemur tyrosine kinase-3 (LMTK3), an oncogenic receptor tyrosine kinase (RTK) implicated in various types of cancer, is primarily involved in regulation of estrogen receptor-α (ERα) by phosphorylation activity (Giamas *et al.*, 2011; Stebbing *et al.*, 2013). Molecular Mechanics/Poisson-Boltzmann Surface Area (MM/PBSA) is a popular method to estimate interaction free energies between biomolecules (Kumari *et al.*, 2014). In this context, recently, Anbarasu and Jayanthi (2018) used a computational-based docking, dynamics, and MM/PBSA approach for the identification of curcumin derivatives, including THC as human LMTK3 inhibitors for breast cancer. It was suggested that future experimental evaluation might prove its role in breast cancer therapeutics.

To further understand the efficacy of THC in breast cancer, Han *et al.* (2016) investigated the antitumor effects and mechanism of THC in human breast cancer cells (MCF-7). It was found that THC exerted marked antiproliferative activity against MCF-7 cells in a dose-dependent manner with IC_{50} of 107.8 µM for 24 h. Tetrahydrocurcumin was shown to mediate cell-cycle arrest at G0/G1 phase and induces apoptosis in MCF-7 cells via the mitochondrial pathway, by activating caspase-9 and caspase-3 cleavage, while increasing Bax expression. Tetrahydrocurcumin treatment also elevated the intracellular ROS, and decreased Bcl-2 and PARP expression. Cytochrome c release to cytosol and the loss of mitochondrial membrane potential was also shown with THC treatment, thus, suggesting that THC may be an excellent chemopreventive agent in the treatment of breast cancer.

Similarly, in an earlier study, Kang *et al.* (2014) also examined the efficacy and the mechanism of action of THC in human breast cancer cells (MCF-7). It was shown that THC exhibited significant cell growth inhibition by inducing mitochondrial apoptosis and G2/M arrest and apoptosis via p38 MAPK in human breast cancer MCF-7 cells. Moreover, co-treatment of MCF-7 cells with THC and p38 MAPK inhibitor, SB203580, effectively reversed the dissipation in mitochondrial membrane potential and blocked THC-mediated Bax up-regulation, Bcl-2 down-regulation, caspase-3 activation as well as p21 up-regulation, suggesting that p38 MAPK might mediate THC-induced apoptosis and G2/M arrest in MCF-7 breast cancer cells. The above findings clearly suggest that THC may potentially serve as a therapeutic agent for breast cancer.

Wright *et al.* (2013) evaluated the pharmacodynamic effects of chemically-complex turmeric extracts (crude extract or essential oil-free curcuminoid fraction) vs. purified curcuminoid-only turmeric extracts normalized to curcuminoid content on human breast cancer cell growth and tumor cell secretion of parathyroid hormone-related protein (PTHrP), an important driver of cancer bone metastasis, using an estrogen-receptor negative human breast cancer cell lines (MDA-MB-231 cells). Sabinsa provided THCs, manufactured by reduction of the naturally occurring mixture of curcuminoids present in turmeric (≥96% pure). The results of this study showed that the isolated essential oils actually increased PTHrP secretion, a potentially adverse biological effect. Similarly, ginger essential oils, analogous to turmeric essential oils, also increased PTHrP secretion. Thus, this study revealed that naturally-occurring mixture of the three curcuminoids was as potent as the individual curcuminoids in inhibiting cancer cell growth and expression of the osteolytic factor PTHrP. The bioactivity of clinically-relevant, chemically-complex botanical extracts underscored by the discovery that the secondary oils of turmeric could have adverse effects in breast cancer, as the essential oils actually enhanced breast cancer cell secretion of osteolytic factors.

In contrast, the authors (Wright *et al.*, 2013) showed that curcumin and BDMC vs. DMC exhibited differential effects on breast cancer cell viability and inhibition of PTHrP secretion and was statistically equipotent to the naturally occurring mixture of curcuminoids. Degradative metabolites (vanillin and ferulic acid) did not inhibit cell growth or PTHrP, while reduced metabolites (THCs) had inhibitory effects on cell growth and PTHrP secretion but only at concentrations ≥10-fold higher than the curcuminoids.

Glioma (Brain and Spinal Cord Tumors)

Glioma is a broad category of brain and spinal cord tumors that come from glial cells, support nerve cells. Recently, Zhang *et al.* (2018b) evaluated the effects of THC on the radiosensitivity of glioma cells and the possible molecular mechanism. It was reported that glioma cells treated with THC in combination with radiation therapy significantly induced G0/G1 cell cycle arrest and decreased S phase cells through the down-regulation of cyclin D1 and proliferative cell nuclear antigen (PCNA) (Fig. 65). In addition, the intracellular GSH was also decreased in THC co-treated glioma (C6) cells. The combination treatment group demonstrated lower cell viability and higher apoptosis rate as compared to radiation group. The *in vivo* efficacy assay also indicated that tumor growth was greatly inhibited by THC in combination with radiation treatment.

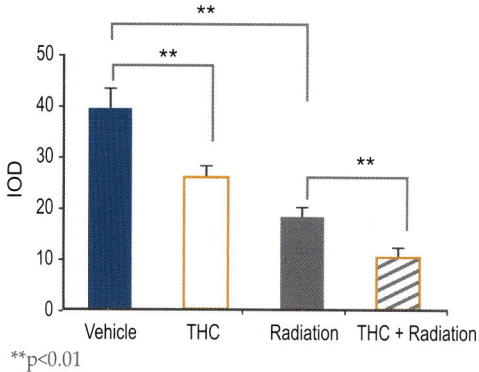

Fig. 65: Effect of THC on the expressions of cell cycle phase-related proteins in C6 cells. Bar graph shows the quantification of immunocytochemical staining of PCNA expressed as integrated optical density (IOD) in glioma (C6) cells. (Adapted from Zhang *et al.*, 2018b)

Lung Carcinoma

Autophagy plays a crucial role in the cellular pathological and physiological processes and in maintaining cellular homeostasis (Wang and Qin, 2013). In carcinogenesis, overexpression of phosphatidylinositol 3-kinase (PI3K/protein kinase B (Akt) and mammalian target of rapamycin (mTOR)) suppress autophagy (Levine and Kroemer, 2008; Zi *et al.*, 2015). Song *et al.* (2018) investigated whether THC inhibits PI3K/Akt/mTOR pathway and induces autophagy in lung cancer cells (A549) *in vitro*. It was found that THC treatment significantly inhibited the proliferation of A549 cells in a dose-dependent manner (Fig. 66). Regarding the effect on molecular targets, THC treatment significantly reduced the levels of p-mTOR, p-Akt and p62, indicating their involvement in THC-induced autophagic cell proliferation inhibition (Song *et al.*, 2018). Moreover, THC treatment activated the levels of the autophagy-associated protein markers LC3II/I (the conjugated forms of LC3) and reduced the p62 expression, a selective autophagy substrate. All the findings of this study suggested that THC inhibition of A549 lung cancer cell proliferation could be achieved through the autophagy pathway mechanisms (Fig. 67).

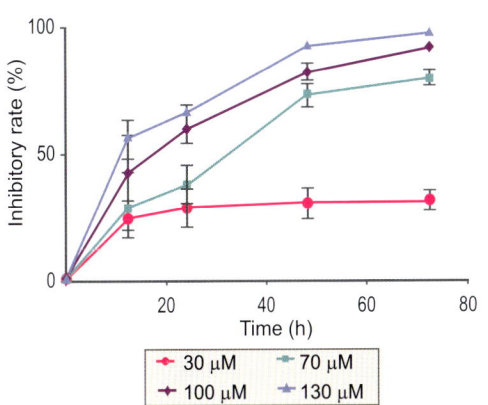

Fig. 66: Effect of THC on A549 cell proliferation. THC 130 μM concentration showed the highest inhibitory effect on A549 cell proliferation, whereas THC 30 μM had the lowest inhibitory effect, thus indicating a dose-dependent effect of THC treatment.
(Adapted from Song *et al.*, 2018)

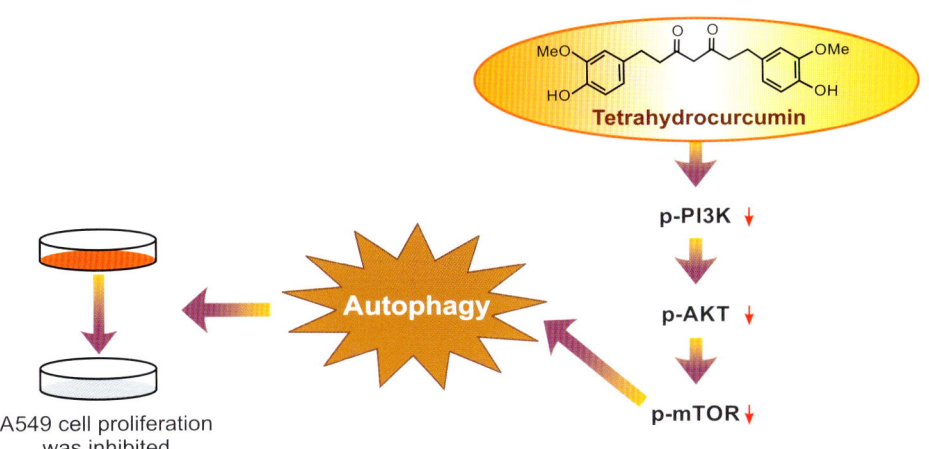

mTOR: Mammalian target of rapamycin, also known as the mechanistic target of rapamycin; Akt: Protein kinase B; PI3K: Phosphatidylinositol 3-kinase.

Fig. 67: Potential mechanisms for THC-induced autophagy.
(Adapted from Song *et al.*, 2018)

Fibrosarcoma

The effect of THC on the invasion and motility of highly-metastatic HT1080 human fibrosarcoma cells was studied. Tetrahydrocurcumin reduced HT1080 cell invasion and migration that was associated with downregulation of matrix metalloproteinase (MMP-2, MMP-9) and uPA, ECM degradation enzymes, inhibition of metalloproteinase (TIMP)-2 and membrane-type 1 matrix metalloproteinase (MT1-MMP), regulators of cell adhesion to ECM proteins (Yodkeeree et al., 2008). The effect of THC in reducing the secretion of MMP-2, MMP-9 and uPA from HT1080 cells supported the inhibitory effect of THC on cancer cell invasion. MMP-2 secreted as pro-MMP-2, a latent zymogen, is activated on the cell surface by MT1-MMP and TIMP-2. After activation, an MT1-MMP proteolytic processing leads to its inactive form and appearance of this form has been strongly correlated with MMP-2 activation. It was found that THC significantly reduces total MT1-MMP and thereby decreases pro-MMP2 activation.

Osteosarcoma (Bone Cancer)

Human osteosarcoma is considered as a malignant tumor with poor prognosis that readily metastasizes. Given the role of THC as a powerful antioxidant, Zhang et al. (2017) investigated the potential mechanisms by which THC may reduce the tumor cell growth, suppress migration and invasion in nude mice lung metastasis model of osteosarcoma. The findings of this study revealed that THC significantly reduced the growth of osteosarcoma cells and suppressed migration and invasion (Fig. 68).

Chapter 3
TETRAHYDROCURCUMIN (THC): THE MAJOR METABOLITE WITH MAJOR BENEFITS

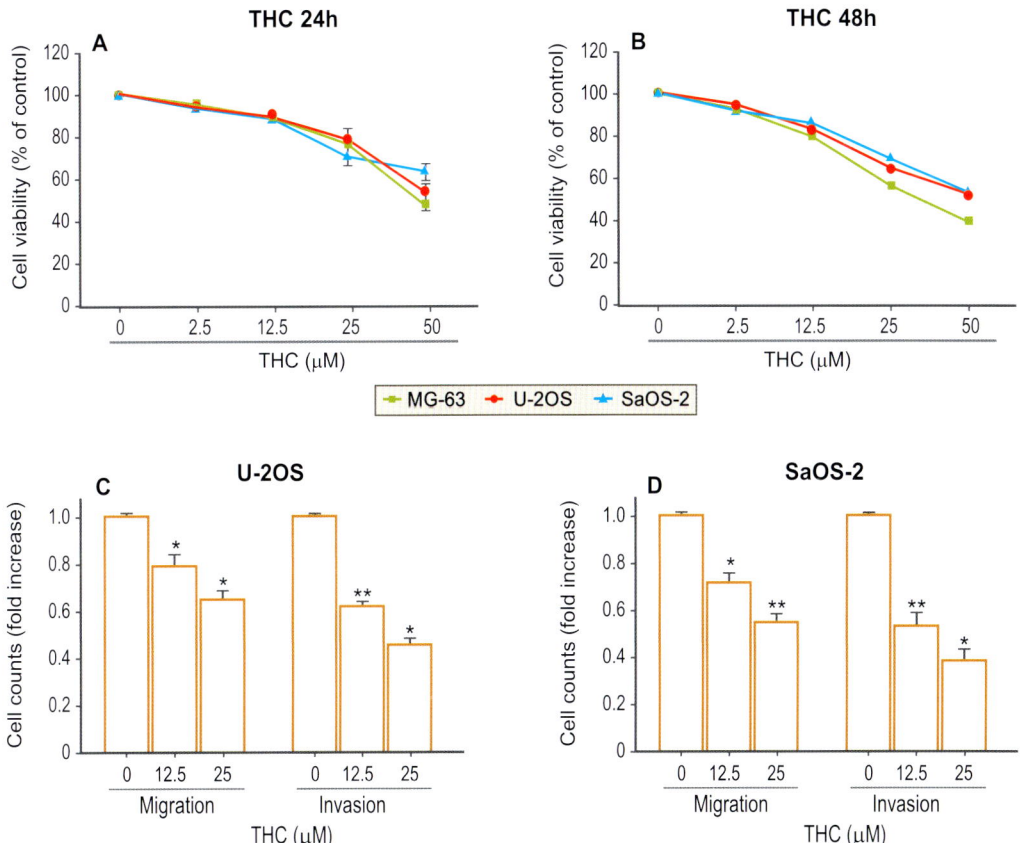

Migration and invasion of cells were assayed for 48 h using Boyden chamber and Matrigel-coated Boyden chamber, respectively; *p< 0.05; **p<0.01; MTT: 3-(4,5-dimethylthiazol-2-yl)-2,5-diphenyltetrazolium bromide.

Fig. 68: Effect of THC on the cell viability, migration and invasion in human osteosarcoma cells.
(Adapted from Zhang *et al.*, 2017)

(A) (B): MG-63, U-2OS, and SaOS-2 human osteosarcoma cells were treated with different concentrations of THC (0–50 μM) in medium for 24 and 48 h, and cell viability was measured by MTT assay.
(C) (D): The bar graphs summarize the effect of THC on migration and invasion assays performed using U-2OS and SaOS-2 cells.

Tetrahydrocurcumin has been reported to have anti-tumor activity in several tumor types. Hypoxia-inducible factor-1α (HIF-1α) has been demonstrated to be associated with tumor metastasis by regulating epithelial-mesenchymal transition (EMT). It was also reported by Zhang *et al.* (2017) that the mesenchymal-epithelial transition (MET) process was facilitated by THC in nude mice studies. Importantly, *in vitro* studies confirmed that HIF-1α expression was downregulated by THC by inhibiting Akt/mTOR and p38 MAPK pathways. In addition, it was suggested that THC exhibited a remarkable inhibitory effect on HIF-1α expression and angiogenesis under hypoxic conditions (Figs. 69 & 70). Furthermore, THC activated autophagy and induced MET and suppressed angiogenesis in a HIF-1α-related manner. The authors suggested that THC potentially provides therapeutic strategies for human osteosarcoma by suppressing angiogenesis and metastasis via downregulating HIF-1α and by promoting autophagy mechanisms.

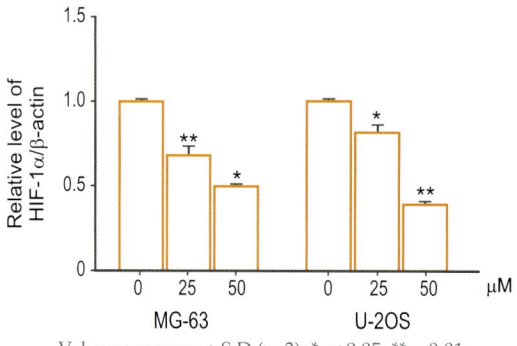

Values are mean ± S.D (n=3); *p< 0.05; **p<0.01.

Fig. 69: Effect of THC on the expression of HIF-1α.
The expression of HIF-1α assessed by western blotting in MG-63 and U-2OS cells treated with different concentrations of THC (0–50 μM). (Adapted from Zhang *et al.*, 2017)

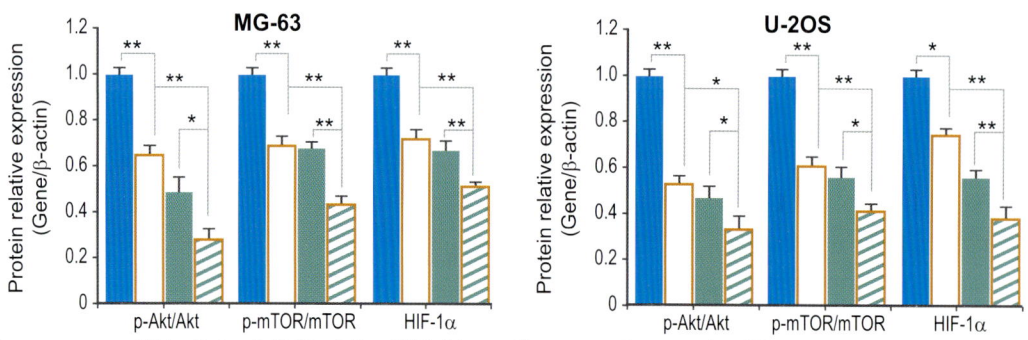

Values are mean ± SD (n=3); *p< 0.05; **p<0.01; mTOR: Mammalian target of rapamycin; HIF-1α: Hypoxia-inducible factor 1-α

Fig. 70: Effect of THC on the expression of HIF-1α by suppressing Akt/mTOR and p38 MAPK signaling pathways.
The bar graph shows the expressions of Akt/mTOR pathway and HIF-1α in MG-63 and U-2OS cells assessed by western blotting (Control, THC 25 μM, Akt inhibitor LY294002 20 μM and THC+LY294002 groups). (Adapted from Zhang *et al.*, 2017)

Leukemia

Bolger *et al.* (2018) evaluated the distribution of curcumin and its metabolism to THC in human PBMCs obtained from healthy individuals and CLL patients following exposure to Lipocurc™ (liposomal curcumin). It was observed that curcumin was metabolized to THC in PBMCs of both healthy individual and CLL patients supplemented with Lipocurc™. However, curcumin distribution into PBMC from CLL patients was higher compared to PBMC from healthy individuals, while metabolism to THC was similar, suggesting potential therapeutic benefit of curcumin and its metabolites in CLL patients.

Autophagy is non-apoptotic form of programmed cell death, functioning as a tumor suppressor mechanism similar to apoptosis and is crucial for maintaining cellular homeostasis (Clarke, 1990). Wu *et al.* (2011) investigated the anticancer effect of curcumin and THC in human acute myelogenous leukemia cells (HL-60) *in vitro*. The findings of this study revealed that THC induced cell death through autophagy but not apoptosis. The authors demonstrated that mechanistically, THC treatment decreased phosphorylation of phosphatidylinositol 3-kinase (PI3K), Akt (protein kinase B) and mammalian target of rapamycin (mTOR) and modulated phosphorylation of mitogen-activated protein kinases (MAPKs) in HL-60 cells. Autophagy is characterized by the formation of numerous acidic vascular organelle (AVO) (Paglin *et al.*, 2001). It was reported that THC remarkably increased the expression of light chain 3 (LC3) and Beclin-1 proteins in HL-60 cells, the regulators of autophagy in mammalian cells followed by AVO formation (Kang *et al.*, 2011; Kimura *et al.*, 2009). The authors recommend that THC could be used as a new anticancer agent for human leukemia because of its prominent effect on HL-60 cells and its new anticancer mechanism of inducing autophagy.

Cervical Cancer

Molecularly targeted therapies are aimed to improve treatment outcomes in cervical cancer patients. In this regard, it may be relevant to point out that the relationship between COX-2, its synthesized product PGE$_2$ and cervical cancer has been already established (Sales et al., 2001). Tetrahydrocurcumin was found to inhibit tumor angiogenesis in CaSki cells (cervical cancer cells)-implanted nude mice by downregulating HIF-1-α, VEGF expression, and its receptors (Yoysungnoen, 2015). Recently, the same group investigated the inhibitory effects of oral administration of THC (100, 300, and 500 mg/kg of THC daily for 30 consecutive days) on COX-2 expression and their signaling pathways associated with cervical cancer using xenografts in nude mice, where CaSki cells were subcutaneously injected in nude mice to establish tumors (Yoysungnoen et al., 2016). It was shown that THC treatment significantly reduced the relative tumor volume (RTV) (Fig. 71). Tetrahydrocurcumin also decreased the cell proliferation index (Ki-67 overexpression) in cervical tumors (Fig. 72). Mechanistically, THC-mediated tumor growth inhibition was associated with attenuation of COX-2, EGFR, p-ERK1 & 2, and p-AKT expression (Fig. 73). These findings provide evidence that THC exerts anticancer effects against cervical cancer modulating multiple molecular targets.

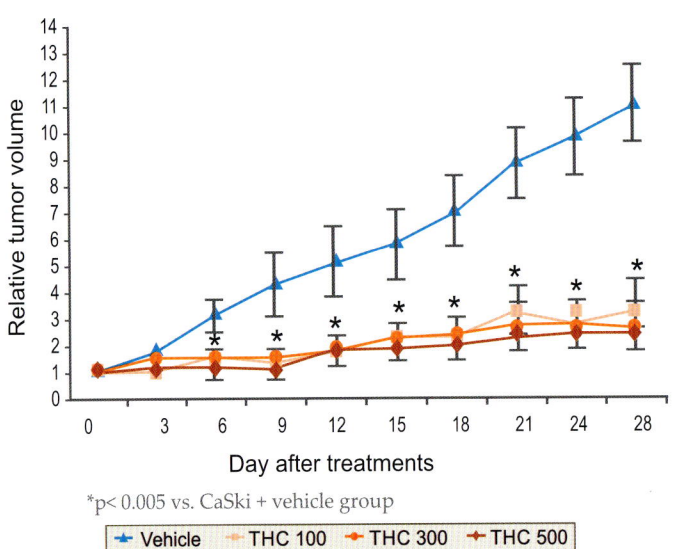

Fig. 71: Effect of THC on the tumor volume in CaSki cells (cervical cancer cells)-implanted nude mice. (Adapted from Yoysungnoen et al., 2016)

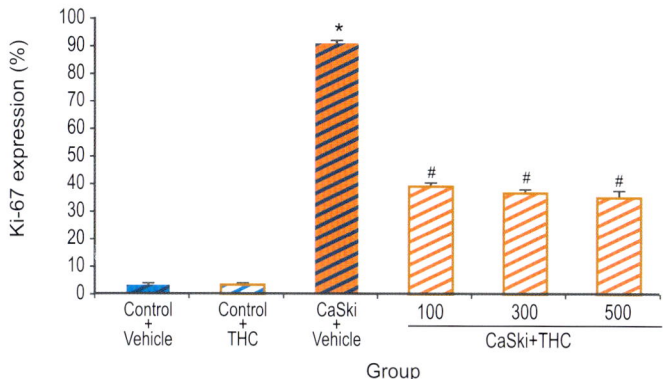

*p< 0.001 vs. Control + vehicle group; #p< 0.001 vs. CaSki + vehicle group.

Fig. 72: Effect of THC on Ki-67 expression in CaSki cells (cervical cancer cells)-implanted nude mice. (Adapted from Yoysungnoen et al., 2016)

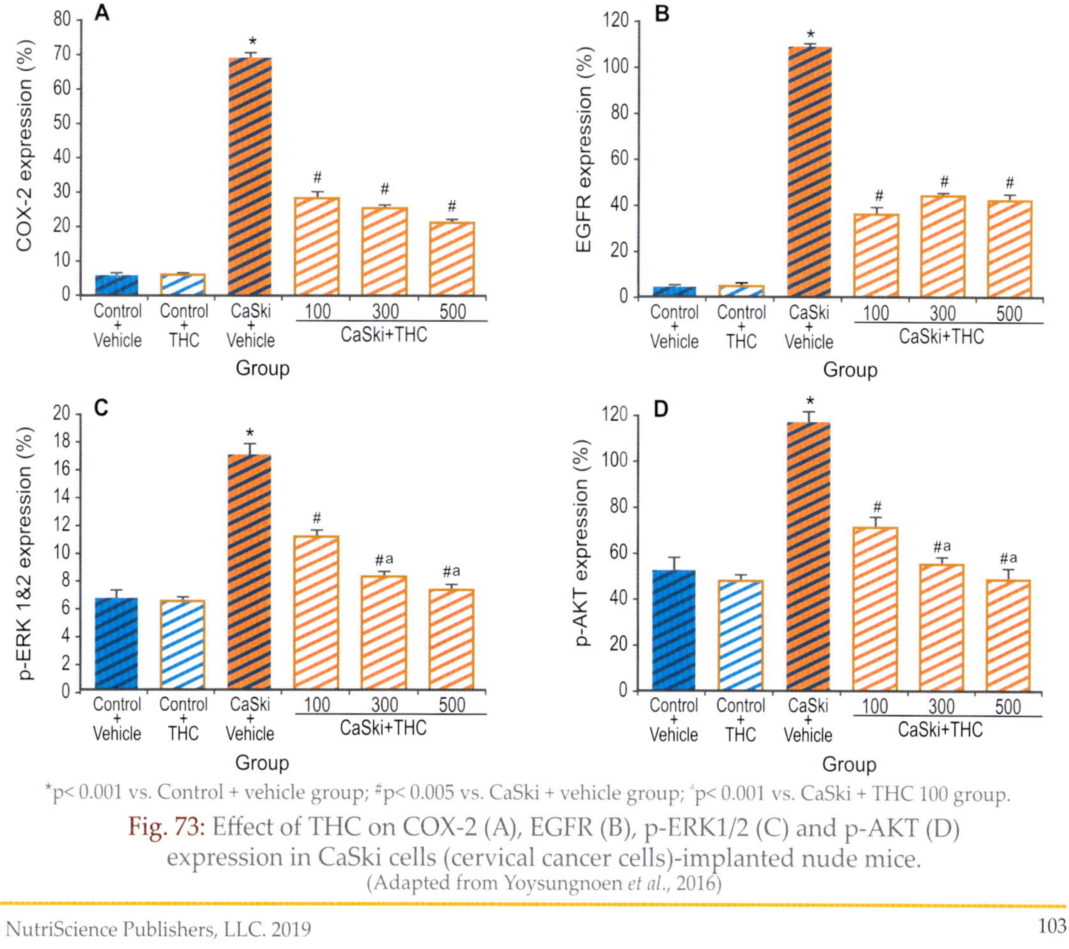

*p< 0.001 vs. Control + vehicle group; #p< 0.005 vs. CaSki + vehicle group; ªp< 0.001 vs. CaSki + THC 100 group.

Fig. 73: Effect of THC on COX-2 (A), EGFR (B), p-ERK1/2 (C) and p-AKT (D) expression in CaSki cells (cervical cancer cells)-implanted nude mice.
(Adapted from Yoysungnoen et al., 2016)

Anti-diabetic Potential

Diabetes is a metabolic disorder primarily defined by elevated blood sugar caused by insufficient production of insulin or inability to utilize the available insulin. In the case of type 1 diabetes, the body requires extraneous insulin since it fails to produce adequate insulin. On the other hand, in type 2 diabetes, there is a combination of an absolute insulin deficiency and failure of the cells to use insulin efficiently (insulin resistance). Genetic defects, cystic fibrosis-related- and gestational-diabetes, high doses of glucocorticoids induced steroid diabetes are variant forms of diabetes.

Amongst various types, type 2 diabetes mellitus is the most common type of diabetes involving insulin receptors. Insulin binding to receptors is the first event signifying the action of insulin, and this first step represents a major control point for the effects of insulin *in vivo*. It is not a fixed biological process but is subjected to modulation by alterations in either the receptor or affinity. Insulin receptors have been demonstrated in cells of a large variety of tissues from different animal species (Murugan et al., 2008). Some of the important features of diabetes also include increased levels of blood glucose, glycosylated haemoglobin, generation of ROS, oxidative damage to liver and kidney, increased lipid peroxidation, alteration in the levels of carbohydrate metabolic enzymes, depletion of antioxidants such as catalase (CAT), glutathione peroxidase (GPx), SOD, GSH, GST, vitamin C, vitamin E etc.

It is reported that the insulin secretory defect could result either from a progressive decline in β-cell function or a defect in β-cell mass. The β-cell failure in type 2 diabetes leads to insulin resistance which is associated with β-cell mass expansion and increased the responsiveness of nutrient-secretion coupling with excessive insulin biosynthesis (Prentki and Nolan, 2006) resulting in obesity finally leading to β-cell degradation.

Decreased insulin levels in the blood lead to an increase in glucose resulting in hyperglycemia. Chronic hyperglycemia leads to glucose auto-oxidation and further onto ROS production. Also, excess glucose level encourages protein glycosylation (Aragno et al., 1999; Bonnefont-Rousselot et al., 2000; Robertson, 2004).

In addition, increased ROS production causes oxidative stress and destruction of critical nonenzymic and enzymic CAT, GSH-Px, and SOD antioxidants and ultimately deleterious for the β islets with the lowest levels of intrinsic antioxidant defenses (Lenzen et al., 1996; West, 2000).

Kim et al. (2009) examined potential anti-diabetic mechanisms of curcumin, Curcumin C3 Complex®, and THCs (both provided by Sabinsa) in H4IIE rat hepatoma and Hep3B human hepatoma cells. Findings of this study showed that curcuminoids increased the phosphorylation of AMP-activated protein kinase (AMPK) and its downstream target acetyl-CoA carboxylase (ACC) in H4IIE and Hep3B cells with 100 times (curcumin) to 100,000 times (THCs) the potency of metformin. Thus, the results of this study suggest that AMPK mediated suppression of hepatic gluconeogenesis may be a potential mechanism mediating glucose-lowering effects of curcuminoids and THCs.

Tetrahydrocurcuminoids were shown to activate pancreatic β-cells involved in the secretion of insulin. In addition, THCs treatment in diabetic animals regulated blood glucose resulting in a significant improvement in enzymes that are associated with carbohydrate metabolism. Furthermore, THCs treatment also significantly improved the catalytic activities of hexokinase, glucose-6-phosphate dehydrogenase (G6PD), glucose-6-phosphatase, fructose-1,6-bisphosphatase, and sorbitol dehydrogenase enzymes, the major hepatic metabolic enzymes involved in carbohydrate metabolism in streptozotocin-induced diabetic rats (Pari and Murugan, 2005).

Tetrahydrocurcuminoids have been shown to have the capability to activate proinsulin synthesis and insulin release and thereby reducing plasma glucose and increasing insulin during diabetes. It was demonstrated that THCs significantly reduced TBARS and hydroperoxides in the liver and kidney of diabetic rats (Table 10). In addition the scavenging of free radicals by increasing the activity of SOD, CAT, GPx, GST, vitamins C and E were also reported (Murugan and Pari, 2006). Tetrahydrocurcumin was also evaluated for its inhibitory response on membrane lipid peroxidation by TBARS using rat liver homogenate. It was shown that THC was effective in preventing membrane lipid peroxidation induced by $FeSO_4$/ascorbate in concentration dependent manner (Prabhu et al., 2011).

Table 10: Influence of THCs and curcumin on the content of TBARS and hydroperoxides in rat liver and kidney. (Adapted from Murugan and Pari, 2006)

Groups	TBARS		Hydroperoxides	
	Liver	Kidney	Liver	Kidney
	(mM/100g tissue)		(mM/100g tissue)	
Normal	0.75 ± 0.05	1.76 ± 0.12	80.15 ± 5.45	55.85 ± 03.80
Diabetic Control	1.85 ± 0.11	3.73 ± 0.22	100.55 ± 5.93	78.66 ± 4.64
Diabetic + THCs (80 mg/kg)	1.06 ± 0.07	1.98 ± 0.14	87.09 ± 4.74	61.39 ± 4.48
Diabetic + Curcumin (80 mg/kg)	1.35 ± 0.08	2.30 ± 0.13	93.86 ± 4.17	68.14 ± 3.87

Karthikesan *et al*. (2010a) evaluated the anti-hyperlipidemic effect of THCs (provided by Sabinsa) and chlorogenic acid (CGA) alone and in combination on alterations in lipids, lipoproteins and enzymes involved in lipid metabolism in STZ-NA-induced type 2 diabetic rats. It was reported that administration of THCs ameliorated lipid abnormalities in experimental type 2 diabetes. In addition, the combination of CGA and THCs remarkably reduced the STZ-induced changes in lipid profile compared to the effects of CGA or THCs alone in diabetic rats.

Streptozotocin-nicotinamide considerably reduced the erythrocyte receptors and the insulin target tissues. It has been shown that THCs exert remarkable anti-hyperglycemic effects. Thus, the above findings imply that the anti-hyperglycemic effect of the THCs is partly due to the release of insulin from the existing pancreatic cells. Tetrahydrocurcuminoids have been demonstrated to activate insulin secretion and thereby significantly reducing blood glucose. Furthermore, in addition to enhancing insulin secretion, THCs also increased insulin binding sites in the STZ–NA diabetic animal model (Murugan and Pari, 2006).

Tetrahydrocurcuminoids (80 mg/kg/bw) (provided by Sabinsa) were administered to STZ–NA-induced diabetic rats orally for 45 days in order to evaluate its effect on insulin-binding sites of erythrocytes and to understand the underlying mechanism by which THCs produce the anti-hyperglycemic effect. The impact of THCs on levels of blood glucose (Fig. 74), plasma insulin (Fig. 75) and insulin-receptor interaction on erythrocyte cell membranes were assessed.

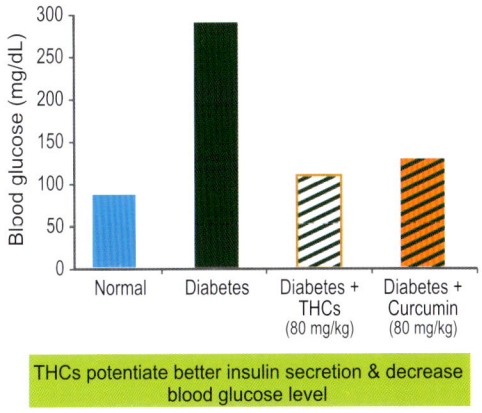

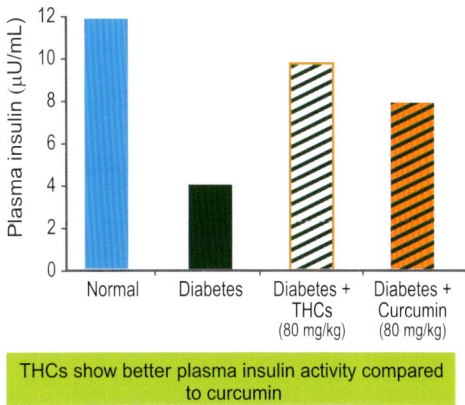

Fig. 74: Effect of THCs on the levels of blood glucose in normal and experimental rats.
(Adapted from Murugan *et al.*, 2008)

Fig. 75: Effect of THCs on the levels of serum insulin in normal and experimental rats.
(Adapted from Murugan *et al.*, 2008)

Mean specific binding of insulin was significantly lowered in diabetic rats with a decrease in plasma insulin. Erythrocytes from diabetic rats showed a decreased ability for insulin–receptor binding when compared with THCs treated diabetic rats. These results suggest that acute alteration of the insulin receptor on the membranes of erythrocytes occurred in diabetic rats. This study suggests the mechanism by which THCs increase the number of total cellular insulin binding sites resulting in a significant increase in plasma insulin. The effect of THCs was found to be more prominent than that of curcumin (Murugan *et al.*, 2008).

Oral THCs treatment at 80 mg/kg/bw for 15 days decreased hepatotoxicity induced by the commonly used antibiotic erythromycin estolate and the anti-malarial drug chloroquine in STZ-NA-induced diabetic rats. Tetrahydrocurcuminoids showed an anti-hyperlipidemic effect after 45 days at the same dose. Tetrahydrocurcuminoids also elevated the membrane-bound antioxidant enzymes, altered the levels of fatty acids, glucose and insulin in the blood of diabetic rats. Based on the findings it was concluded that THCs effectively decreased lipid peroxidation in several other tissues of the diabetic rats. All the above findings revealed that THCs exert higher antidiabetic effects than curcumin at similar doses (Anand *et al.*, 2008).

Similarly, oral administration of THCs at 80 mg/kg/bw to diabetic rats for 45 days resulted in a significant reduction in blood glucose and significant increase in plasma insulin levels. In addition, THCs caused significant increase in the activities of SOD, CAT, GPx, GST and reduced glutathione in the brains of diabetic rats with significant decrease in the lipid peroxidative markers TBARS and hydroperoxides in brain, suggesting efficacy for protection against lipid peroxidation-induced membrane damage. The effect of THCs was greater than that of curcumin. The study concluded that during diabetes, brain tissue is more vulnerable to oxidative stress and increased lipid peroxidation. Results of the present study suggest that THCs may contribute to its protective action against lipid peroxidation and enhancement of cellular antioxidant defense in addition to its anti-diabetic effect in type 2 diabetic rats (Pari and Murugan, 2007c).

The individual and synergistic effect of THCs and CGA on glycoprotein levels in plasma, liver and kidney of normal and STZ-NA-induced diabetic rats were evaluated (The principle behind combination therapy was to use drugs with different mechanisms of action). Streptozotocin when administered intraperitoneally at 45 mg/kg/bw, leads to a significant increase in plasma glucose and glycoproteins while decreasing plasma insulin. Tetrahydrocurcuminoids (80 mg/kg/bw) and CGA (5 mg/kg/bw) as individual and combined dose were administered to diabetic rats for a period of 45 days. The combination of THCs/CGA was more effective in decreasing plasma glucose, glycoproteins and increased insulin levels. The combination of THCs/CGA showed significant protection of membrane proteins against STZ-NA-induced diabetic rats (Karthikesan *et al.*, 2010b; Pari *et al.*, 2010; Pari and Karthikesan, 2009; Pari and Murugan, 2007d).

Streptozotocin-nicotinamide-induced diabetic rats showed significant increase in the concentration of palmitic acid (16:1), stearic acid (18:0) and oleic acid (18:1) in the tissues of liver, kidney and brain and decrease in the concentrations of linolenic acid (18:3) and arachidonic acid (20:4). The oral administration of THCs (80 mg/kg/bw) for 45 days to these diabetic rats decreased the concentrations of fatty acids, viz., palmitic, stearic, and oleic acid and elevated the levels of linolenic and arachidonic acid thereby suggesting that THCs have anti-diabetic and anti-hyperlipidemic effects. These effects of THCs were more potent than that of curcumin at the same dose (Murugan and Pari, 2007a & 2007c).

Karthikesan *et al.* (2010a) reported that the treatment with THCs or CGA significantly reduced the concentrations of tissue lipids (total cholesterol, triglycerides, free fatty acids (FFAs) and phospholipids (Pls)), in diabetic rats as compared to the normal rats, suggesting increased lipoprotein lipase (LPL) activity following administration of THCs/CGA might be due to increased insulin secretion. Further, combined treatment with THCs/CGA dramatically decreased the concentrations of tissue lipids compared to individual treatment with THCs or CGA and thus can potentially ameliorate lipid abnormalities in experimental type 2 diabetes.

Chen *et al.* (2018) demonstrated that THC simultaneously increased glucose uptake and activated insulin signaling in an unsaturated fatty acid, oleic acid-treated HepG2 cells, suggesting that THC may be able to reverse insulin resistance in steatosis in liver cells that may lead to obesity and diabetes.

Kim *et al.* (2018) reported that THC increased glucose-induced insulin secretion than the islets cultured in the medium without THC (Fig. 76). Also, after treatment with cytokine cocktail (CTK - containing IL-1β, IL-1α and TNF-α), THC-treated islets showed significant improvement in glucose-induced insulin release (Fig. 77A), GSH content (Fig. 77B), along with reduction of NO production (Fig. 77C) as compared with islets not treated with THC. Thus, the authors suggest that

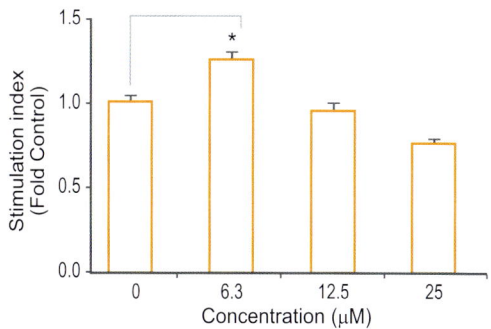

*p<0.05 vs. Control group

Fig. 76: Effect of THC on islet cell function.
(Adapted from Kim *et al.*, 2018)

preoperative THC administration enhances islet function before transplantation and attenuates the cytokine-induced damage associated with apoptosis.

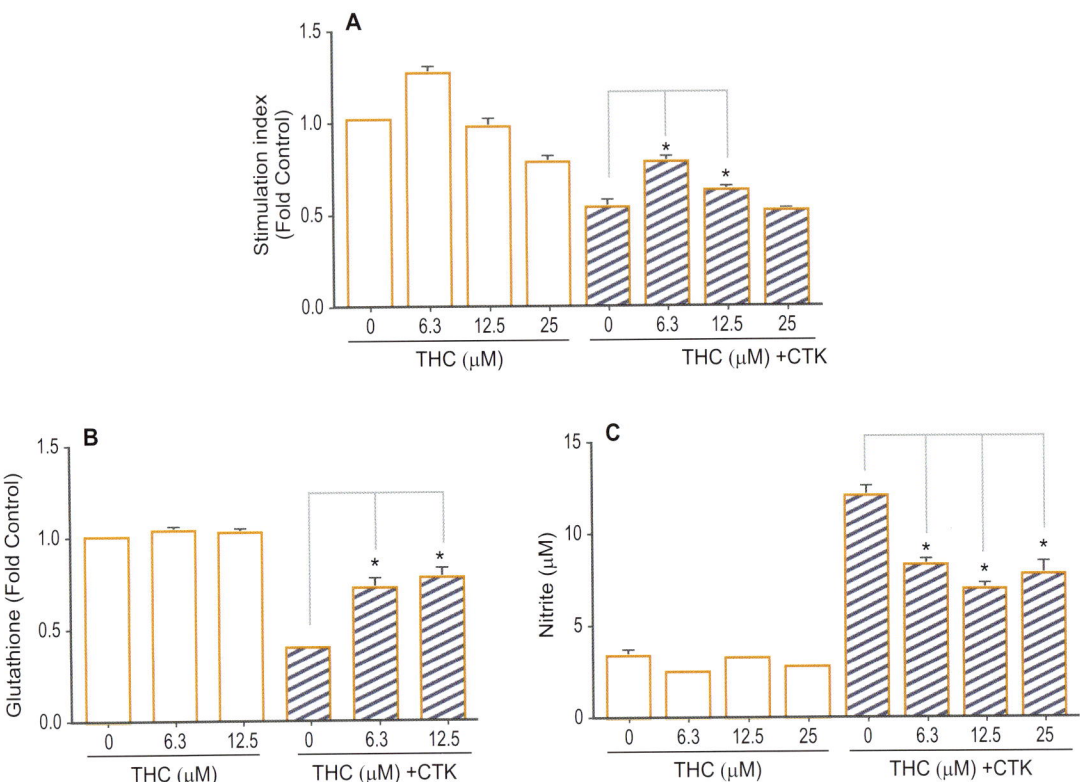

Data show mean (SE) values (p<0.05). *p<0.05 vs. CTK-only treatment.

Fig. 77: Effect of THC on islet cell function (A), GSH (B) and NO (C) in response to cytokines.
(Adapted from Kim *et al.*, 2018)

Anti-obesity Activity

Neyrinck *et al*. (2013) investigated whether *C. longa* extract (provided by Sabinsa) rich in curcumin with outer coat removed black pepper at doses compatible with human use, could modulate systemic inflammation in diet-induced obese mice. This study assessed the potential relevance of changes in adiposity and gut microbiota effect on obesity. Mice were fed with either a control diet, a high fat diet (HFD) or a HFD containing *C. longa* extract (0.1% of curcumin) with outer coat removed black pepper (0.01%), at the doses that can be extrapolated to human exposure, for four weeks. The results of this study revealed that oral administration of curcumin with outer coat removed black pepper improved pro-inflammatory disorders in the subcutaneous tissue following HFD feeding. In addition, *C. longa* extract and outer coat removed black pepper decreased HFD-induced proinflammatory cytokines expression in the subcutaneous adipose tissue, an effect independent of adiposity, immune cells recruitment, angiogenesis, or modulation of gut bacteria controlling inflammation. Based on the results, it was suggested that combination of curcumin and outer coat removed black pepper might be a natural alternative in the prevention of inflammatory disorders occurring early in the development of HFD-induced obesity. Interestingly, this study showed substantial levels of THC, but not curcumin accumulation in the subcutaneous adipose tissue, suggesting that THC, the metabolite of curcumin accumulated inside white adipose tissue might be responsible for the anti-inflammatory effect observed after administration of *C. longa* extract added in the HFD.

In a recent study, Pan *et al*. (2018) evaluated the therapeutic effect of THC, on high fat diet (HFD)-induced obesity associated with non-alcoholic fatty liver disease (NAFLD) and insulin resistance using C57BL/6 mice. For 10 weeks, mice were fed with HFD and then received THC (20 or 100 mg/kg) with continuation on a HFD for another 10 weeks. Findings from the study showed that THC significantly decreased final body weight, weight gain, and also relative epididymal and mesenteric weights compared with those in the HFD alone group (Table 11). In addition, it also reduced the adipocyte size (Figs. 78A & 78B) significantly in THC group compared with that of the HFD alone group.

Table 11: Effect of THC on body weight gain, relative organ weights and serum parameters in HFD-fed obese mice. (Adapted from Pan *et al.*, 2018)

	ND	HFD	HFD + THC (20 mg/kg)	HFD + THC (100 mg/kg)	ND + THC (100 mg/kg)
Body weight gain					
Initial weight (g)	25.9 ± 1.1[a]	34.0 ± 1.2[a]	33.4 ± 2.2[a]	33.8 ± 2.9[a]	26.8 ± 0.5[a]
Final weight (g)	28.0 ± 1.2[c]	43.0 ± 2.2[a]	38.4 ± 3.4[b]	39.5 ± 2.9[b]	29.0 ± 2.0[c]
Weight gain (g)	2.2 ± 0.7[c]	9.0 ± 0.4[a]	5.0 ± 2.7[b]	5.7 ± 3.3[b]	2.2 ± 1.1[c]
Relative adipose tissue and organ weights					
Epididymal fat	1.1 ± 0.4[c]	6.6 ± 0.4[a]	5.3 ± 0.8[b]	5.6 ± 0.7[b]	0.9 ± 0.7[c]
Retroperitoneal fat	0.3 ± 0.2[b]	2.4 ± 0.3[a]	2.1 ± 0.3[a]	2.2 ± 0.4[a]	0.2 ± 0.1[b]
Mesenteric fat	0.7 ± 0.4[bc]	2.3 ± 0.4[a]	1.4 ± 0.4[bc]	1.5 ± 0.3[b]	0.9 ± 0.3[c]
Liver (%)	4.4 ± 0.1[b]	5.6 ± 0.9[a]	3.9 ± 0.1[b]	4.0 ± 0.2[b]	4.1 ± 0.2[b]
Kidney (%)	1.3 ± 0.1[c]	1.7 ± 0.1[a]	1.6 ± 0.1[b]	1.5 ± 0.1[b]	1.3 ± 0.2[c]
Serum biochemical parameters					
GOT (U/L)	88.0 ± 9.9[b]	130.0 ± 18.9[a]	88.8 ± 10.2[b]	73.0 ± 20.6[bc]	60.5 ± 14.9[c]
GPT (U/L)	32.3 ± 1.5[b]	42.5 ± 7.9[a]	32.0 ± 4.6[b]	38.5 ± 6.8[ab]	31.7 ± 1.5[b]
TG (mg/dL)	52.8 ± 3.9[b]	67.0 ± 9.8[a]	52.3 ± 2.2[b]	42.5 ± 5.9[c]	51.0 ± 3.6[bc]
TCHO (mg/dL)	71.8 ± 2.9[cd]	129.3 ± 6.6[a]	93.8 ± 10.2[b]	81.0 ± 5.0[c]	61.7 ± 7.6[d]

ND: Normal Diet; HFD: High Fat Diet.

Values are expressed as the mean ± SE (n = 8 per group). Mean values within each column with different labels (a–d) are significantly different (p<0.05) according to one-way analysis of variance and Duncan's multiple range test. The relative organ weight was expressed as a percentage of body weight (liver weight/body weight × 100).

Chapter 3
TETRAHYDROCURCUMIN (THC): THE MAJOR METABOLITE WITH MAJOR BENEFITS

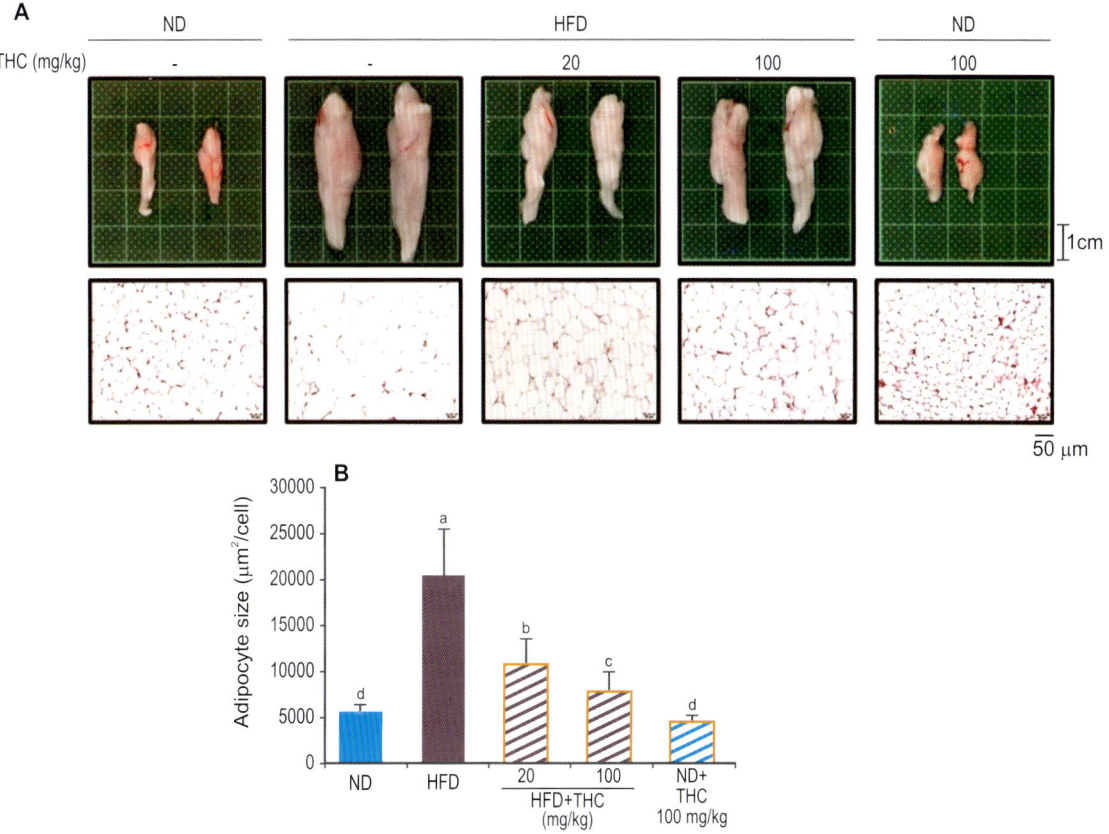

Values are expressed as mean ± SEM. Mean values with different letters indicate significantly different (p<0.05). ND: Normal Diet; HFD: High Fat Diet.

Fig. 78: Effect of THC intervention on HFD-induced adiposity and adipocyte size.
(A) Epididymal adipose tissue images (200 x) with H & E staining after 20 weeks of treatment (n=8)
(B) Quantification of adipocyte size (n=6)

(Adapted from Pan *et al.*, 2018)

Also, THC reduced adipogenic markers and activated AMPK (a key regulator of cellular and whole-body energy balance) signaling in adipose tissue. Further, HFD feeding resulted in downregulation of phospho-AMPK, which was dramatically increased by THC treatment, followed by inactivation of its downstream target acetyl-CoA carboxylase (ACC) (Fig. 79). Subsequently, inflammatory macrophage infiltration and polarization were decreased by THC in mouse epididymal adipose tissues.

Chapter 3
TETRAHYDROCURCUMIN (THC): THE MAJOR METABOLITE WITH MAJOR BENEFITS

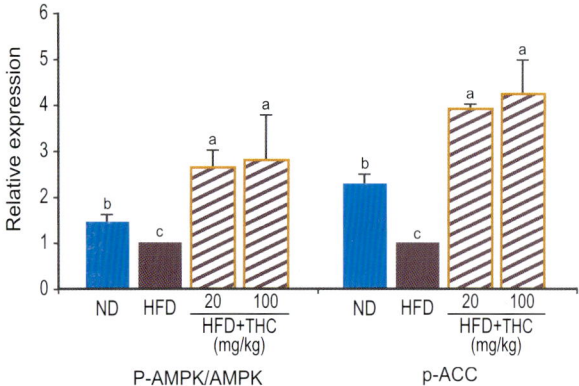

Fig. 79: Effect of THC on the proteins associated with adipogenesis, lipid metabolism and AMPK signaling in HFD-fed mice.

Western Blot analysis with protein-specific antibody was used to determine the protein levels of p-AMPK (Thr172), AMPK, p-ACC (Ser79) and ACC of the adipose tissues. (Adapted from Pan *et al.*, 2018)

In the liver, THC treatment showed a reduction in liver size, relative liver weight and hepatic triglycerides (Figs. 80A & 80B and Table 11). In addition, it showed markedly alleviated steatosis via the down regulation of lipogenesis, activation of AMP-activated protein kinase (AMPK) and increase of fatty acid oxidation.

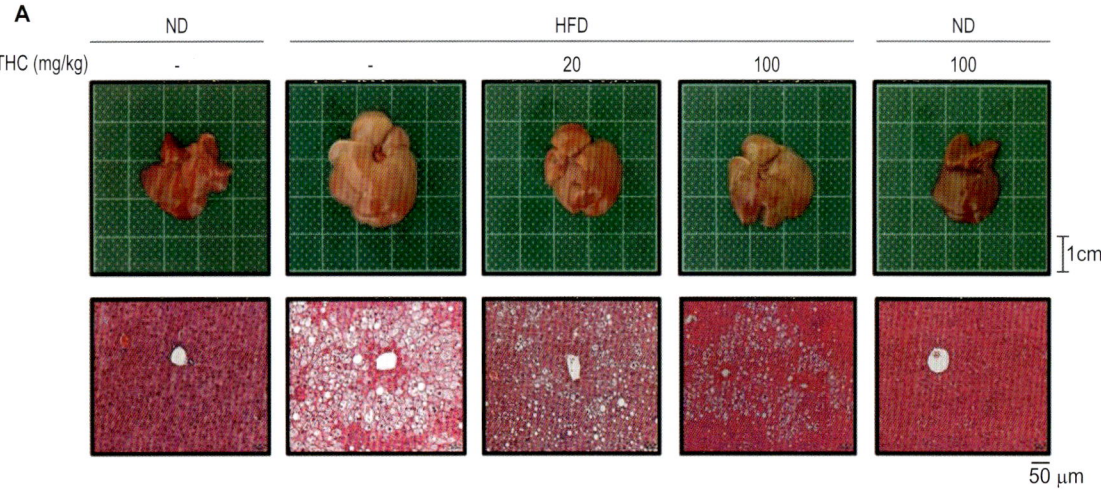

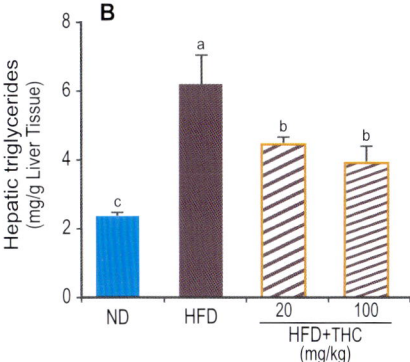

Values are expressed as mean ± SEM. Mean values with different letters indicate significantly different (p<0.05). ND: Normal Diet; HFD: High Fat Diet.

Fig. 80: Effect of THC on hepatic steatosis and inflammation in HFD-fed mice.
(A) The gross morphology (upper) and histological examination of the livers stained with H&E (magnification × 200)
(B) Hepatic triglycerides (n=5) (Adapted from Pan *et al.*, 2018)

Administration of THC at both dosages for 10 weeks reversed the abnormal serum glucose and insulin concentrations, and thus effectively decreased the homeostatic model assessment of insulin resistance (HOMA-IR) index compared to the HFD alone group (Figs. 81A, 81B & 81C). It showed significant improvement in glucose tolerance capacity, plasma glucose level at 30, 60 and 120 min and also AUCs were significantly lower in THC-treated group compared to the HFD alone group (Figs. 81D & 81E).

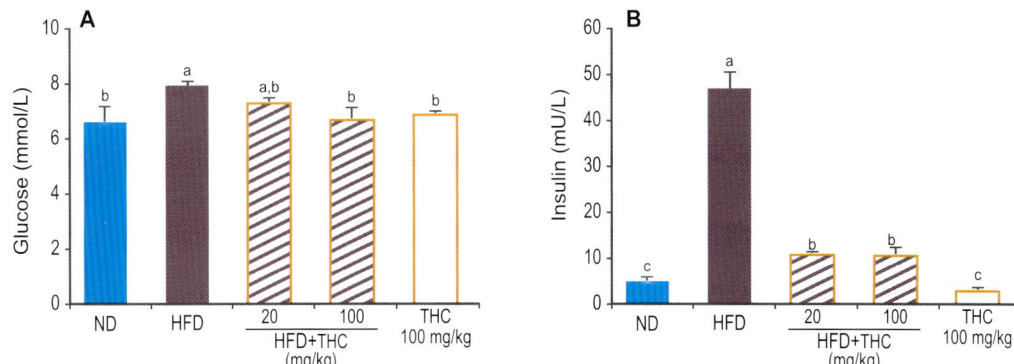

Values are expressed as mean ± SEM with n = 8 animals per group.
Mean values with different letters indicate significantly different (p<0.05).
ND: Normal Diet; HFD: High Fat Diet.

TETRAHYDROCURCUMIN (THC): THE MAJOR METABOLITE WITH MAJOR BENEFITS

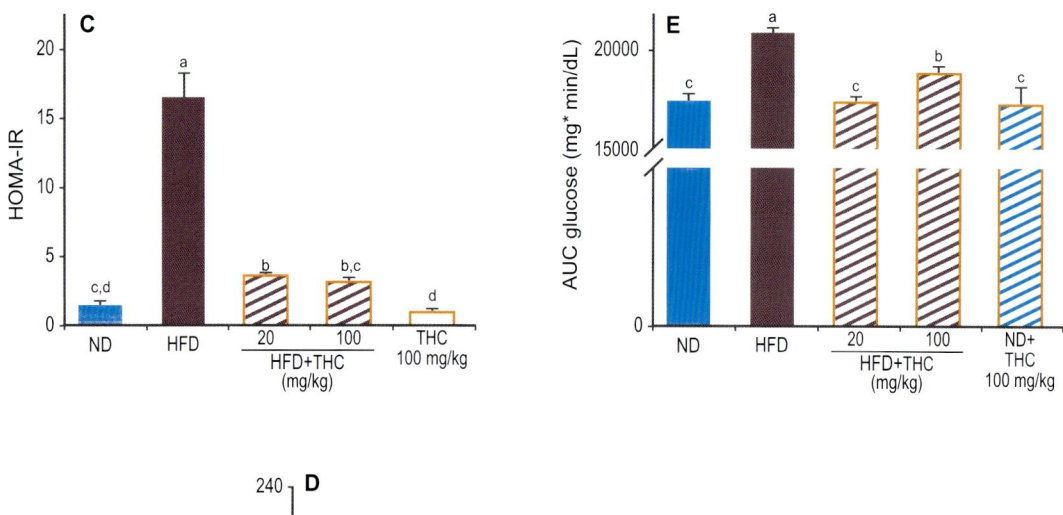

Values are expressed as mean ± SEM with n = 8 animals per group.
Mean values with different letters indicate significantly different ($p<0.05$).
ND: Normal Diet; HFD: High Fat Diet.

Fig. 81: Effect of THC intervention on glucose tolerance and insulin resistance.
(A) Fasting serum glucose
(B) Insulin
(C) HOMA-IR index were measured in each group. Oral glucose tolerance test (OGTT) was performed at the end of week 20 to evaluate glucose tolerability.
Blood samples were collected for glucose measurement at 0, 30, 60, 90 and 120 min after glucose administration (1g/kg)
(D) Blood glucose concentration-time course curves
(E) Area under the curve of OGTT (Adapted from Pan *et al.*, 2018)

Tetrahydrocurcumin improved blood glucose level and insulin resistance by altering a cascade of genes associated with glucose metabolism and by decreasing the macrophage infiltration into the liver and adipose tissues of the HFD-fed mice.

The study concluded that THC intervention showed potential therapeutic effects against obesity and hepatic steatosis, and suggesting that application of THC may act as a novel therapeutic approach for the treatment of obesity and NAFLD in obese subjects (Pan *et al.*, 2018).

Neuroprotective Potential

Anti-Alzheimer Potential

The hallmarks of Alzheimer's disease are the formation of amyloid plaques, neurofibrillary tangles and neuro-inflammation. The mediators of inflammation IL-1β, ROS, iNOS and lipid peroxidation products are among the predominant inflammatory cascade contributing to both neurodegenerations and production and accumulation of the β-amyloid peptide (Aβ) (Akiyama *et al.*, 2000). Considerable attention has been directed towards identifying compounds with neuroprotective properties.

Tetrahydrocurcumin treatment significantly inhibited the mRNA and protein levels of iNOS and IL-1β in the LPS associated inflammation-mediated brain tissue of mice. Soluble amyloid-β appears to relate with synaptic loss and neurodegeneration in Alzheimer's (Frautschy *et al.*, 2001) and THC reduced it by 75% (Begum *et al.*, 2008).

The advantages of THC in preventing neuronal damage against amyloid-β induced toxicity have been reported by several researchers recently. The authors showed that THC decreased amyloid-β-induced (i) ROS activity, (ii) reduction of mitochondrial membrane potential and (iii) caspase activation and concluded that THC protects against amyloid-β-induced toxicity potential through its antioxidant activity (Mishra et al., 2011).

A recent study, Randino et al. (2016) analyzed curcuminoid molecules, all the single components (curcumin, DMC, BDMC and cyclocurcumin (CYC)) and their metabolites (THC, HHC, OHC) in the C. longa extract in a liposomal solution, composed of 1,2-dioleoyl-sn-glycero-3-phospho-rac-(1-glycerol) (DOPG), for their ability to interact with the amyloid-β fragment (Aβ). It was reported that the "semi-folded" conformation of CYC is poorly present in curcumin (not present at all in its predominant keto-enol form) but still significantly present in the case of THC. Interestingly, it was reported that the more flexibility by THC shows a different behavior in DOPG bilayer or in the hexafluoro-2-propanol (HFIP)/water mixture, by shifting the conformational equilibrium of Aβ to the helical structure in DOPG. However, it was stated that this ability of THC was not preserved in the HFIP/water solution. Hence, THC could adopt a reactive conformation similar to CYC with better ability to interact with Aβ.

Anti-Parkinson's Disease Potential

Parkinson's disease (PD) is a neurodegenerative disorder associated with aging and is most prevalent in individuals over the age of 85 (de Lau et al., 2004). Aging is associated with rapid metabolism of dopamine (DA) into 3,4-dihydroxyphenylacetaldehyde (DOPAL) by monoamine oxidase (MAO) in intra-neuronal spaces (Goldstein et al., 2013). The DOPAL damages the dopaminergic neurons and contributes to the loss of DA-containing terminals, both characteristics of PD. 1-Methyl-4-phenyl-1,2,3,6-tetrahydropyridine (MPTP), a synthetic compound, is known to induce Parkinson's-like symptoms (Mandel et al., 2007). Rajeswari and Sabesan (2008) have demonstrated that Swiss albino mice treated intraperitoneally with MPTP show a significant degradation of DA compared with a control group. In an MPTP-induced Parkinson's model, THC increased the levels of DA in mice after MPTP treatment through the inhibition of MAO-B activity. Thus, THC may have the potential to be used as a therapeutic agent for the prevention or treatment of PD.

Chapter 3
TETRAHYDROCURCUMIN (THC): THE MAJOR METABOLITE WITH MAJOR BENEFITS

Brain Ischemia and Reperfusion (I/R) Injury Protection

Brain ischemia is among the leading cause of death with majority of the cases associated with ischemic strokes. High levels of homocysteine (Hcy) or hyperhomocysteinemia (HHcy) causes increased oxidative stress and generation of excessive free radicals during I/R injury in genetic HHcy condition contributing to autophagy (Cheng *et al*., 2011; Tyagi *et al*., 2005). Tetrahydrocurcumin, one of the major metabolites of curcumin, has a wide range of beneficial effects, including neuroprotective properties.

Tyagi *et al*. (2012) evaluated the neuroprotective effects of THC against homocysteinylated cyto-c mediated autophagy in the cystathionine-β-synthase heterozygote knockout (CBS+/−) mice, a well-characterized genetic model of severe HHcy in mice after cerebral ischemia.

It has been reported that the administration of THC (25 mg/kg) remarkably decreased the infarct volume and the neurological outcome (neuroscore, Fig. 82) in HHcy mice after I/R injury. In addition, THC also improved post-ischemic brain injury by decreasing the vascular permeability and edema measured by brain water content as the index for edema (Figs. 83A & 83B). Overall, it was shown that THC can prevent I/R induced brain injury and improve the blood-brain barrier integrity.

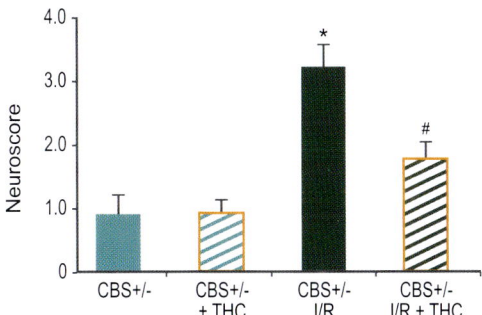

*$p<0.05$ values significantly different from CBS+/− mice,
#$p<0.05$ values significantly different from CBS+/− I/R mice; n=4 animals/group

Fig. 82: Neuroprotective effect of THC against ischemia/reperfusion insult.
Bar graph represents neuroscore of vehicle and THC-treated mice measured 3 days after middle cerebral artery occlusion. (Adapted from Tyagi *et al*., 2012)

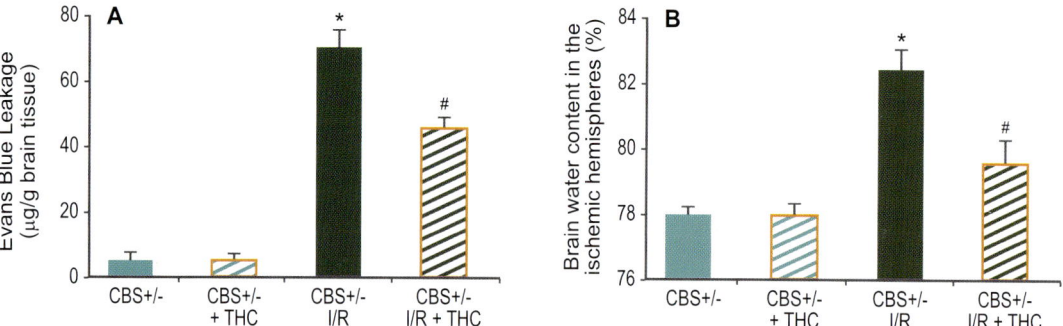

*$p<0.05$ values are significantly different from CBS+/− mice, #$p<0.05$ values are significantly different from CBS+/− I/R mice; n=4 animals/group

Fig. 83: Effect of THC on Blood Brain Barrier Integrity.
(A) Quantitative analysis of the extravasation of Evans blue dye showing integrity of the blood–brain barrier after 45 min of maximum allowable carry over (MACO) and 72 h of reperfusion.
(B) Brain edema formation after 45 min of MACO and 72 h of reperfusion
(Adapted from Tyagi *et al.*, 2012)

Stress decreases Hcy metabolic enzyme methylenetetrahydrofolate reductase (MTHFR) and increases S-adenosyl-L-homocysteine hydrolases (SAHH) echelons, thus causing an increase in total Hcy levels in the tissue. It was shown that THC supplementation up-regulated MTHFR and down-regulated SAHH genes in CBS+/− mice, retaining *trans*-sulfuration and remethylation pathways, thereby reducing the total Hcy levels in tissues (Fig. 84).

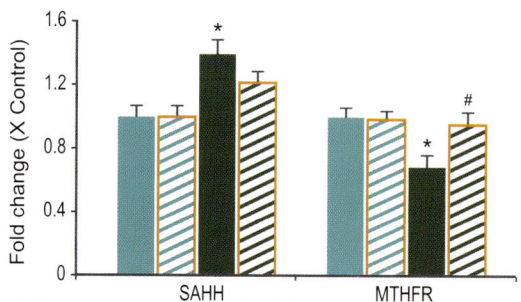

*$p<0.01$ values are significantly different from CBS+/− mice;
#$p<0.01$ values are significantly different from CBS+/− I/R mice; n=4 animals/group.

Fig. 84: Effect of THC on Hcy metabolism and levels.
Bar graph represents densitometric analysis of semi-quantitative expression of SAHH and MTHFR mRNA. Total mRNA was isolated from the brain of all experimental groups from CBS+/− mice and the mRNA levels of MTHFR and SAHH were measured by quantitative real-time PCR (QRT-PCR).
(Adapted from Tyagi *et al.*, 2012)

Homocysteine causes oxidative stress (Tyagi *et al.*, 2005 & 2006), generation of excessive free radicals (ROS) during I/R injury in genetic HHcy condition, which plays a major role in brain injury associated with stroke. It was reported that consistent with earlier observations, THC treatment significantly decreased oxidative stress by down-regulating oxidant enzyme (p47phox) and up-regulating antioxidant enzyme (catalase) expression after I/R injury (Fig. 85). In addition, findings from the study also demonstrated that THC prevented homocysteinylation of cyto-c by decreasing oxidative stress, which in turn initiate MMP-9 activation (Fig. 86).

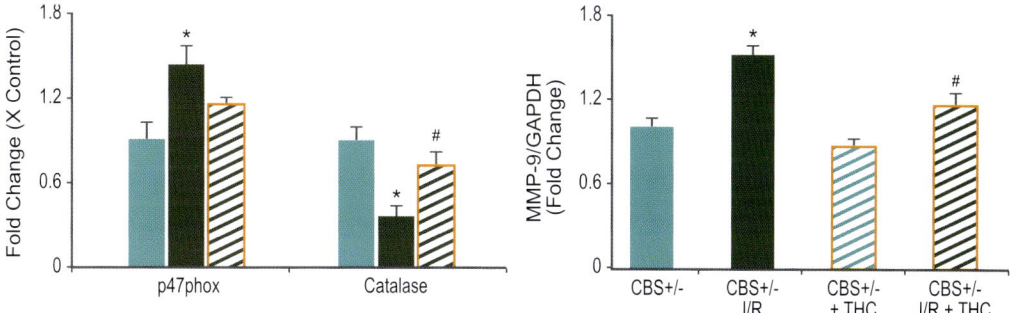

*$p<0.05$ values are significantly different from CBS+/− mice; #$p<0.05$ values are significantly different from CBS+/− I/R mice; n=4.

Fig. 85: Effect of THC on oxidative stress. Bar graph represents p47phox and catalase protein expressions. (Adapted from Tyagi *et al.*, 2012)

Fig. 86: Effect of THC on MMP-9. Bar graph represents MMP-9 protein expressions. (Adapted from Tyagi *et al.*, 2012)

Furthermore, Tyagi *et al.* (2012) showed that microtubule associated protein 1 light chain LC3-I to LC3-II and damage regulated autophagy modulator (DRAM) protein expressions were increased in CBS+/− ischemic mice. The authors demonstrated that THC ameliorated the conversion of LC3-I to LC3-II (Fig. 87A) and the occurrence of autophagy associated increase in the DRAM protein level (Fig. 87B) in a genetical model of severe HHcy mice after cerebral I/R injury, in part, by homocysteinylation of cyto-c and activation of MMP-9. It was concluded that THC may be an effective prophylactic agent in the prevention of Hcy induced HHcy, one of the neurodegenerative disorders (stroke) that contributes to autophagy and (I/R) injury.

Chapter 3
TETRAHYDROCURCUMIN (THC): THE MAJOR METABOLITE WITH MAJOR BENEFITS

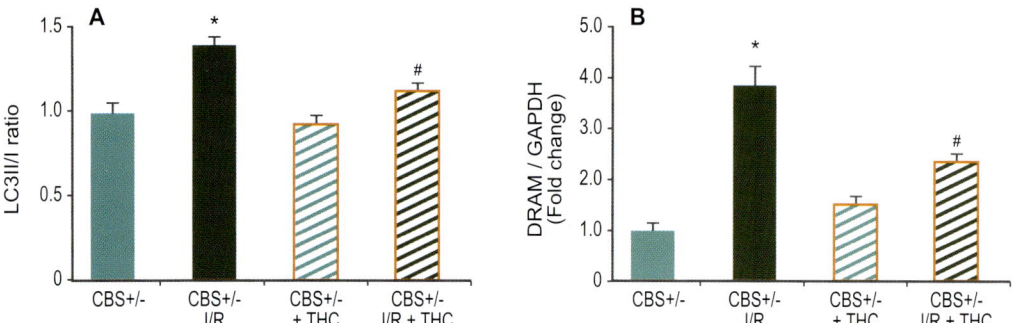

*$p<0.05$ values significantly different from CBS+/− mice; #$p<0.05$ values significantly different from CBS+/− I/R mice; n=4 animals/group.

Fig. 87: Effect of THC on autophagy.
(A) LC3II/I protein expression ratio; (B) DRAM protein expression (Adapted from Tyagi *et al.*, 2012)

Elevated levels of Hcy, causes endothelial dysfunction by inducing oxidative stress in most of the neurodegenerative disorders and is highly correlated with mitochondrial dynamics such as fusion and fission, the two opposing processes involved in the mitochondrial dynamics. In a most recent mechanistic study, Vacek *et al.* 2018 investigated whether increased levels of Hcy impaired the balance of mitochondrial fission and fusion in mouse brain endothelial cells (bEnd3) that may result in mitochondrial remodeling and the protective effect of THC was explored on Hcy-mediated modulation of mitochondrial dynamics. It was shown that pre-treatment of bEnd3 with THC (15 µM) ameliorated Hcy-induced oxidative damage, mitochondrial fission/fusion, and mitophagy. The findings of this study strongly suggest that THC has beneficial effects on mitochondrial remodeling and could be developed as a potential therapeutic agent against HHcy-induced mitochondrial dysfunction in neurodegenerative disorders.

Vacek *et al.* (2018) observed that Nip-like protein X (NIX), an atypical BH3-only protein, which localizes to the mitochondrial outer membrane (Zhang and Ney, 2009), recruits LC3 and were co-localized with each other in the Hcy-treated group, thus causing mitochondrial damage and affecting the mitochondrial integrity. On the other hand, THC treatment protects the mitochondrial integrity by decreasing the co-localization of NIX and LC3. Findings from the study demonstrated that Hcy resulted in cell toxicity in a dose-dependent manner; and supplementation of THC prevented the detrimental effects of Hcy on cell survival. It was shown that Hcy-induced the protein levels of mitochondria fission and fusion markers, dynamin related protein 1 (DRP1) and mitofusin 2 (Mfn2), respectively, and autophagy marker (LC3), whereas the levels of the above proteins in Hcy-treated cells were significantly decreased by treatment with THC (Fig. 88).

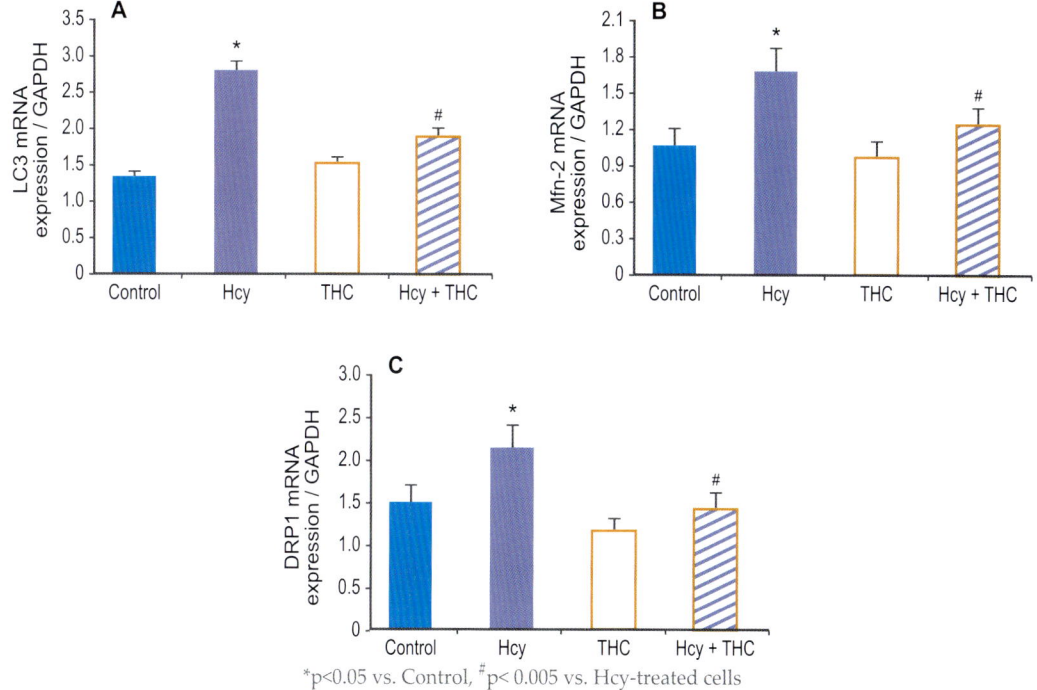

$*p<0.05$ vs. Control, $^{\#}p< 0.005$ vs. Hcy-treated cells

Fig. 88: Effect of THC on Hcy-induced mitochondrial dynamics and autophagy. Bar graphs represent the protein intensity of LC3 (A), Mfn-2 (B) and DRP-1 (C) in different bEnd3 cells treated groups with or without THC. (Adapted from Vacek *et al.*, 2018)

This study concluded, that pre-treatment of bEnd3 cells with THC ameliorated Hcy-induced oxidative damage, mitochondrial fission/fusion, and mitophagy, suggesting that THC has beneficial effects on mitochondrial remodeling and could be developed as a potential therapeutic agent against HHcy-induced mitochondrial dysfunction.

Lin *et al.* (2016) assessed the neuroprotective effects of THC in a mouse model of cerebral I/R injury and investigated the involvement of golgi reassembly and stacking protein 65 (GRASP65) and the extracellular signal regulated kinase (ERK) signaling pathway. The ERK signaling pathway has an important role in cerebral I/R injury. Golgi reassembly and stacking protein (GRASPs) are membrane proteins involved in the regulation of Golgi assembly, cell migration, division and apoptosis. The findings from Lin *et al.* (2016) showed that THC exerted dose-dependent protective effects by suppressing the ERK pathway followed by reducing the phosphorylation of GRASP65 in cerebral I/R injury (Fig. 89), thus provided new mechanistic insight on the protective effect of THC against cerebral I/R injury.

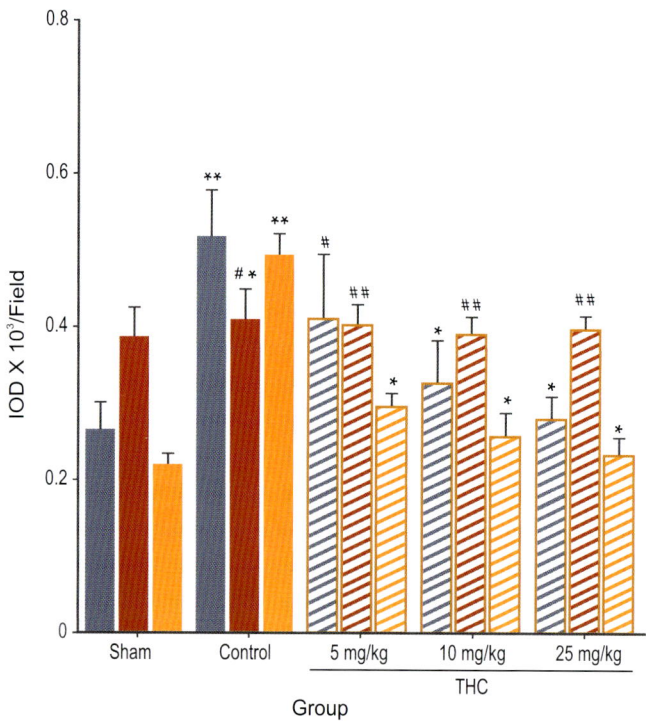

Values are mean ± SD; **p<0.01 vs. Sham group; *#p<0.05 vs. Sham group; #p<0.05 vs. Control group; *p<0.01 vs. Control group; ##p>0.05 vs. Control group; ERK: Extracellular Signal Regulated Kinase; p: Phosphorylated; GRASP65: Golgi Reassembly and Stacking Protein 65.

Fig. 89: ERK, pERK, GRASP65 and pGRASP65 protein expression in mice from each group following reperfusion for 24 h treated with or without THC.
(Adapted from Lin *et al.*, 2016)

Chapter 3
TETRAHYDROCURCUMIN (THC): THE MAJOR METABOLITE WITH MAJOR BENEFITS

Traumatic Brain Injury (TBI) Protection

Traumatic brain injury (TBI), defined as a mechanical injury accompanied by serious complications, has high morbidity and mortality rates and remains a primary cause of disability and other health issues for people worldwide. After the primary injury, the secondary insult, which involves apoptosis, free-radical production and inflammation, aggravates the damage produced by TBI (Kabadi and Faden, 2014). Autophagy was shown to occur concurrently with apoptosis contributing to the functional loss in brain injury models (Lockshin and Zakeri, 2004). Tetrahydrocurcumin has been shown to ameliorate autophagy by reducing homocysteinylation of cyto-c in HHcy pathologic conditions in the ischemia and/or reperfusion injury (Tyagi *et al.*, 2012). Gao *et al.* determined the mechanistic actions, modulation of PI3K/AKT pathway and autophagy (Fig. 90), associated with the neuroprotective effect of THC after TBI in a rat model (Gao *et al.*, 2016). It was reported that intraperitoneal injection of THC (25 or 50 mg/kg) alleviated brain edema, attenuated TBI-induced neuron cell death,

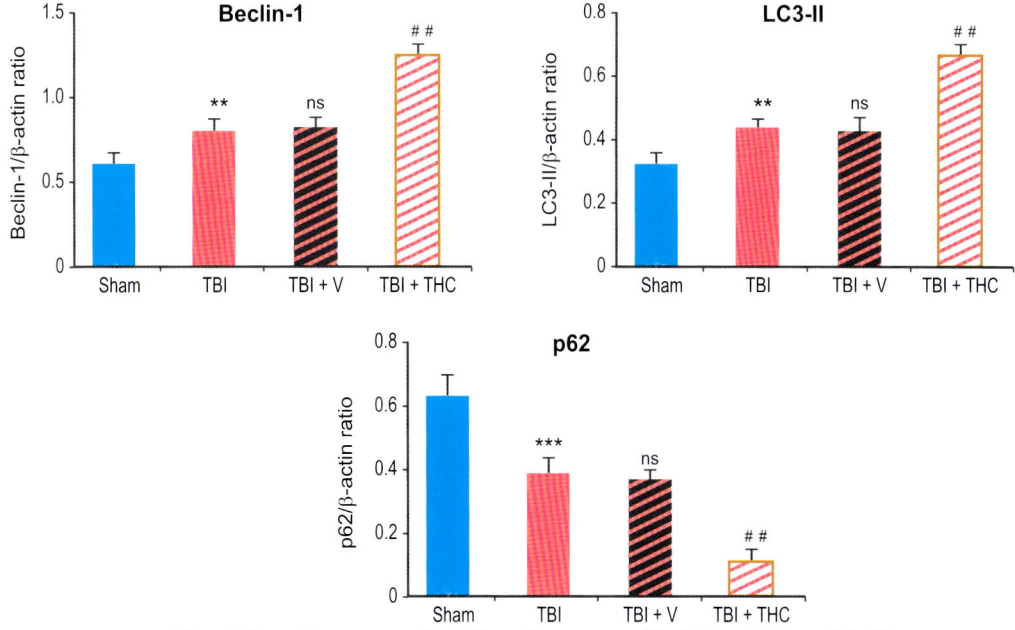

***$p < 0.001$ vs. Sham group; **$p < 0.01$ vs. Sham group; ##$p < 0.01$ vs. TBI + vehicle (V) group; ns: Not Significant; TBI: Traumatic Brain Injury.

Fig. 90: The effect of THC on autophagy at the molecular level following TBI. THC treatment significantly increased the expressions of autophagy-associated proteins (Beclin-1 and LC3-II) and decreased the expression of p62. (Adapted from Gao *et al.*, 2016)

Chapter 3
TETRAHYDROCURCUMIN (THC): THE MAJOR METABOLITE WITH MAJOR BENEFITS

decreased the degree of apoptosis and improved neurobehavioral function, which were accompanied by enhanced autophagy (Fig. 90). The findings of this study suggest that THC may be an attractive neuroprotective agent for TBI therapy.

Recently, Gao *et al.* (2017) investigated the neuroprotective effects of THC on mitochondrial apoptosis and autophagy using the same rat model of TBI. The autophagy activation associated with the mitochondrial apoptotic pathway was examined using autophagy inhibitor 3-methyladenine (3-MA) on the expression of mitochondrial apoptosis-associated protein markers, Beclin-1 and LC3-II. Tetrahydrocurcumin + 3-MA treatment significantly reduced Beclin-1 and LC3-II, as well as the expression of Bax, a protein associated with the mitochondrial apoptotic pathway compared to THC in TBI rats. In addition, THC + 3-MA also increased the level of cleaved caspase-3 in TBI rats (Fig. 91). Thus, finding of this study

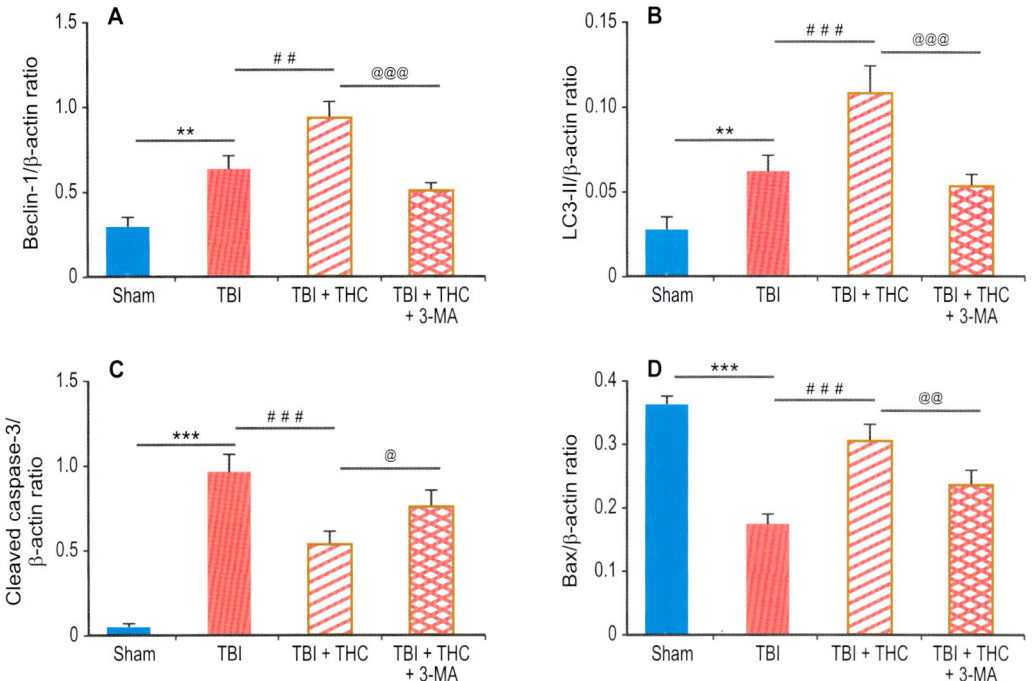

**$p<0.01$, ***$p<0.001$ vs. Sham group; ##$p<0.01$, ###$p<0.001$ vs. TBI group;
@$p<0.05$, @@$p<0.01$, @@@$p<0.001$ vs. TBI + THC group; TBI: Traumatic Brain Injury; 3-MA: 3-methyladenine.

Fig. 91: Effect of THC on mitochondrial apoptotic associated proteins after autophagy inhibitor 3-MA treatment.
Bar graphs represent quantitative analysis: the ratios of Beclin-1 (A), LC3-II (B), the expression of cleaved caspase-3 (C) and Bax (D) (Adapted from Gao *et al.*, 2017)

provided evidence that THC suppresses the mitochondrial apoptotic pathway by activating autophagy and provides neuroprotection after TBI in rats.

Nuclear factor erythroid 2-related factor 2 (Nrf2), a transcription factor, plays an important role in protecting TBI-induced secondary brain injury, regulating inflammatory cytokines and inducing antioxidant and detoxifying enzyme (Jin *et al.*, 2009). Wei *et al.* (2017) investigated whether THC exerts neuroprotective effects and its potential mechanisms, in a rat model of TBI. The findings of this study revealed that THC treatment protected neuronal cells, reduced oxidative stress alleviating the oxidative insult of TBI through the activation of the Nrf2 pathway. It was shown that rather than the upregulation of protein expression, THC promoted translocation of Nrf2 from the cytoplasm to the nucleus and enhanced Nrf2 binding (Fig. 92). Thus, the results of this study suggest that THC improves neurological outcome after TBI insult, possibly by activating the Nrf2 signaling pathway.

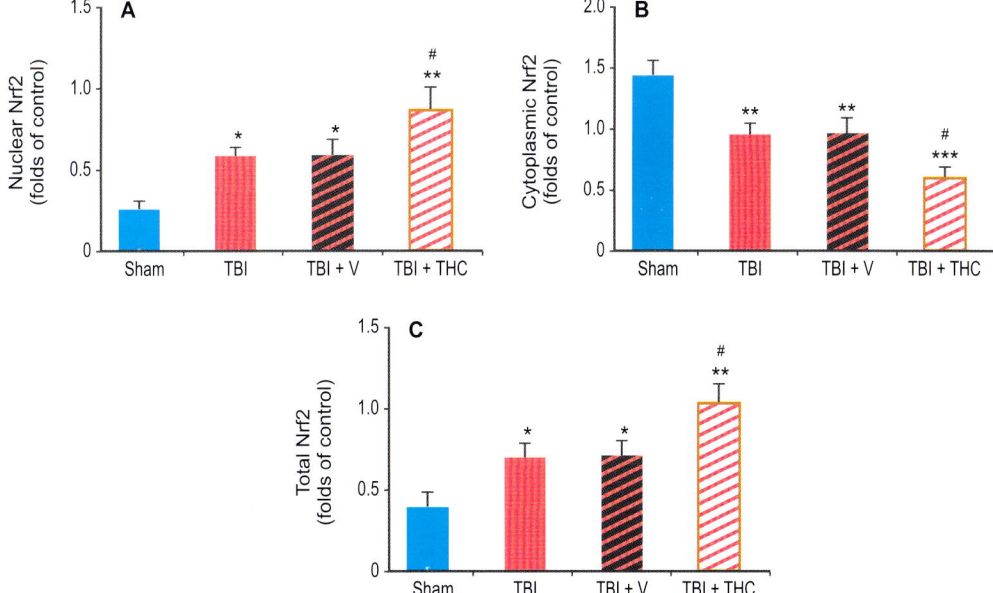

*$p<0.05$, **$p<0.01$ and ***$p<0.001$ vs. Sham group; #$p<0.05$ vs. TBI + vehicle (V) group; TBI: Traumatic Brain Injury.

Fig. 92: Effect of THC on translocation of Nrf2 from cytoplasm to nucleus and enhanced Nrf2 binding. (Adapted from Wei *et al.*, 2017)

(A) Nuclear Nrf2 expression after THC treatment in rats post-TBI
(B) Cytoplasmic protein Nrf2 expression after THC treatment post-TBI
(C) Total protein Nrf2 expression after THC treatment post-TBI

Protection Against Chemotherapy-induced Peripheral Neuropathy (CIPN)

Chemotherapy-induced peripheral neuropathy (CIPN) is a common side effect, varying from 30 to 70% of patients receiving chemotherapy, leading to a poor quality of life and discontinuation of useful anticancer treatment (Brown *et al.,* 2014). Vincristine is one of the most common chemotherapeutic agents used to treat several types of malignancies, such as leukemias, lymphomas, and sarcomas; however, uniformly all patients experienced neurotoxic side effect of vincristine treatment. Thus, its anticancer efficacy is limited by the development of a mixed sensorimotor neuropathy. Vincristine exerts neurotoxicity by binding to neuronal cytoskeleton protein (β-tubulin) and causes disruptive action in polymerization of microtubules, oxidative stress and release inflammatory mediators which lead to axonal degeneration and slowing of motor nerve conduction velocity (Jaggi and Singh, 2012).

Greeshma *et al*. (2015) investigated the protective efficacy of THCs (provided by Sabinsa) on vincristine-induced neuropathic pain in male Wistar rat model. Pregabalin, a selective voltage-gated calcium (Ca^{2+}) ion channels (Cav) N-type (Cav 2.2) antagonist was used as a positive control. Rats injected with vincristine exhibited evidence of CIPN. Tetrahydrocurcuminoids administration protected the vincristine-induced decrease in functional (sciatic functional index) loss and conduction velocity in a dose-dependent manner. Tetrahydrocurcuminoids at 80 mg/kg treatment significantly improved the motor nerve conduction velocity comparable to pregabalin (Fig. 93). Tetrahydrocurcuminoids at 80 mg/kg significantly attenuated the neuropathic pain manifestations by increasing the nociceptive threshold, decreasing the oxidative stress, inflammatory mediators and total calcium levels in sciatic nerve in vincristine injected rats. The results were comparable to pregabalin (positive control) used in this study. It was shown that THCs 80 mg/kg exhibited superior antioxidant activity than pregabalin, suggesting that THCs attenuated the vincristine-induced behavioral, biochemical, neurophysiological and histological changes in rats.

Chapter 3
TETRAHYDROCURCUMIN (THC): THE MAJOR METABOLITE WITH MAJOR BENEFITS

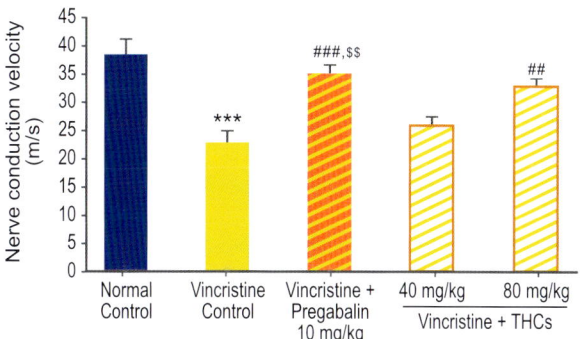

Values are as mean ± SD (n=6 animals per group); ***$p<0.001$ in comparison to normal control group; ##, ###$p<0.01$ and $p<0.001$ respectively in comparison to vincristine- treated group; $$$p<0.01$ in comparison to THCs 40 mg/kg treated group

Fig. 93: Effect of THCs (40 and 80 mg/kg) on motor nerve conduction velocity in vincristine-induced neuropathic pain rat model.
(Adapted from Greeshma *et al.*, 2015)

It was concluded that the effects of THCs may be attributed to multiple actions, namely antinociceptive, anti-inflammatory, calcium inhibitory, TNF-α inhibition, neuroprotective and antioxidant activity, and thus, THCs can be the promising candidates for the prevention of CIPN caused by chemotherapeutic agents.

Anti-aging Potential

To date, several studies have acknowledged the potential anti-aging benefits of THCs for its use both in nutritional and topical applications. More importantly, THC was shown to improve the life span in animals. A preliminary study showed that THC (0.2%) administered to mice at the age of 13 months had a longer life span than the control mice (Kitani *et al.*, 2007). Further, a growing number of studies provide evidence for the safety and versatility of THCs in supporting healthy aging and longevity. Tetrahydrocurcuminoids, the major metabolites of curcuminoids, provide more appealing options for the manufacturers aiming to revitalize their anti-aging supplement formulations.

Xiang et al. (2011) evaluated the role of THC on regulation of the O-type forkhead domain transcription factor (FOXO), which is involved in many biological processes such as aging, the oxidative stress response, and growth regulation using primary mouse embryonic fibroblast cells (NIH 3T3) and *Drosophila melanogaster* as a model organism. The authors demonstrated that THC promotes translocation of FOXO4 to the nucleus at least in part through inhibition of Akt phosphorylation in NIH 3T3 cells.

Next, to demonstrate whether FOXO mediates the effect of THC on oxidative stress *in vivo*, Xiang et al. (2011) performed a sequence of experiments using *Drosophila* as a model organism. Wild-type (WT) *D. melanogaster* (Oregon-R) and a second control line, *yellow white* flies (*yw*), were used as controls. First, oxidative stress was induced in wild-type *D. melanogaster* flies by adding paraquat (7.5 mM), a superoxide-generating agent in the food. All wild-type flies in the control group died after 12 days. On the other hand, THC (50-150 µM) repressed the oxidative stress response and led to a significant restoration of survival (~28%) in the experimental group. Resveratrol was also found to prolong the lifespan of *Drosophila*, although the effect was smaller than that was seen with THC. However, at the same dose levels (50–150 µM) curcumin did not increase the tolerance of flies to oxidative stress (Figs. 94 & 95). In addition, life-span analysis on the effect of THC and

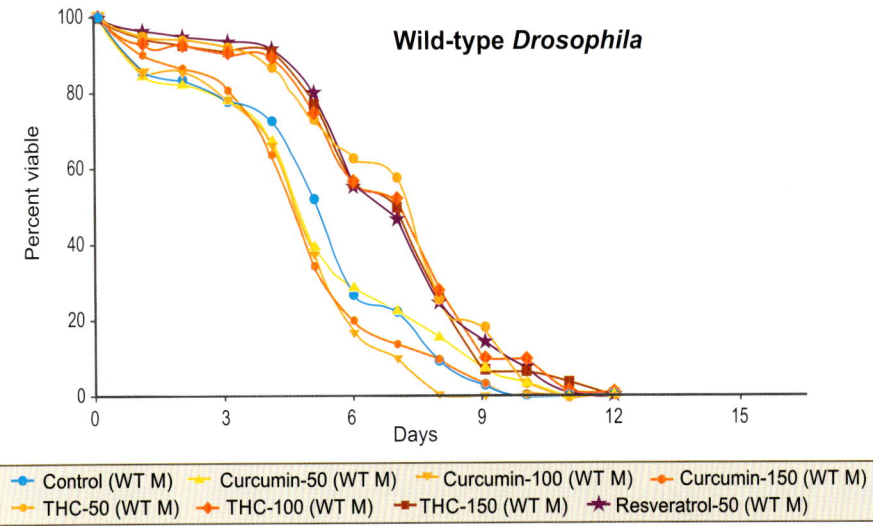

Fig. 94: Effect of THC, resveratrol and curcumin on the life span of wild type *Drosophila* flies under oxidative stress conditions. (Adapted from Xiang et al., 2011)

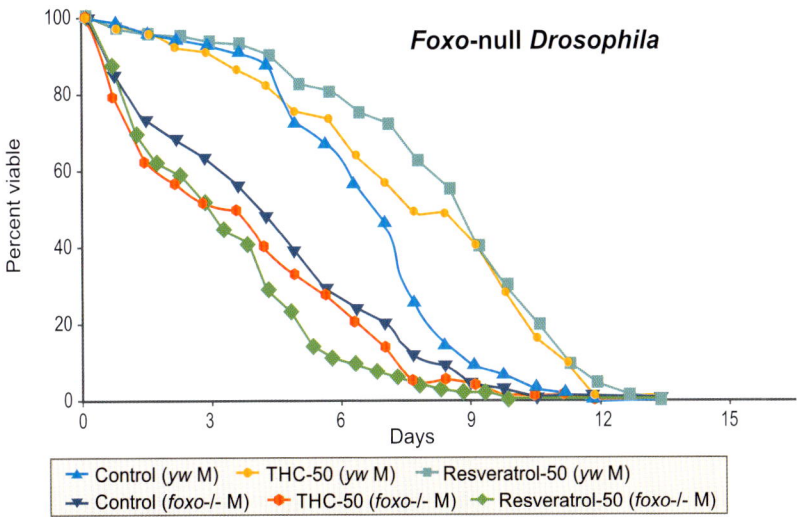

Fig. 95: Effect of THC and resveratrol on the life span of *foxo*-null mutant flies under oxidative stress conditions. (Adapted from Xiang *et al.*, 2011)

curcumin in flies with *yw* background and Oregon-R (WT) also showed that THC, but not curcumin extended the life span in *Drosophila* under normal conditions (Xiang *et al.*, 2011).

To determine whether FOXO mediates the effect of THC on oxidative stress response, *Drosophila* flies with *yw* background was used to generate *foxo*-null mutant background flies. The *foxo*-null mutant flies were created by crossing *yw; FRT82B, foxo25/TM6B* with *yw; foxo21/TM6B*. Both male and female offspring were analyzed in these experiments. Oxidative stress was induced by adding paraquat (7.5 mM), a superoxide-generating agent in food. Although THC extended the life span of wild-type *Drosophila*, THC, including resveratrol could not extend the life span of *foxo*-null flies under oxidative stress conditions (Fig. 95) (Xiang *et al.*, 2011). Thus, it was evident that the effect of antioxidant THC on life span may not be attributable to an effect on scavenging of ROS, suggesting that the effect of THC on the life span extension of *Drosophila* under oxidative stress conditions was *foxo*-dependent.

In addition, sirtuins family of proteins are highly conserved NAD^+-dependent deacetylases and well known for regulating the acetylation state of FOXO and affecting the nuclear

Chapter 3
TETRAHYDROCURCUMIN (THC): THE MAJOR METABOLITE WITH MAJOR BENEFITS

localization of FOXO under oxidative stress in mammalian cells (Wang *et al.*, 2007). Sir2, a homolog in mammals is known as SIRT1. Therefore, whether *Drosophila Sir2*, a homolog of mammalian SIRT1 is required for THC to affect life span was evaluated. For these experiments *Sir2*-null mutant flies, *yw; Sir217/CyO* was created by crossing with *yw; Df(2L)BSC30/CyO* strains. The *yw* flies were used as a control line. It was shown that *Sir2*-null mutants were short-lived, and that THC did not extend their life span (Fig. 96). These results suggest that THC regulates aging processes via an evolutionarily conserved regulatory network of genes that includes both *foxo* and *Sir2* (Wang *et al.*, 2007; Xiang *et al.*, 2011).

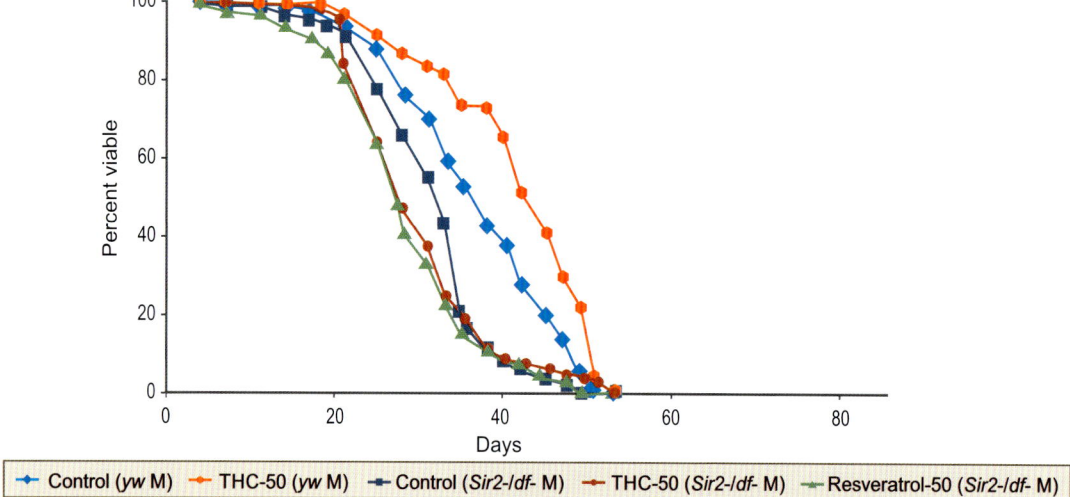

Fig. 96: Effects of THC or resveratrol (50 μM) on the life span of *Sir2-/df* mutant *Drosophila* under natural conditions.
Life span studies were carried out at 25 °C with a total of around 80 newly enclosed male (M) flies (*yw* background). (Adapted from Xiang *et al.*, 2011)

Chapter 3
TETRAHYDROCURCUMIN (THC): THE MAJOR METABOLITE WITH MAJOR BENEFITS

Anti-osteoarthritic Potential

Park *et al.* (2016) investigated whether long-term administration of THCs and curcumin (provided by Sabinsa) may exert protection against osteoarthritis in ovariectomized (OVX) obese rats with osteoarthritis induced by intra-articular injection of monoiodoacetate (MIA). The MIA injection was used to generate a similar pathology as osteoarthritis by disrupting glycolysis at the site of the injection resulting in the eventual death of chondrocytes by increased inflammation (Guzman *et al.*, 2003). The OVX rats with MIA injection into the knee were treated with 0.4% curcumin or 0.4% THCs, or 17 β-estradiol (30 μg/kg) + dextrin (0.4%) that served as positive controls. Rats treated with 0.4% dextrin served as control, and saline injection into the knee and 0.4% dextrin served as normal control.

It was shown that serum glucose levels were elevated up to 40–50 min after the oral glucose challenge and decreased slowly in all rats subsequently (Fig. 97A). An oral glucose tolerance test (OGTT) performed in overnight feed deprived rats showed higher OGTT in control than the positive control. The AUC of glucose in THCs group was similar to the positive control, whereas the AUC of curcumin and THCs groups had insulin similar to the positive control (Figs. 97B & 97C), suggesting, curcumin- and THCs-treated rats had greater insulin sensitivities than control rats.

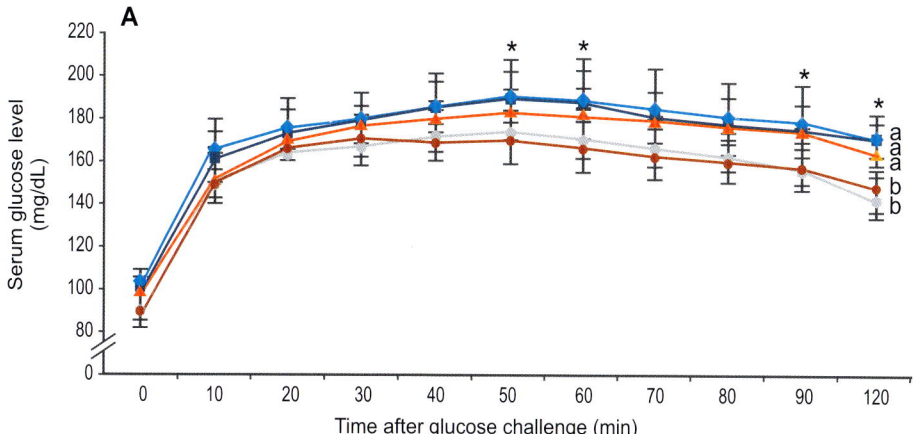

Asterisks represent the significant treatment effect by repeated measures of a two-way ANOVA test at p<0.05 (a, b)

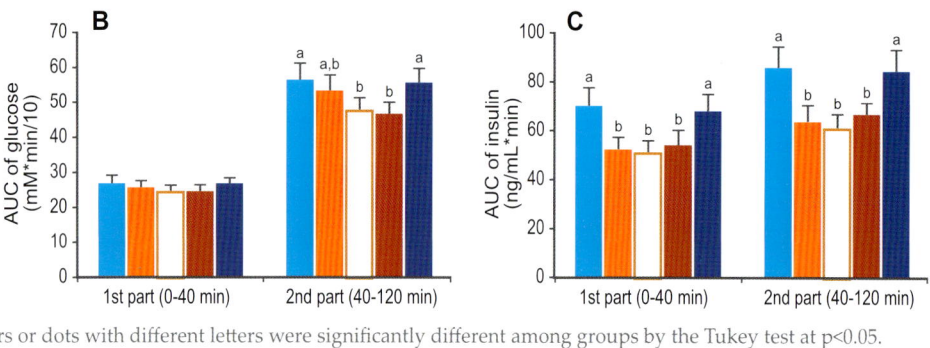

The bars or dots with different letters were significantly different among groups by the Tukey test at p<0.05.

■ Control ■ Curcumin ☐ THCs ■ Positive control ■ Normal control

Fig. 97: The area under the curve of serum glucose and insulin during oral glucose tolerance test.
(A) Serum glucose levels measured at selected time points
(B), (C) Area under the curve of glucose and insulin levels, respectively

(Adapted from Park *et al.*, 2016)

It was shown that curcumin and THCs reduced osteoarthritis symptoms and pain related behaviors (Fig. 98) in estrogen-deficient rats fed with HFD. Monoiodoacetate is also known to initiate osteoarthritis by activating MMPs by inducing inflammation and elevating

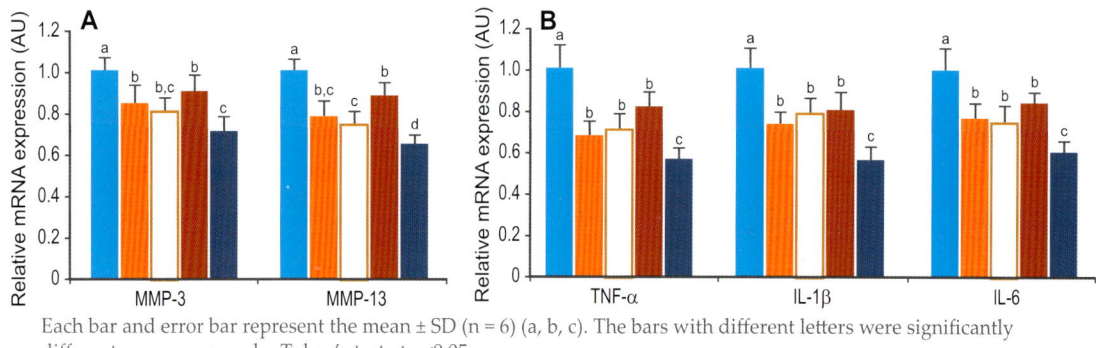

Each bar and error bar represent the mean ± SD (n = 6) (a, b, c). The bars with different letters were significantly different among groups by Tukey's test at p<0.05.

■ Control ■ Curcumin ☐ THCs ■ Positive control ■ Normal control

Fig. 98: Bar graph representation of the expression of MMPs and pro-inflammatory cytokines at the mRNA levels in the articular cartilage after intra-articular injection of monoiodoacetate (MIA) for 21 days. (Adapted from Park *et al.*, 2016)

cytokine release. Although curcumin and THCs suppressed the expressions of MMP3 and MMP13 compared to the control group, it was reported that THCs decreased their expression slightly better than curcumin (Fig. 98A). Also, curcumin and THCs suppressed the expressions of pro-inflammatory cytokines (TNF-α, IL-1β, and IL-6) compared to the control group (Fig. 98B).

It was concluded that although curcumin and THCs increased insulin concentration, only THCs improved glucose tolerance, which might indirectly delay the long-term progression of osteoarthritis. Though THCs and curcumin are potential new candidates for treating postmenopausal symptoms and osteoarthritis in humans, THCs may have advantages over curcumin for long-term treatment.

Anti-allergic Activity

Reactive oxygen species (ROS) generated in macrophages produce PGE_2, NO, cytokine IL-1β, IL-6, and TNF-α, together leading to the development of inflammation (Haddad *et al.*, 2001). Curcumin was reported to depress the release of ROS from macrophages and inhibit histamine release from rat mast cells, suggesting the anti-allergic activities of curcumin. In this context, Suzuki *et al.* (2005) investigated the underlying active mechanisms and structural features of curcumin in exerting these activities. The anti-allergic activities were assessed by the measurement of histamine release from rat basophilic leukemia cells, RBL-2H3. Curcumin and THC caused a marked decrease in histamine release. Glycosides of curcumin, BDMC and THC also inhibited the release of histamine, though less potently than curcumin did. Findings from this study revealed that all compounds with potent radical scavenging activities caused a definite decrease in histamine release therefore could play a significant role in exerting both the anti-oxidative and anti-allergic activities.

Anti-asthmatic Activity

Recently, Chen *et al.* (2018) investigated the efficacy of dietary THC on allergic asthma compared to curcumin in an ovalbumin-induced asthmatic mouse model. It has been reported that both THC and curcumin exerted beneficial effects on asthmatic related to nasal symptoms in mice. Also, THC decreased the pathological conditions (eosinophils and mucus hyper-production), oxidative stress (malondialdehyde), cytokine production (IL-13), Th-17 and cytotoxic T cell subsets. In addition, THC attenuated Th2 responses and suppressed the IL-4Rα-Jak1-STAT6 and Jagged1/Jagged2-Notch1/Notch2 axis activity in asthmatic mice. Interestingly, THC found to be more effective than curcumin in suppressing the tissue eosinophilia, mucus production and IL-4Rα-Jak1-STAT6 pathway activity. In addition, THC inhibited peripheral eosinophil level, Th2 cytokines (IL-4 and IL-5), and Th2 cell subsets and enhanced glutathione, an antioxidant enzyme. Chen *et al.* (2018) concluded that THC was superior to curcumin in modulating allergic asthmatic phenotypes, especially attenuating the Th2 response, suggesting that THC might be a potentially effective agent for asthma treatment.

Anti-viral Potential

The epidemic of Ebola virus (EBOV) that occurred in 2014 in West Africa has been the largest outbreak since the first report of the disease in 1976 (Schieffelin *et al.*, 2014). Unlike most viral infections, which remain asymptomatic and subclinical for quite some time, EBOV contrastingly shows high pathogenicity. Ebola virus first disables immune system and then attacks the vascular system as well as other organs. In severe conditions, patients develop hypovolemic shock and multiorgan failure. There is no specific treatment for EBOV. Anti-viral drugs such as brincidofovir and flavipiravir have been identified. ZMapp is another experimental treatment for Ebola viral disease which consists of monoclonal antibodies that serve as antiviral therapy (Qiu *et al.*, 2014). Baikerikar (2017) reported that curcumin, curcuminoids as well as THC show potential inhibitory action against all viral proteins (VPs) of EBOV as evidenced by the docking scores. Comparing the docking scores of all target proteins, it was observed that BDMC shows better binding affinity than curcumin. Interestingly, metabolite THC shows comparable binding affinity as curcumin, thus throwing some light on the possibility to explore this compound as an anti-viral agent against EBOV. It was suggested that curcumin, curcuminoids, and metabolite THC can be potential compounds for developing a new therapy for Ebola viral disease.

Tetrahydrocurcumin was proposed as an alternative to curcumin for prevention of HIV-1 infection. Recently, a group of researchers (Mirani *et al.*, 2019) investigated the equivalency between curcumin and THC (provided by Sabinsa) for their gp120-CD4 binding inhibitory activity against HIV-1 infection using in silico study, *in vitro*. The findings of this study concluded that THC exhibited equivalent gp120-CD4 binding inhibitory activity as compared with curcumin due to its stable hydrophobic interactions with residues Asp368 and Trp427 deeper in the Phe43 cavity of CD4 receptor. It was also suggested that THC-loaded oil-in-water microemulsion gel exhibited increased efficacy as compared with conventional THC and may be a potential candidate for the prevention of HIV-1 infection.

Oral Health

THCs for Gingival Tissue Health

Antioxidant supplements with their anti-inflammatory properties exert beneficial effects and may play a potential role in the prevention and successful treatment of disorders associated with gingival tissues and other supporting structures of the teeth (Battino *et al.*, 2005).

San Miguel *et al.* (2011) attempted to provide cytotoxicity, proliferation and migration data on the *in vitro* effects of bioactive antioxidant mixtures on human oral fibroblast cells,

TETRAHYDROCURCUMIN (THC): THE MAJOR METABOLITE WITH MAJOR BENEFITS

obtained from human gingival (HG) and human periodontal ligament-like (HPDL) tissues. To evaluate the effect of antioxidant, each of these oral fibroblasts was treated with bioactive pure polyphenol and turmeric derivative mixtures; resveratrol (R), ferulic acid (F), phloretin (P) and THCs (T); mixtures: RFT, PFR, and PFT. Cell viability, proliferation, morphology and migratory behavior were analyzed.

It was reported that resveratrol, ferulic acid and THCs (RFT) mixture decreased the cell number at higher concentrations (10^{-3} M), whereas increased the cell number at lower concentrations (10^{-5} M) in HGF cells. High and low concentrations (10^{-3}-10^{-5} M) of the antioxidants, including resveratrol, ferulic acid and THCs (RFT); and phloretin, ferulic acid, resveratrol (PFR) may have beneficial effects on functional mechanisms of regulating fibroblast migration and proliferation during gingival healing or periodontal repair.

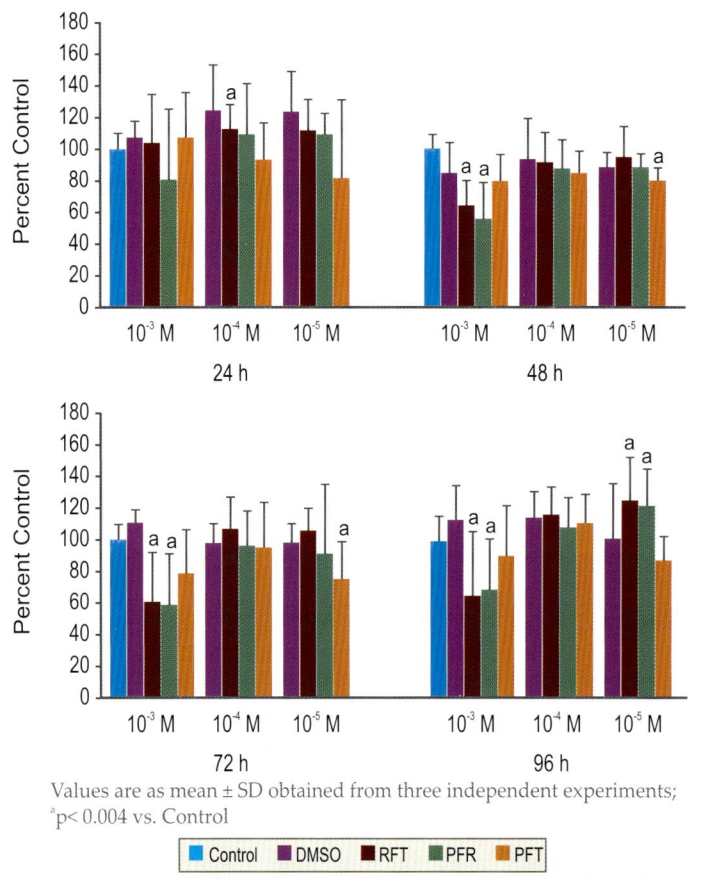

The authors observed that only one triple combination (PFT) showed a significant antioxidant effect associated with cell viability in HGF cells with little effect on HPDL cells (Figs. 99A & 99B).

In an extended study, the same authors (San Miguel *et al*., 2012) investigated the effects of the bioactive antioxidant mixtures on the stressors, such as hydrogen peroxide (H_2O_2),

Values are as mean ± SD obtained from three independent experiments; $^a p < 0.004$ vs. Control

Fig. 99A: Effect of antioxidant mixtures on HGF cell viability. (Adapted from San Miguel *et al*., 2011)

Chapter 3
TETRAHYDROCURCUMIN (THC): THE MAJOR METABOLITE WITH MAJOR BENEFITS

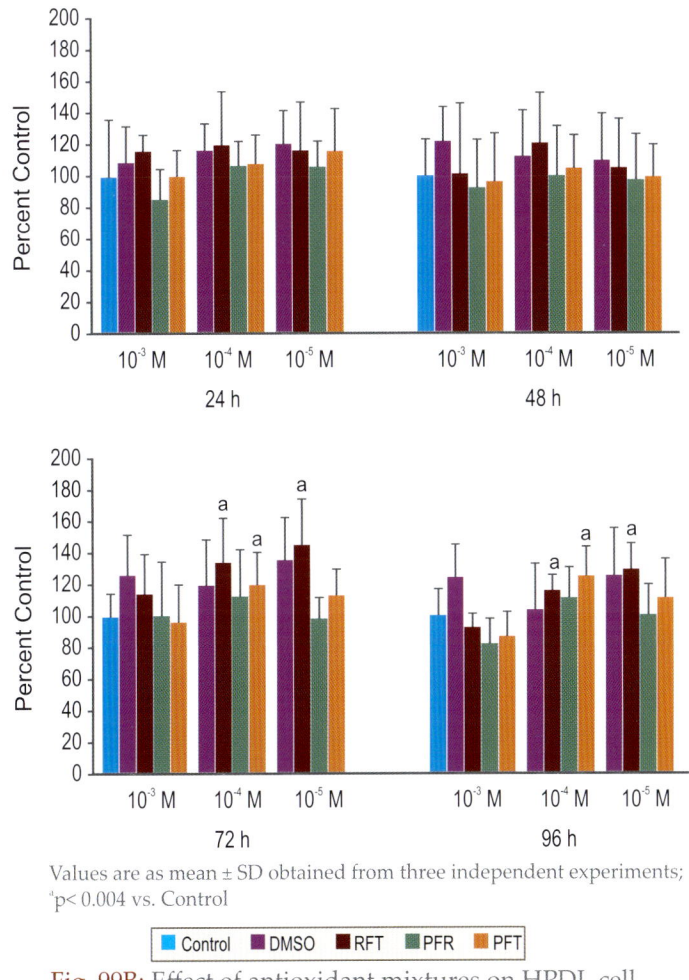

Values are as mean ± SD obtained from three independent experiments; ^{a}p< 0.004 vs. Control

Fig. 99B: Effect of antioxidant mixtures on HPDL cell viability. (Adapted from San Miguel *et al.*, 2011)

ethanol (EtOH) and nicotine (Nic) on cultured oral fibroblast viability, DNA synthesis and ROS activity. It was shown that common oral stressors have the potential to increase gingival cellular damage by decreasing cell viability and proliferation while increasing ROS. On the other hand, the natural antioxidant combinations, namely RFT, PFR and PFT applied complementary or synergistic mechanisms protected the oral fibroblasts from the detrimental toxic effects of stressors (H_2O_2, EtOH and Nic) by decreasing total ROS and increasing cell viability and DNA synthesis.

In dentistry, the use of metals in fillings, braces, implants, bridges and other prosthodontic restorations is a common practice. The use of zinc (Zn) and copper (Cu) released from gold alloys, and nickel (Ni) released from nickel–chromium alloys may have the potential of inducing ROS that activate signaling molecules to change cellular responses leading high cytotoxic effect on fibroblast. In a subsequent study, San Miguel *et al.* (2013) investigated whether specific antioxidant combinations counteract the effects of Cu, Ni and Zn on cultured oral fibroblast proliferation and oxidative damage. Oral fibroblasts were pre-treated with Cu, Ni and Zn for 60 min and were treated with 10^{-5} M combinations of bioactive antioxidant mixtures (RFT, PFR, PFT) for 24 h. Findings from this study indicate that metal stressors may increase gingival cellular damage by decreasing cell viability, and proliferation while increasing ROS. The antioxidant products may have complementary or synergistic mechanisms to counteract the detrimental effects of the metal stressors to decrease ROS and increase cell viability and DNA synthesis.

THCs for Canker Sore and Gingivitis Management

Canker sore, also called recurrent aphthous stomatitis (mouth ulcer), is one of the most common oral mucosal disorder. Most canker sores are characterized by multiple, recurrent, small, round, or ovoid ulcers with circumscribed margins, erythematous haloes, and yellow or grey floors that occur both in children and adults (Scully and Porter, 2008). Gingivitis, the mildest form of periodontal disease affects about 50% of the adult population, is characterized by inflammation of the gums caused by the bacterial biofilm (dental plaque) that accumulates on teeth adjacent to the gingiva (gums) (Pihlstrom *et al.*, 2005; Sculley and Langley-Evans, 2003). Turmeric is being used to offer relief from gingivitis and periodontitis (Cikrikci *et al.*, 2008) and 2% whole turmeric gel being used as an adjunct to scaling and root planning (Behal *et al.*, 2011). Recent studies provide evidence that isolated turmeric fraction and its components, curcuminoids, may be useful for controlling dental biofilms and subsequent dental caries formation (Pandit *et al.*, 2011). However, effect of THC in the management of canker sore or gingivitis is unknown.

Recently, Sami Labs carried out a prospective, open label, two arm, clinical trial to study the efficacy and safety of THCs (C3 Reduct® ODN) in canker sore and gingivitis (Sami Labs, 2017; Manuscript submitted for publication in 2019). The aim was to reduce pain associated with ulcers through topical applications or reduce outbreak frequency with systemic medications, most of them having serious adverse effects. Findings from this study showed a significant improvement in the throat relief score. Safety analysis showed that there was no adverse effect experienced by the patients during the study period. Thus, the current study showed that THCs could be effective in decreasing the symptoms of canker sore and gingivitis.

THCs in the Treatment of Oral Leukoplakia

A recent study evaluated the efficacy and safety of THCs in the treatment of oral leukoplakia. Patients, 40 to 70 years (mean age of 56 years), with oral mucosal lesions with clinical features of leukoplakia were given 2% THCs gel with advice to apply the gel to the affected areas, 5 times daily for 12 weeks. Tetrahydrocurcuminoids gel (2%) was formulated by Sami Labs, Bengaluru, India. The lesion was examined, and its characteristics were documented in a standard manner at baseline, 3, 6, 9, and 12 weeks. All the patients reported a reduced burning sensation within 3 weeks of THCs treatment and were completely asymptomatic by the end of the study. Similarly, there was a decrease in the size of the lesion during the follow-up period. The authors concluded that THCs when topically applied in gel form are remarkably effective in alleviating clinical symptoms of leukoplakia (Chhaparwal *et al.*, 2018).

Summary

As metabolites of curcuminoids, THCs mediate the several biological activities through antioxidant activity *in vivo*. In fact, recent studies show that THCs exert greater antioxidant activity than curcumin both *in vitro* and *in vivo*. Tetrahydrocurcuminoids also show very high DPPH scavenging activity and inhibition of both AAPH-induced linoleic acid oxidation activity and AAPH-induced RBC hemolysis activity.

Tetrahydrocurcuminoids reduced the formation of advanced glycation products and cross linking of collagen in diabetic rats. Tetrahydrocurcuminoids have been reported to stimulate pancreatic beta cells which play a key role in the production and secretion of insulin.

Tetrahydrocurcuminoids showed potent anti-inflammatory effect in animal studies. The β-diketone moiety in THCs is probably responsible for this.

Chapter 3
TETRAHYDROCURCUMIN (THC): THE MAJOR METABOLITE WITH MAJOR BENEFITS

Tetrahydrocurcuminoids decreased the concentrations of tissue lipids in experimental animals and thus, can potentially ameliorate lipid abnormalities in type 2 diabetes. In addition, THCs can increase glucose uptake and activate insulin simultaneously, suggesting that THCs may be able to reverse insulin resistance in steatosis in liver cells that may lead to obesity and diabetes.

The suppression of oxidative stress by THCs seems to be responsible for its cardioprotective and renal protective activities.

Tetrahydrocurcuminoids provided significant hepatoprotective effects in rats. They also reduced the pathological changes of the liver such as inflammatory infiltration of hepatocytic nuclei and cell infiltration. Both curcumin and THCs have shown to produce anti-proliferation and anti-angiogenesis effects.

It is demonstrated that the anti-angiogenic properties of curcumin and THCs represent a common mechanism for their anticancer activities. It is quite clear from several studies described that THCs have tremendous anticancer potential against various cancers. Tetrahydrocurcuminoids activate the mitochondrial apoptosis pathways in liver cancer cells and have been shown to activate autophagy mediated cell death in lung and osteosarcoma. Furthermore, THCs activate metalloprotease and inhibit tumor metastasis in fibrosarcomas and potentiate rotation and chemotherapy in breast and glioma tumors. Thus, THCs seem to have multiple mechanisms of anticancer activities and show potential to be used as an adjuvant therapy for several cancers.

- **Hepatocellular carcinoma:** Tetrahydrocurcumin was more effective than curcumin in inducing apoptosis of H22-induced ascites tumor cells by activating the mitochondrial apoptosis pathway, suggesting THC could be a potentially effective agent for hepatocellular carcinoma treatment
- **Colon cancer:** Tetrahydrocurcumin was found to be more effective than curcumin in preventing azoxymethane-induced colon carcinogenesis

- **Breast cancer:** Tetrahydrocurcumin exerted marked anti-proliferative activity against MCF-7 cells in a dose-dependent manner, suggesting that THC may be an excellent chemopreventive agent in the treatment of breast cancer

- **Glioma (brain and spinal cord tumors):** Tetrahydrocurcumin in combination with radiation therapy significantly decreased the proliferation of glioma cells and inhibited tumor growth

- **Lung carcinoma:** Tetrahydrocurcumin treatment inhibited A549 lung cancer cell proliferation through the autophagy pathway

- **Fibrosarcoma:** Tetrahydrocurcumin reduced invasion and migration of highly-metastatic HT1080 human fibrosarcoma cells by reducing total MT1-MMP and decreasing pro-MMP2 activation

- **Osteosarcoma (bone cancer):** Tetrahydrocurcumin significantly reduced the growth of osteosarcoma cells and suppressed migration and invasion, suggesting that THC provides potential therapeutic strategies for human osteosarcoma by suppressing angiogenesis and metastasis via downregulating HIF-1α and by promoting autophagy mechanisms

- **Leukemia:** Tetrahydrocurcumin remarkably increased the expression of LC3 and Beclin-1 proteins in human PBMC obtained from healthy individuals and chronic lymphocytic leukemia (CLL) patients, suggesting potential therapeutic benefit of THC in CLL patients

- **Cervical cancer:** Tetrahydrocurcumin treatments significantly reduced the relative tumor volume (RTV) CaSki cells (cervical cancer cells)-implanted nude mice that was associated with attenuation of COX-2, EGFR, p-ERK1/2, and p-AKT expression indicating that THC exerts anticancer effects against cervical cancer via multiple molecular targets

Chapter 3
TETRAHYDROCURCUMIN (THC): THE MAJOR METABOLITE WITH MAJOR BENEFITS

Tetrahydrocurcumin, one of the major metabolites of curcumin, has a wide range of beneficial neuroprotective properties.

- Tetrahydrocurcumin increased DA in animal model of PD, decreased MAO-B activity, attenuated neuronal cell death, and decreased oxidative stress induced by HHcy suggesting that THC may be an attractive neuroprotective agent. Tetrahydrocurcumin reduces the amyloid-β-plaque formation thus potentially useful for treatment of Alzheimer's disease

- Tetrahydrocurcumin increased the levels of DA after MPTP treatment in the animal model of PD through the inhibition of MAO-B activity. Thus, THC may have the potential to be used as a therapeutic for the prevention of PD

- High level of Hcy or HHcy causes increased oxidative stress and generation of excessive free radicals (ROS) during I/R injury. Tetrahydrocurcumin was shown to prevent I/R induced brain injury and improve the blood-brain barrier integrity

- Traumatic brain injury (TBI) has high morbidity and mortality rates worldwide. Tetrahydrocurcumin alleviated brain edema, attenuated TBI-induced neuron cell death, decreased the degree of apoptosis and improved neurobehavioral function, which were accompanied by enhanced autophagy, suggesting that THC may be an attractive neuroprotective agent for TBI therapy

- Chemotherapy induced peripheral neuropathy (CIPN) is a common side effect in cancer patients. Tetrahydrocurcumin significantly attenuated the neuropathic pain manifestations by increasing the nociceptive threshold, decreasing the oxidative stress, inflammatory mediators and total calcium levels in sciatic nerve in vincristine injected rats, indicating THC can be a promising candidate for the prevention of CIPN caused by chemotherapeutic agents

Tetrahydrocurcumin regulated many transcription factors (FOXO, SIRT1) involved in the biological activities associated with the aging process. As natural metabolites of the curcuminoids, THCs present an attractive option to supplement manufacturers seeking to revitalize their anti-aging formulations.

Curcumin and THC reduced osteoarthritis symptoms and pain related behaviors in estrogen-deficient rats with osteoarthritis induced by intra-articular injection of MIA. The MIA is known to initiate osteoarthritis by activating MMPs by inducing inflammation and elevating cytokine release. Tetrahydrocurcumin decreased the expressions of MMP3 and MMP13 slightly better than curcumin.

Tetrahydrocurcumin inhibited the release of histamine, though less potently than curcumin and could play a significant role in exerting both the antioxidative and anti-allergic activities.

Tetrahydrocurcumin was superior to curcumin in modulating allergic asthmatic phenotypes, especially attenuating the Th2 response, suggesting that THC might be a potentially effective agent for asthma treatment.

Tetrahydrocurcumin exerts beneficial effects and may play a potential role in oral health.

- A bioactive pure polyphenol and turmeric derivative mixtures containing THC decreased the cell number at lower concentrations in HGF cells. In addition, a combination of resveratrol, ferulic acid, phloretin and THCs counteracted the detrimental effects of the metal stressors and reduced gingival cellular damage by decreasing cell viability, and proliferation while increasing ROS

- Recent prospective, open label, two arm, clinical study conducted by Sami Labs on the efficacy and safety of THCs (C3 Reduct® ODN) in canker sore and gingivitis, showed that THCs could be effective in decreasing the symptoms of canker sore and gingivitis

From numerous research being done on THCs, it is clear that THCs could help in slowing down the aging process thus leading to prolonged healthy life style.

Cosmetic Applications

THCs in Cosmetic Formulations

The role of curcuminoids as topical antioxidants has been validated in laboratory experiments. Curcuminoids are reported to protect normal human keratinocytes from hypoxanthine/xanthine oxidase injury in *in vitro* studies (Bonte et al., 1997). Curcuminoids, because of their yellow color are not preferred for cosmetics, since they stain clothing, skin, etc. Tetrahydrocurcuminoids being white in color, are preferred in topical preparation.

Free radical chain reactions are implicated in most degenerative biological reactions. Free radicals on the surface of the skin generated through exposure to ultraviolet (UV) radiation, chemicals or other environmental stress factors catalyze aging of the skin. Tetrahydrocurcuminoids scavenge and inhibit propagation of free radicals. They also help to improve the shelf life of fat-based topical formulations by inhibiting the autoxidation of fats. The anti-inflammatory effects of THCs combined with their efficient antioxidant action render them useful as ingredients in anti-aging formulations and in topical formulations designed to maintain general skin health and integrity.

Sabinsa's patent (Majeed, 2007) demonstrated the role of THCs in contributing to post-translational modification, cross-linking and optimization of cell electric potential in physiologic states characterized by poor morphological functional differentiation of cells. e.g. premalignant states or malignancy. The patent discloses that THCs would prevent undesired cross linking by attaching to amino and carboxy groups of the protein amino acids. This would effectively stop the chain reaction which otherwise would lead to deterioration of cell homeostasis, premature aging and premature cell death.

The invention proposed in the patent demonstrates use of THCs in *in vivo* experimental conditions such as preventing UV sunburn and cross-linking in the skin cells exposed to UV radiation. Cross-linking was measured based on the percent of thymine dimer cells in presence or absence of THCs. This activity appears to be different from the antioxidant characteristic of THCs.

Experiments on the effect of topical application of THCs on female SKH-1 mice (8-9 weeks old) showed significant decrease in the percent of thymine dimer cells and sunburn cells compared to non-treated group (Tables 12 & 13).

Table 12: Effect of topical application of THCs on UV-B light-induced formation of thymine dimers in mouse epidermis. (Adapted from Majeed, 2007)

Treatment	Number of mice /group	% Thymine dimer cells	% Protection
No UVB	3	0	-
Acetone + UVB	7	8.9 ± 0.02	0
THCs (10 µmol) + UVB	6	7.3 ± 0.03	24.7
THCs (20 µmol) + UVB	6	1.6 ± 1.30	82.0

Table 13: Effect of topical application of THCs on UV-B induced formation of skin sunburn cells in mouse epidermis. (Adapted from Majeed, 2007)

Treatment	Number of mice /group	% Sunburn cells	% Inhibition
No UVB	5	0.1	-
Acetone + UVB (60 mJ/cm^2)	5	3.0	-
Dibenzoylmethane (10 µmol)	5	1.2	60
Dibenzoylmethane (20 µmol)	5	0.9	70
THCs (10 µmol) + UVB	5	1.6	47
THCs (20 µmol) + UVB	5	1.4	53

Chapter 3
TETRAHYDROCURCUMIN (THC): THE MAJOR METABOLITE WITH MAJOR BENEFITS

Also, the patent provides a practical and safe solution to regulate functions of tyrosinase activity by use of THCs. Based on *in vitro* experimental data, THCs were found to have considerable potential in inhibiting the process of melanogenesis, and this effect was related to their inhibitory activity on tyrosinase.

For cosmetic applications, encapsulation of THCs in phosphatidylcholine liposomes offers an aqueous dispersion for addition to cosmetic formulations (Arunothayanun *et al.*, 2005). Fig. 100 shows that antioxidant activity of THCs, vitamin E, or a mixture of THCs and vitamin E, when prepared as alcoholic solutions, were low and occurred only for short period. There was no further reduction of ABTS free radicals after 10 minutes which was in contrast to liposomal dispersions. Therefore, phosphatidylcholine liposomes possess a sustained antioxidant activity and improve the activity of their encapsulated compounds.

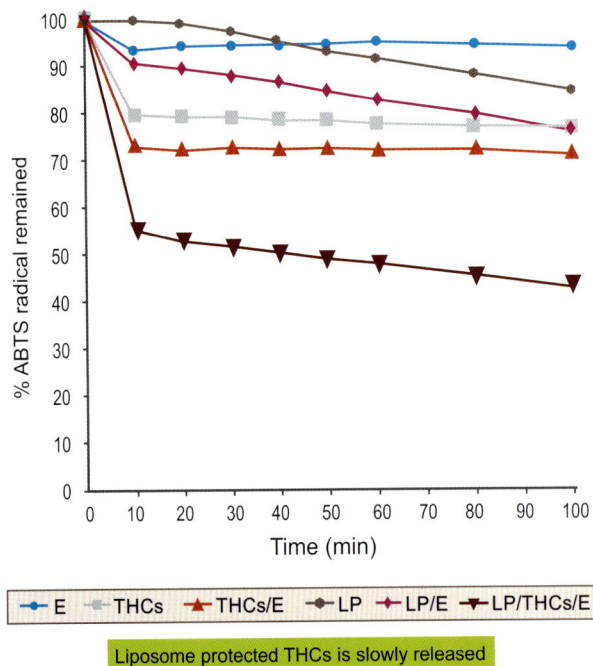

E: Vitamin E 1000 µg/mL alcoholic solution; THCs: Alcoholic solution of THCs 500 µg/mL; THCs/E: Alcoholic solution of THCs 500 µg/mL and vitamin E 1000 µg/mL; LP: Phosphatidyl choline liposomes; LP/E: Vitamin E 1000 µg/mL in liposomes; LP/THCs/E: THCs 500 µg/mL and vitamin E 1000 µg/mL in liposomes

Fig. 100: ABTS (%) radical cation remained following addition of 1:3 dilution of vitamin E, alcoholic solution of THCs, phosphatidyl choline liposomes and THCs and vitamin E combination.

The results show immediate reaction by the free radicals on THC molecules in the ethanolic solution, whereas, liposomes protected THCs have delayed free radicals access to THCs in the lamellae.

THC Against Skin Disorders

Tetrahydrocurcumin exhibits a broad spectrum of therapeutic activities without any side effects and hence it has been used in the cosmetic products. Earlier studies reported that THC protects skin by minimizing the inflammation, free radical quenching, impaired wound-healing, improved collagen deposition, improved fibroblast and vascular density (Wu *et al.*, 2014). The anti-angiogenic properties of THC help to improve the accumulation of extracellular matrix (ECM) components through remodeling of the wound repair.

Recently, Trivedi *et al.* (2017) evaluated the effect of THC on a wide range of skin rejuvenating parameters and its implication in wound healing, at the *in vitro* settings, using human foreskin fibroblast (HFF-1) and melanoma (B16-F10) cell lines. The results of the MTT assay on the cytotoxic effect of THC on these two cell lines in term of % cell viability of L-ascorbic acid at concentration of 10 µM reveal that THC at all the tested concentrations (up to 10 µg/mL) was found to be safe and nontoxic and showed dose-dependent effects.

Next, in order to determine the effects of THC on skin strength, hydration level and overall suppleness, the authors evaluated the ECM components synthesis such as collagen, elastin and hyaluronic acid in HFF-1 cell line. The results of this study revealed that THC improved the level of collagen (37.90%), elastin (90.1%), and hyaluronic acid (74.19%) at 1 µg/mL (Figs. 101-103), suggesting that THC may be a potential phytoconstituent in cosmetic formulations.

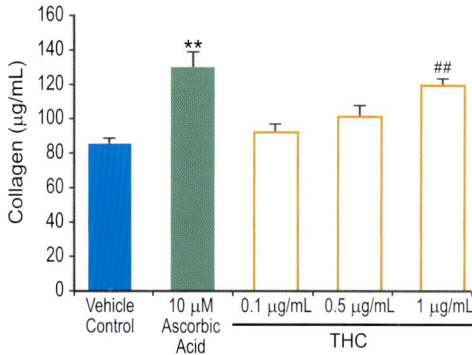

**p<0.01 vs. Vehicle control; ##p<0.01 vs. Ascorbic acid

Fig. 101: Effects of THC on ECM component collagen in HFF-1 cells. (Adapted from Trivedi *et al.*, 2017)

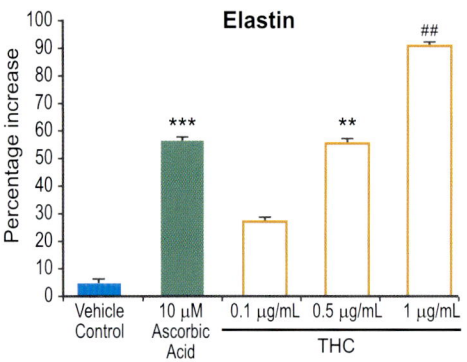

***p<0.001 and **p< 0.01 vs. Vehicle control;
##p<0.01 vs. Positive control (ascorbic acid) group.

Fig. 102: Effects of THC on ECM component elastin. (Adapted from Trivedi *et al.*, 2017)

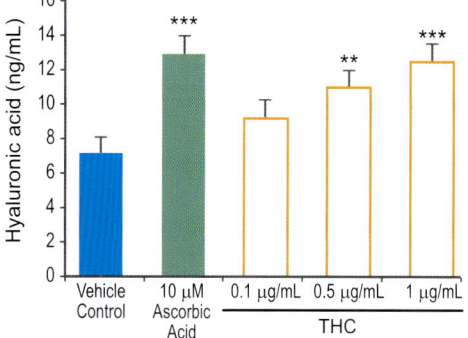

***p<0.001 and **p<0.01 all statistical comparison with respect to vehicle control.

Fig. 103: Influence of THC on the synthesis of ECM component hyaluronic acid against UVB-induced stress in HFF-1 cells. (Adapted from Trivedi *et al.*, 2017)

The mouse melanoma (B16-F10) cells were used to determine the effect of THC on melanin synthesis. Kojic acid, a standard skin whitening cosmetic products, was used in this study for comparing the skin whitening effect of THC. It was reported that THC reduced the cellular content of melanin in a dose-dependent manner (Fig. 104). In addition, THC significantly decreased α-MSH melanin synthesis at the lowest concentration (0.1 µg/mL) by 78.5%

(p<0.001) compared to kojic acid, suggesting that THC efficiently inhibited melanin production in the B16-F10 melanoma cells.

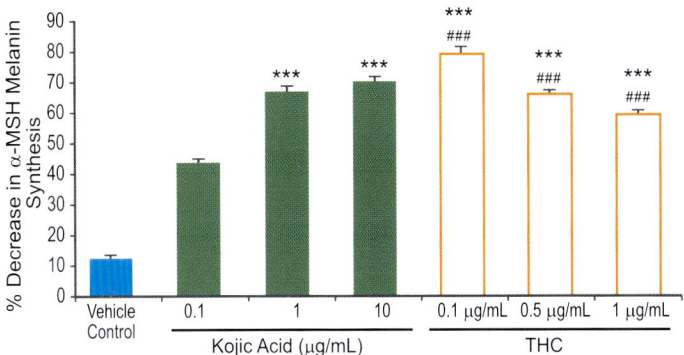

***p<0.001 vs. Vehicle control; ###p<0.001 vs. Positive control (ascorbic acid).

Fig. 104: Effect of THC on inhibition of melanogenesis (skin whitening potential) in B16-F10 cells. (Adapted from Trivedi et al., 2017)

Further, to determine the effect of THC on UV-protection (photoaging), the effect of THC was measured in UVB-induced stress (UVB-irradiation, 200 mJ/cm^2) HFF-1 cells and percentage of cell viability was assessed. Tetrahydrocurcumin was reported with dose-dependent increased effect on cell viability and the percentage UVB-protection rate (Fig. 105).

In addition, to evaluate the effect of THC on wound healing, cell migration assay was performed in HFF-1 cells. The percent migration of HFF-1 fibroblasts cells in response to THC treatment was found to be

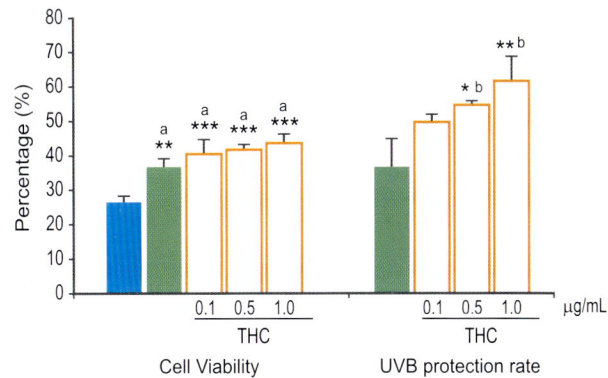

L-AC: L-ascorbic acid; ***p< 0.001, **p< 0.01 and *p< 0.05; a and b represent statistical comparison with vehicle control and ascorbic acid group respectively

Fig. 105: Anti-wrinkling potential and cytoprotective effect of THC against UVB-induced stress in HFF-1 cell lines. (Adapted from Trivedi et al., 2017)

significant, 78.51% at the end of 48 h compared to the untreated control (41.11%). The percentage of cell migration in response to THC treatment (78.51%) was very effective similar to the ascorbic acid (positive control) (80.90%) (Fig. 106).

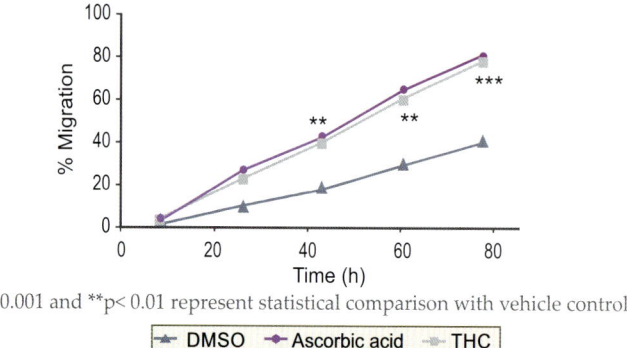

Fig. 106: Effect of THC on percentage of cell migration rate of HFF-1 cells after induction of a scratch 0-48 h. (Adapted from Trivedi *et al.*, 2017)

In summary, THC can protect the skin matrix by enhancing the synthesis of extracellular component and improving the skin elasticity and tightness by enabling wound healing through collagen synthesis. Overall, THC can be applied as a safe skin lightening, wound healing agent and for the treatment of various skin disorders.

Chapter 3
TETRAHYDROCURCUMIN (THC): THE MAJOR METABOLITE WITH MAJOR BENEFITS

In vitro Studies for Cosmetic Application

In vitro Studies (Sami Labs, 2009)

Tetrahydrocurcuminoids were found to be effective skin lightening agent with multifunctional topical benefits and no sensitization side effects. The products act on several of the major targets that cause undesirable pigmentation, age spots, freckles and other related skin conditions.

Tetrahydrocurcuminoids have shown good efficacy in these *in vitro* studies for lightening skin tone.

Antioxidant Assay Using Cell Lines by ROS Scavenging Method

A cell permeable, non-fluorescent dye, dichloro fluorescein diacetate (DCFH-DA) after intracellularly getting de-esterified is converted to dichloro fluorescein upon oxidation by the ROS. The scavenging activity of the sample is indicated by the decrease in fluorescence (wavelength 485/520 nm).

Reactive oxygen species generated in the body due to stress conditions like UV exposure, pollution, aging etc affect melanocytes of the skin. The melanocytes under these stress conditions are stimulated to produce more melanin as a defense mechanism. This condition is called UV-induced melano-genesis which results in hyperpigmentation.

Chapter 3
TETRAHYDROCURCUMIN (THC): THE MAJOR METABOLITE WITH MAJOR BENEFITS

Tetrahydrocurcuminoids have an IC_{50} value of 1.5 µg/mL which implies that concentrations as low as 1.5 µg/mL can reduce generation of ROS in Swiss 3T3 mouse fibroblast cell line by 50% (Fig. 107). A comparison on the efficacy of THCs and green tea extract by ROS scavenging method is shown in Fig. 108.

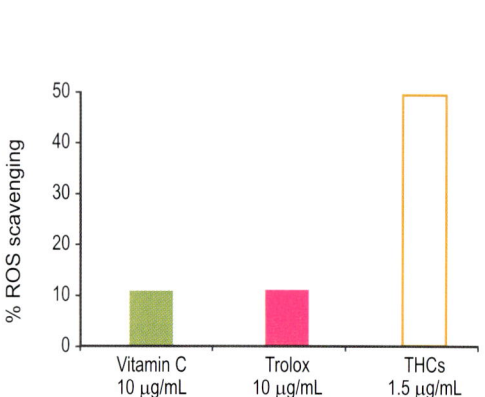

Fig. 107: Comparison of ROS scavenging of THCs with Vitamin C and trolox.

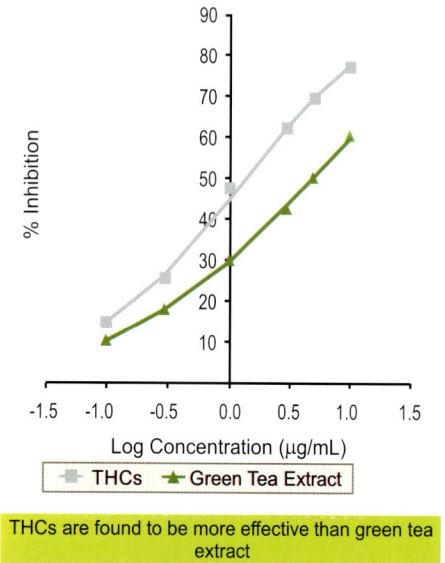

THCs are found to be more effective than green tea extract

Fig. 108: Comparative efficacy of THCs and green tea extract by ROS scavenging method.

Antioxidant Assay by Lipid Peroxidation Method

Lipid peroxidation was assessed by measuring TBARS concentration by a spectrophotometric method. The product of lipid peroxidation like malondialdehyde forms a diadduct with thiobarbituric acid, which is a pink chromogen that has maximum absorption at 535 nm. Inhibition of lipid peroxidation of melanocyte membranes also augments depigmentation process. Efficacy of THCs to inhibit lipid peroxidation has been compared with coffee bean extract (Fig. 109) and IC_{50} values of THCs were also determined (Fig. 110).

TETRAHYDROCURCUMIN (THC): THE MAJOR METABOLITE WITH MAJOR BENEFITS

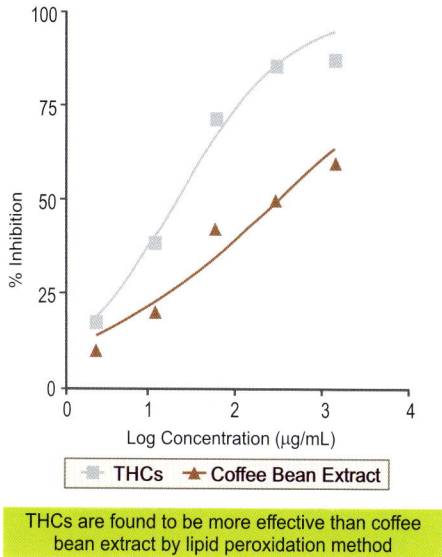

Fig. 109: Comparative efficacy of THCs and coffee bean extract on inhibition of lipid peroxidation.

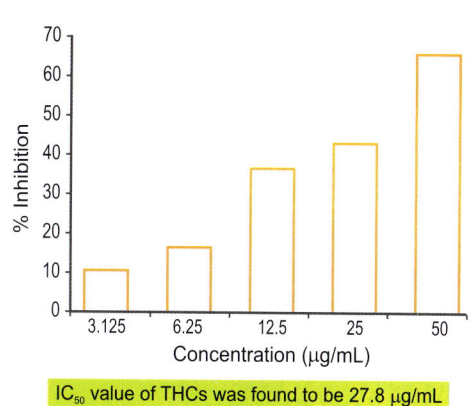

Fig. 110: Lipid peroxidation inhibition of THCs.

Antioxidant Assay by DPPH Method

The free radical scavenging activity is determined based on the stable free radical DPPH with antioxidant in organic/aqueous organic media resulting in bleaching of the DPPH due to its quenching by the interaction with the analytes. The decrease of absorbance of DPPH compared to blank measured spectrophotometrically at 516 nm is related to the concentration of antioxidant in the test solution (Fig. 111). Generation of free radicals in skin due to various stress conditions such as UV exposure, pollution, aging etc, results in induction of melanin synthesis.

Chapter 3
TETRAHYDROCURCUMIN (THC): THE MAJOR METABOLITE WITH MAJOR BENEFITS

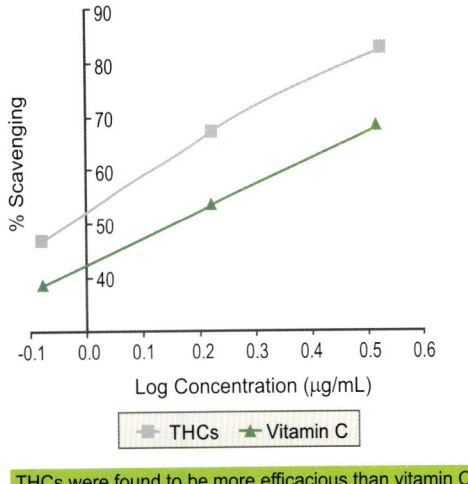

THCs were found to be more efficacious than vitamin C

Fig. 111: Comparative efficacy of THCs and vitamin C by DPPH method.

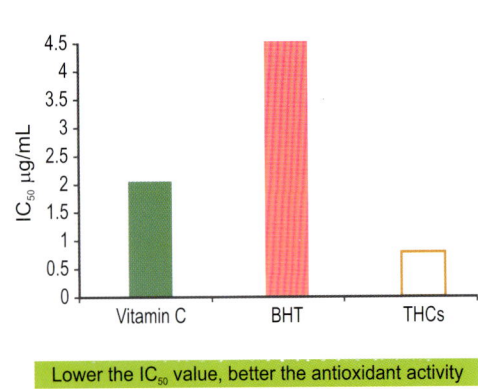

Lower the IC_{50} value, better the antioxidant activity

Fig. 112: Comparison of antioxidant activity of THCs with BHT and vitamin C.

Tetrahydrocurcuminoids are effective in scavenging the stable free radical DPPH with an IC_{50} value of 0.8 µg/mL, implying that concentrations as low as 0.8 µg/mL can inhibit generation of free radicals by 50% (Fig. 112).

Antioxidant Assay by ORAC Method

The oxygen radical absorbance capacity (ORAC) assay depends on the free radical damage to a fluorescent probe through the change in its fluorescence intensity. The change of fluorescence intensity is an index of the degree of free radical damage. In the presence of antioxidant, inhibition of free radical damage reflected in the protection against the change of probe fluorescence, is a measure of its antioxidant capacity against the free radical.

The ORAC value is a measure of inhibition of peroxyl radicals. It is represented as trolox equivalents where the product is compared with trolox (vitamin E analogue), a standard inhibitor of peroxyl radicals. Higher the ORAC value, better is the peroxyl radical inhibition.

Tetrahydrocurcuminoids have high ORAC value of 10,786 ± 490 μM trolox equivalents/g (Fig. 113) and thus THCs are effective in inhibiting the peroxyl radicals.

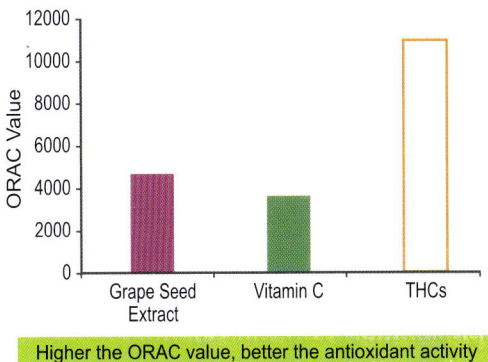

Fig. 113: Comparison of ORAC values of THCs with vitamin C and grape seed extract.

Antioxidant Assay by HORAC Method

The hydroxyl radical averting capacity (HORAC) value is a measure of inhibition of hydroxyl radicals. The HORAC value is represented as gallic acid equivalents where the product is compared with gallic acid, a standard inhibitor of hydroxyl radicals. Higher the HORAC value, better is the hydroxyl radical inhibition.

Hydroxyl radical prevention capacity is assessed using fluorescein (FL) as the fluorescent probe. The hydroxyl radical is generated by a Co(II)-mediated reaction. The fluorescent decay curve of FL is monitored in the presence and absence of the inhibitor and the AUC is integrated. Net AUC is calculated which is an index of hydroxyl radical prevention capacity expressed in Gallic acid equivalents.

Tetrahydrocurcuminoids have a high HORAC value of 2715 ± 80 μM gallic acid equivalents/g. Hence, THCs are effective in inhibiting the hydroxyl radicals.

Chapter 3
TETRAHYDROCURCUMIN (THC): THE MAJOR METABOLITE WITH MAJOR BENEFITS

Melanogenesis Inhibitory Activity

The intracellular melanin in B16F1 mouse melanoma cells treated with varying concentrations of the sample is extracted by 1N NaOH. The brown colored melanin thus extracted is estimated at 405 nm. This brown color intensity of the melanin is quenched in the presence of the inhibitor.

Hyperpigmentation, the darkening of skin is due to uncontrolled melanogenesis in the melanocytes of skin. Hence, inhibition of melanin production helps in lightening the skin tone. Tetrahydrocurcuminoids were shown to inhibit melanogenesis in melanoma cell models. Tetrahydrocurcuminoids at a concentration as low as 3.0 ± 0.5 μg/mL can inhibit 50% melanogenesis in melanoma cells (Fig. 114).

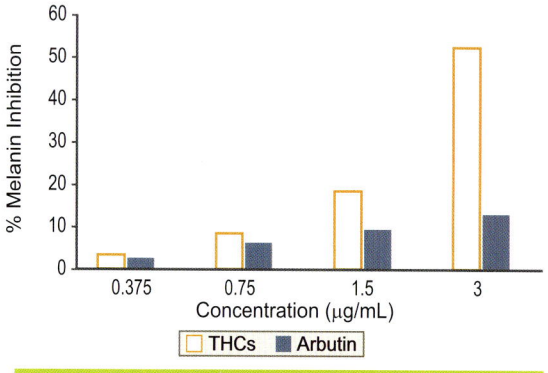

Melanin inhibition by THCs was found to be better than arbutin

Fig. 114: Melanin inhibition in B16F1 mouse melanoma cell line.

Cyclooxygenase (COX) Inhibitory Activity

The enzyme COX-1 or COX-2 is allowed to react on substrate arachidonate in presence and absence of the inhibitor. The amount of prostaglandins (PGF2α) produced by stannous chloride reduction of COX-derived $PGFH_2$ are estimated by EIA (Cayman) using a broadly specific antibody that binds to the entire major prostaglandin compounds. The decrease in prostaglandins released in presence of inhibitor is directly proportional to inhibition. Tetrahydrocurcuminoids have an IC_{50} value of 100 μg/mL which implies that concentration as low as 100 μg/mL can inhibit 50% cyclooxygenase activity (Fig. 115).

Chapter 3
TETRAHYDROCURCUMIN (THC): THE MAJOR METABOLITE WITH MAJOR BENEFITS

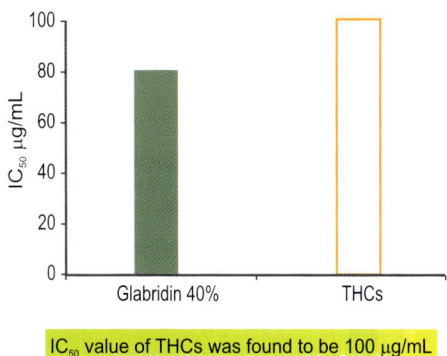

Fig. 115: COX-1 inhibitory activity of THCs in comparison with glabridin 40%.

Summary

Excessive tyrosinase production, melanogenesis, oxidation of tissue lipids, ROS, peroxyl and hydroxyl free radicals generated under stress conditions such as UV exposure, pollution, aging etc., result in undesirable skin conditions such as pigmentation, age spots and freckles.

Tetrahydrocurcuminoids are potentially good antioxidants and significantly help to scavenge ROS, hydroxyl and peroxyl radicals. They inhibit peroxidation of lipids and cyclooxygenase enzyme – which has a significant role in inflammation.

Tetrahydrocurcuminoids also have significant skin lightening property, as they are potent inhibitors of melanogenesis. They are recommended over other colored compounds which cause undesirable color deposit on the skin after topical application.

Chapter 3
TETRAHYDROCURCUMIN (THC): THE MAJOR METABOLITE WITH MAJOR BENEFITS

Toxicity Studies

Acute Toxicity Studies *(Sami Labs, 2003, 2015)*

The acute oral toxicity of THCs was investigated in two separate studies using two strains of rats, namely Sprague-Dawley (SD) rats and Wistar rats. In the first study, the male and female SD rats (6-8 weeks of age) were administered with a single oral (gavage) dose of THCs, at a dosage of >2000 mg/kg/bw. No mortality was observed at the end of the study period of 4 days. It was concluded that the cut off median lethal dose of THCs after single oral administration to male or female rats was found to be >2000 mg/kg/bw. In a subsequent study with female Wistar rats (9-11 week of age), it was shown that the median lethal dose of THCs after single oral administration was >5000 mg/kg/bw. No mortality was observed in these animals throughout the study period. Based on the results of these studies, it was concluded that the cut off median lethal dose of THCs after single oral administration to female rats was found to be >5000 mg/kg/bw and can be classified to Category 5 or Unclassified as per globally harmonized classification system.

Recently, Zhang *et al*. 2018a estimated the median lethal dose (LD_{50}) of THC in male and female ICR mice weighing 18–22 g. The authors reported that the animals in the THC group showed no abnormal behavioral change. No convulsions and deaths were observed during the 14 days of behavioral study. It was reported that the LD_{50} value of graded dose of THC in mice was greater than 10,000 mg/kg. The above study supports the previous findings that THC possesses a wide margin of safety.

Salmonella typhimurium Reverse Mutation Assay *(Sami Labs, 2010a)*

The AMES test was conducted using *Salmonella typhimurium* strain. The study showed that the mean numbers of revertant colonies counted at different concentrations were comparable to that of the controls for both the experiments, in the absence and presence of metabolic activation. It was concluded that THCs did not induce mutations in *S. typhimurium* up to the maximum concentration of 5000 µg/plate.

Repeated Insult Patch Test (RIPT) on Human Subjects *(Sami Labs, 2010b)*

The study was designed by repetitive epidermal contact on the primary or cumulative irritation and/or allergic contact sensitization potential of RIPT/THCs. It was concluded that THCs did not produce any reaction as well as challenge phase in all the 50 patients.

Subchronic Oral Toxicity Studies

Repeated dose subchronic oral toxicity of THCs in Wistar rats was performed for 90 days with 14 days recovery. Rats were administered with the vehicle or THCs via oral route at doses of 0, 100, 200 and 400 mg/kg/bw for a consecutive period of 90 days with 14-day recovery period to evaluate the potential reversibility of any findings. All rats survived until scheduled euthanasia. All the animals appeared normal from day 1 to the end of observation period. In conclusion, oral administration of THCs once daily had no adverse effect on general health, haematological, clinical chemistry parameters, urine parameters, organ weights and gross appearance of the tissues/organs of the rats. Thus, THCs administration was tolerated by the rats of both sex up to the level of 400 mg/kg/bw/day. Hence it reveals that THCs in rats have no toxicity up to 400 mg/kg/bw. Based on these results, the no observed adverse effect level (NOAEL) of THCs in rats, following oral administration for 90 days was found to be 400 mg/kg/bw/day *(Majeed et al., 2019)*.

Reproductive/Developmental Toxicity/Embryotoxicity

To assess the reproduction/developmental toxicity, THCs were administered through oral gavage to Wister rats for a consecutive period of 54 days. Both male and female rats were administered with vehicle or THCs via oral route at doses of 0, 100, 200 and 400 mg/kg/bw for a consecutive period of 90 days. Oral administration of THCs once daily up to 55 days can be well tolerated in rats of both the sex at levels up to 400 mg/kg/bw. Based on these results, the NOAEL was considered to be 400 mg/kg/bw/day for reproductive parameters (Majeed *et al.*, 2019).

Summary

- The cut off median lethal dose of THCs after single oral administration to rats was found to be >5000 mg/kg/bw
- The independent research highlights that LD_{50} value of THC in mice was greater than 10,000 mg/kg
- THCs did not produce any skin irritation and/or allergic reaction
- NOAEL of THCs in rats, following oral administration for 90 days was found to be 400 mg/kg/bw/day
- NOAEL of THCs was considered to be 400 mg/kg/bw/day for reproductive parameters

Chapter 3
TETRAHYDROCURCUMIN (THC): THE MAJOR METABOLITE WITH MAJOR BENEFITS

Safety Study

A 28-day Safety Assessment of THCs *(Sami Labs/ClinWorld Ltd, 2010)*

Though several efficacy studies on THCs are carried out in animals, no safety data is available for consumption of THCs as a supplement. In this regard, Sabinsa conducted a single centered, open labeled clinical trial in humans for establishing safety of oral supplementation of THCs.

The study involved 20 healthy human volunteers who were given 300 mg of THCs once daily for 28 days. Laboratory parameters analyzed at the baseline and at the end of the study showed no significant difference in haematological parameters (such as leukocyte count, erythrocyte count, haemoglobin, hematocrit, platelets etc.) and in serum components (like aspartate aminotransferase, alanine aminotransferase, γ-glutamyl transferase, total bilirubin, total protein, uric acid, total cholesterol, high density lipoprotein, low density lipoprotein, triglycerides, etc.) (Table 14). No significant change in the body mass index (BMI) was observed and no adverse event was reported during the study.

Chapter 3
TETRAHYDROCURCUMIN (THC): THE MAJOR METABOLITE WITH MAJOR BENEFITS

Table 14: Results of 28-day safety study of THCs.

Parameters	Initial (Before administration of THCs)	Final (After 28 days administration of THCs)
Hb (g%)	14.06	14.10
PCV (%)	43.05	43.14
RBC (Million/mm^3)	4.94	4.96
WBC (/mm^3)	7155	7130
Platelet Count (/mm^3)	275400	274950
Total Cholesterol (mg/dL)	175.68	176.55
HDL (mg/dL)	47.84	47.82
LDL (mg/dL)	110.79	112.16
Triglycerides (mg/dL)	85.20	83.00
Total Protein (g/dL)	7.04	7.03
Total Bilirubin (mg/dL)	0.75	0.75
SGPT (IU/L)	22.51	23.43
SGOT (IU/L)	19.96	20.92
GGTP (IU/L)	7.91	7.80
Uric Acid (mg/dL)	3.89	3.89

Thus, it can be concluded that THCs when given at the dose of 300 mg once daily for 28 days are safe.

Chapter 3
TETRAHYDROCURCUMIN (THC): THE MAJOR METABOLITE WITH MAJOR BENEFITS

Conclusion

Tetrahydrocurcumin, a major metabolite of curcumin is an outstanding anti-oxidant with excellent safety margin with LD_{50} values greater than 10 g/kg/bw. Tetrahydrocurcumin also possesses more efficient absorption across intestinal tissues.

Tetrahydrocurcuminoids (THCs) possess a dazzling array of pharmacological properties such as anti-inflammatory, anti-diabetic, anticancer and anti-allergic, as well as hepatoprotective, cardioprotective, neuroprotective and nephroprotective activities surpassing curcuminoids in some of these activities. Tetrahydrocurcuminoids could help in slowing down the aging process.

The colorless nature of Tetrahydrocurcuminoids readily recommend their use in oral and skin care products where it may not stain the tissue, a problem usually associated with curcumin.

Suggested use levels of THCs:
200 to 400 mg in two divided doses

References

Aggarwal BB, Deb L, Prasad S. 2014. Curcumin differs from tetrahydrocurcumin for molecular targets, signaling pathways and cellular responses. *Molecules*. 20(1):185-205.

Akbaraly TN, Kumari M, Head J, Ritchie K, Ancelin ML, Tabak AG *et al*. 2013. Glycemia, insulin resistance, insulin secretion, and risk of depressive symptoms in middle age. *Diabetes Care*. 36(4):928-934.

Akiyama H, Barger S, Barnum S, Bradt B, Bauer J, Cole GM *et al*. 2000. Inflammation and Alzheimer's disease. *Neurobiol Aging*. 21(3):383-421.

Ali MS, Mudagal MP, Goli D. 2009. Cardioprotective effect of tetrahydrocurcumin and rutin on lipid peroxides and antioxidants in experimentally induced myocardial infarction in rats. *Pharmazie*. 64(2):132-136.

Anand P, Thomas SG, Kunnumakkara AB, Sundaram C, Harikumar KB, Sung B *et al*. 2008. Biological activities of curcumin and its analogues (Congeners) made by man and Mother Nature. *Biochem Pharmacol*. 76(11):1590-1611.

Anbarasu K, Jayanthi S. 2018. Identification of curcumin derivatives as human LMTK3 inhibitors for breast cancer: a docking, dynamics, and MM/PBSA approach. *3 Biotech*. 8(5):228.

Aragno M, Tamagno E, Gatto V, Brignardello E, Parola S, Danni O *et al*. 1999. Dehydroepiandrosterone protects tissues of streptozotocin-treated rats against oxidative stress. *Free Radic Biol Med*. 26(11-12):1467-1474.

Arunothayanun P, Wirachwong P, Burananon V, Phisalphong C, Hokputsa S, Suvathi Y, *et al*., 2005. Development of tetrahydrocurcuminoid liposomes as an ingredient for cosmetic products, Proc 7th Scientific Conference of the Asian Society of Cosmetic Scientists. pp. 51-57.

Baikerikar S. 2017. Curcumin and natural derivatives inhibit Ebola viral proteins: An *In silico* approach. *Pharmacogn Res*. 9(Suppl 1):S15-S22.

Battino M, Bompadre S, Politi A, Fioroni M, Rubini C, Bullon P. 2005. Antioxidant status (CoQ10 and Vit. E levels) and immunohistochemical analysis of soft tissues in periodontal diseases. *Biofactors*. 25(1-4):213-217.

Begum AN, Jones MR, Lim GP, Morihara T, Kim P, Heath DD *et al*. 2008. Curcumin structure-function, bioavailability, and efficacy in models of neuroinflammation and Alzheimer's disease. *J Pharmacol Exp Ther*. 326(1):196-208.

Behal R, Mali AM, Gilda SS, Paradkar AR. 2011. Evaluation of local drug-delivery system containing 2% whole turmeric gel used as an adjunct to scaling and root planing in chronic periodontitis: A clinical and microbiological study. *J Indian Soc Periodontol*. 15(1):35-38.

Chapter 3
TETRAHYDROCURCUMIN (THC): THE MAJOR METABOLITE WITH MAJOR BENEFITS

Bolger GT, Licollari A, Tan A, Greil R, Pleyer L, Vcelar B et al. 2018. Distribution of curcumin and THC in peripheral blood mononuclear cells isolated from healthy individuals and patients with chronic lymphocytic leukemia. *Anticancer Res*. 38(1):121-130.

Bolger GT, Licollari A, Tan A, Greil R, Vcelar B, Majeed M et al. 2017. Distribution and metabolism of Lipocurc™ (liposomal curcumin) in dog and human blood cells: species selectivity and pharmacokinetic relevance. *Anticancer Res*. 37(7):3483-3492.

Bonnefont-Rousselot D, Bastard JP, Jaudon MC, Delattre J. 2000. Consequences of the diabetic status on the oxidant/antioxidant balance. *Diabetes Metab*. 26(3):163-176.

Bonte F, Noel-Hudson MS, Wepierre J, Meybeck A. 1997. Protective effect of curcuminoids on epidermal skin cells under free oxygen radical stress. *Planta Med*. 63(3):265-266.

Brown MRD, Ramirez JD, Farquhar-Smith P. 2014. Pain in cancer survivors. *Br J Pain*. 8(4):139-153.

Browning DD. 2008. Protein kinase G as a therapeutic target for the treatment of metastatic colorectal cancer. *Expert Opin Ther Targets*. 12(3):367-376.

Chen BL, Chen YQ, Ma BH, Yu SF, Li LY, Zeng QX *et al*. 2018. Tetrahydrocurcumin, a major metabolite of curcumin, ameliorates allergic airway inflammation by attenuating Th2 responses and suppressing the IL-4Rα-Jak1-STAT6 and Jagged1/Jagged2-Notch1/Notch2 pathways in asthmatic mice. *Clin Exp Allergy*. 48(11):1494-1508.

Chen JW, Kong ZL, Tsai ML, Lo CY, Ho CT, Lai CS. 2018. Tetrahydrocurcumin ameliorates free fatty acid-induced hepatic steatosis and improves insulin resistance in HepG2 cells. *J Food Drug Anal*. 26(3):1075-1085.

Cheng Z, Jiang X, Kruger WD, Pratico D, Gupta S, Mallilankaraman K et al. 2011. Hyperhomocysteinemia impairs endothelium-derived hyperpolarizing factor-mediated vasorelaxation in transgenic cystathionine beta-synthase–deficient mice. *Blood*. 118(7):1998-2006.

Chhaparwal Y, Pai, KM, Kamath, MS, Carnelio S, Chhaparwal S. (2018). Efficacy and safety of tetrahydrocurcuminoid in the treatment of oral leukoplakia: a pilot study. *Asian J Pharmaceut Clin Res*. 11 (12):194-196.

Cikrikci S, Mozioglu E, Yilmaz H. 2008. Biological activity of curcuminoids isolated from *Curcuma longa*. *Rec Nat Prod*. 2(1):19-24.

Clarke PG. 1990. Developmental cell death: morphological diversity and multiple mechanisms. *Anat Embryol* (Berl). 181(3):195-213.

de Lau LM, Giesbergen PC, de Rijk MC, Hofman A, Koudstaal PJ, Breteler MM. 2004. Incidence of parkinsonism and Parkinson disease in a general population: the Rotterdam Study. *Neurology*. 63(7):1240-1244.

Fleck C, Appenroth D, Jonas P, Koch M, Kundt G, Nizze H *et al*. 2006. Suitability of 5/6 nephrectomy (5/6NX) for the induction of interstitial renal fibrosis in rats–influence of sex, strain, and surgical procedure. *Exp Toxicol Pathol*. 57(3):195-205.

Frautschy SA, Hu W, Kim P, Miller SA, Chu T, Harris-White ME et al. 2001. Phenolic anti-inflammatory antioxidant reversal of Aβ-induced cognitive deficits and neuropathology. *Neurobiol Aging*. 22(6):993-1005.

Friesen JB, Liu Y, Chen SN, McAlpine JB, Pauli GF. 2019. Selective Depletion and Enrichment of Constituents in "Curcumin" and Other *Curcuma longa* Preparations. *J Nat Prod*. 82(3):621-630.

Gao Y, Li J, Wu L, Zhou C, Wang Q, Li X et al. 2016. Tetrahydrocurcumin provides neuroprotection in rats after traumatic brain injury: autophagy and the PI3K/AKT pathways as a potential mechanism. *J Surg Res*. 206(1):67-76.

Gao Y, Zhuang Z, Gao S, Li X, Zhang Z, Ye Z et al. 2017. Tetrahydrocurcumin reduces oxidative stress-induced apoptosis via the mitochondrial apoptotic pathway by modulating autophagy in rats after traumatic brain injury. *Am J Transl Res*. 9(3):887-899.

Giamas G, Filipovic A, Jacob J, Messier W, Zhang H, Yang D et al. 2011. Kinome screening for regulators of the estrogen receptor identifies LMTK3 as a new therapeutic target in breast cancer. *Nat Med*.17(6):715-719.

Girija CR, Begum NS, Syed AA, Thiruvenkatam V. 2004. Hydrogen-bonding and C—H··· π interactions in 1,7-bis(4-hydroxy-3-methoxyphenyl)heptane-3,5-dione (tetrahydrocurcumin). *Acta Crystallogr C*.60(Pt 8):o611-o613.

Goldstein DS, Sullivan P, Holmes C, Miller GW, Alter S, Strong R et al. 2013. Determinants of buildup of the toxic dopamine metabolite DOPAL in Parkinson's disease. *J Neurochem*. 126(5):591-603.

Greeshma N, Prasanth KG, Balaji B. 2015. Tetrahydrocurcumin exerts protective effect on vincristine induced neuropathy: Behavioral, biochemical, neurophysiological and histological evidence. *Chem Biol Interact*. 238:118-128.

Guzman RE, Evans MG, Bove S, Morenko B, Kilgore K. 2003. Mono-iodoacetate-induced histologic changes in subchondral bone and articular cartilage of rat femorotibial joints: an animal model of osteoarthritis. *Toxicol Pathol*. 31(6):619-624.

Haddad JJ, Lauterbach R, Saade NE, Sasieh-Garabedian B, Land SC. 2001. α-Melanocyte-related tripeptide, Lys-D-Pro-Val, ameliorates endotoxin-induced nuclear factor κB translocation and activation: evidence for involvement of an interleukin-1β-193–195 receptor antagonism in the alveolar epithelium. *Biochem J*. 355(1):29-38.

Han JS, Lee S, Kim HY, Lee CH. 2015. MS-based metabolite profiling of aboveground and root components of *Zingiber mioga* and *officinale*. *Molecules*. 20(9):16170-16185.

Han X, Deng S, Wang N, Liu Y, Yang X. 2016. Inhibitory effects and molecular mechanisms of tetrahydrocurcumin against human breast cancer MCF-7 cells. *Food Nutr Res*. 60:30616.

Hassaninasab A, Hashimoto Y, Tomita-Yokotani K, Kobayashi M. 2011. Discovery of the curcumin metabolic pathway involving a unique enzyme in an intestinal microorganism. *Proc Natl Acad Sci USA*. 108(16):6615-6620.

Chapter 3
TETRAHYDROCURCUMIN (THC): THE MAJOR METABOLITE WITH MAJOR BENEFITS

Helson L, Bolger G, Majeed M, Vcelar B, Pucaj K, Matabudul D. 2012. Infusion pharmacokinetics of Lipocurc™ (liposomal curcumin) and its metabolite tetrahydrocurcumin in beagle dogs. *Anticancer Res*. 32(10):4365-4370.

Howard BV, Savage PJ, Bennion LJ, Bennett PH. 1978. Lipoprotein composition in diabetes mellitus. *Atherosclerosis*. 30(2):153-162.

Hung WL, Ho CT, Hwang LS. 2011. Inhibitory activity of natural occurring antioxidants on Thiyl radical-induced trans-arachidonic acid formation. *J Agric Food Chem*. 59(5):1968-1973.

Ireson CR, Jones DJ, Orr S, Coughtrie MW, Boocock DJ, Williams ML *et al*. 2002. Metabolism of the cancer chemopreventive agent curcumin in human and rat intestine. *Cancer Epidemiol Biomarkers Prev*. 11(1):105-111.

Itokawa H, Shi Q, Akiyama T, Morris-Natschke SL, Lee KH. 2008. Recent advances in the investigation of curcuminoids. *Chin Med*. 3:11.

Jager R, Lowery RP, Calvanese AV, Joy JM, Purpura M, Wilson JM. 2014. Comparative absorption of curcumin formulations. *Nutr J*. 13:11.

Jaggi AS, Singh N. 2012. Mechanisms in cancer-chemotherapeutic drugs-induced peripheral neuropathy. *Toxicology*. 291(1-3):1-9.

Jia S, Du Z, Song C, Jin S, Zhang Y, Feng Y, *et al*. 2017. Identification and characterization of curcuminoids in turmeric using ultra-high performance liquid chromatography-quadrupole time of flight tandem mass spectrometry. *J Chromatogr A*. 1521:110-122.

Jin W, Wang HD, Hu ZG, Yan W, Chen G, Yin HX. 2009. Transcription factor Nrf2 plays a pivotal role in protection against traumatic brain injury-induced acute intestinal mucosal injury in mice. *J Surg Res*.157(2): 251-260.

Kabadi SV, Faden AI. 2014. Neuroprotective strategies for traumatic brain injury: improving clinical translation. *Int J Mol Sci*. 15(1):1216-1236.

Kamiya S, Sakai Y, Kawasaki H, Osawa T. 1999. Production of tetrahydrocurcumins. Patent:JP11235192 A.

Kang N, Wang MM, Wang YH, Zhang ZN, Cao HR, Lv YH *et al*. 2014. Tetrahydrocurcumin induces G2/M cell cycle arrest and apoptosis involving p38 MAPK activation in human breast cancer cells. *Food Chem Toxicol*. 67: 193-200.

Kang R, Zeh HJ, Lotze MT, Tang D. 2011. The Beclin 1 network regulates autophagy and apoptosis. *Cell Death Differ*. 18(4):571-580.

Karthikesan K, Pari L, Menon VP. 2010a. Antihyperlipidemic effect of chlorogenic acid and tetrahydrocurcumin in rats subjected to diabetogenic agents. *Chem-Biol Interact*. 188(3):643-650.

Karthikesan K, Pari L, Menon VP. 2010b. Protective effect of tetrahydrocurcumin and chlorogenic acid against streptozotocin–nicotinamide generated oxidative stress induced diabetes. *J Funct Foods*. 2(2):134-142.

Chapter 3
TETRAHYDROCURCUMIN (THC): THE MAJOR METABOLITE WITH MAJOR BENEFITS

Kim JM, Araki S, Kim DJ, Park CB, Takasuka N, Baba-Toriyama H et al. 1998. Chemopreventive effects of carotenoids and curcumins on mouse colon carcinogenesis after 1,2-dimethylhydrazine initiation. *Carcinogenesis*. 19(1):81-85.

Kim T, Davis J, Zhang AJ, He X, Mathews ST. 2009. Curcumin activates AMPK and suppresses gluconeogenic gene expression in hepatoma cells. *Biochem Biophys Res Commun*. 388(2):377-382.

Kim SS, Jang HJ, Oh MY, Lee JH, Kang KS. 2018. Tetrahydrocurcumin enhances islet cell function and attenuates apoptosis in mouse islets. *Transplant Proc*. 50(9):2847-2853.

Kimura S, Fujita N, Noda T, Yoshimori T. 2009. Monitoring autophagy in mammalian cultured cells through the dynamics of LC3. *Methods Enzymol*. 452:1-12.

Kitani K, Osawa T, Yokozawa T. 2007. The effects of tetrahydrocurcumin and green tea polyphenol on the survival of male C57BL/6 mice. *Biogerontology*. 8(5):567-573.

Kumari R, Kumar R, Consortium OSDD, Lynn A. 2014. g-mmpbsa- a GROMACS tool for high-throughput MM-PBSA calculations. *J Chem Inf Model*. 54(7):1951-1962.

Lai CS, Wu JC, Yu SF, Badmaev V, Nagabhushanam K, Ho CT et al. 2011. Tetrahydrocurcumin is more effective than curcumin in preventing azoxymethane-induced colon carcinogenesis. *Mol Nutr Food Res*. 55(12):1819-1828.

Lau WL, Khazaeli M, Savoj J, Manekia K, Bangash M, Thakurta RG et al. 2018. Dietary tetrahydrocurcumin reduces renal fibrosis and cardiac hypertrophy in 5/6 nephrectomized rats. *Pharmacol Res Perspect*. 6(2):e00385.

Lee WM. 2017. Acetaminophen (APAP) hepatotoxicity-Isn't it time for APAP to go away? *J Hepatol*. 67(6):1324-1331.

Lenzen S, Drinkgern J, Tiedge M. 1996. Low antioxidant enzyme gene expression in pancreatic islets compared with various other mouse tissues. *Free Radic Biol Med*. 20(3):463-466.

Levine B, Kroemer G. 2008. Autophagy in the pathogenesis of disease. *Cell*. 132(1):27-42.

Li N, Wang L, Zu L, Wang K, Di L, Wang Z. 2012. Antioxidant and cytotoxic diarylheptanoids isolated from *Zingiber officinale* rhizomes. *Chin J Chem*. 30(6):1351-1355.

Liedtke C, Luedde T, Sauerbruch T, Scholten D, Streetz K, Tacke F et al. 2013. Experimental liver fibrosis research: update on animal models, legal issues and translational aspects. *Fibrogenesis Tissue Repair*. 6(1):19.

Lin B, Yu H, Lin Y, Cai C, Lu H, Zhu X. 2016. Suppression of GRASP65 phosphorylation by tetrahydrocurcumin protects against cerebral ischemia/reperfusion injury via ERK signaling. *Mol Med Rep*. 14(5):4775-4780.

Lin JK, Pan MH, Lin-Shiau SY. 2000. Recent studies on the biofunctions and biotransformations of curcumin. *Biofactors*. 13(1-4):153-158.

Liu A, Lou H, Zhao L, Fan P. 2006. Validated LC/MS/MS assay for curcumin and tetrahydrocurcumin in rat plasma and application to pharmacokinetic study of phospholipid complex of curcumin. *J Pharm Biomed Anal*. 40(3): 720-727.

Chapter 3
TETRAHYDROCURCUMIN (THC): THE MAJOR METABOLITE WITH MAJOR BENEFITS

Liu W, Zhang Z, Lin G, Luo D, Chen H, Yang H *et al*. 2017. Tetrahydrocurcumin is more effective than curcumin in inducing the apoptosis of H22 cells via regulation of a mitochondrial apoptosis pathway in ascites tumor-bearing mice. *Food Funct*. 8(9):3120-3129.

Lockshin RA, Zakeri Z. 2004. Apoptosis, autophagy, and more. *Int J Biochem Cell Biol*. 36(12):2405-2419.

Luo DD, Chen JF, Liu JJ, Xie JH, Zhang ZB, Gu JY *et al*. 2019. Tetrahydrocurcumin and octahydrocurcumin, the primary and final hydrogenated metabolites of curcumin, possess superior hepatic-protective effect against acetaminophen-induced liver injury: Role of CYP2E1 and Keap1-Nrf2 pathway. *Food Chem Toxicol*. 123:349-362.

Maehara S, Ikeda M, Haraguchi H, Kitamura C, Nagoe T, Ohashi K *et al*. 2011. Microbial conversion of curcumin into colorless hydroderivatives by the endophytic fungus *Diaporthe sp*. associated with *Curcuma longa*. *Chem Pharm Bull (Tokyo)*. 59(8):1042-1044.

Maheshwari RK, Singh AK, Gaddipati J, Srimal RC. 2006. Multiple biological activities of curcumin: a short review. *Life Sci*. 78(18):2081-2087.

Majeed M. 2007. Use of tetrahydrocurcuminoids to regulate physiological and pathological events in the skin and mucosa. Patent:EP1171144B1.

Majeed M, Badmaev V, Shivakumar U, Rajendran R. 1995. Curcuminoids: antioxidant phytonutrients. Sabinsa Coorporation, NJ, USA.

Majeed M, Natarajan S, Pandey A, Bani S, Mundkur L. 2019. Subchronic and reproductive/developmental toxicity of tetrahydrocurcumin in rats. *Toxicol. Res*. 35 (1): 65-74.

Mandel SA, Sagi Y, Amit T. 2007. Rasagiline promotes regeneration of substantia nigra dopaminergic neurons in post-MPTP-induced Parkinsonism via activation of tyrosine kinase receptor signaling pathway. *Neurochem Res*. 32(10):1694-1699.

Matabudul D, Pucaj K, Bolger G, Vcelar B, Majeed M, Helson L. 2012. Tissue distribution of (Lipocurc™) liposomal curcumin and tetrahydrocurcumin following two-and eight-hour infusions in beagle dogs. *Anticancer Res*. 32(10):4359-4364.

Matsuda H, Tewtrakul S, Morikawa T, Nakamura A, Yoshikawa M. 2004. Anti-allergic principles from Thai zedoary: structural requirements of curcuminoids for inhibition of degranulation and effect on the release of TNF-alpha and IL-4 in RBL-2H3 cells. *Bioorg Med Chem*. 12(22):5891-5898.

Mimura, A, Takahara, Y, Osawa, T, 1993. Method for making tetrahydrocurcumin and a substance containing the antioxidative substance tetrahydrocurcumin. Patent:US 5266344.

Mirani A, Kundaikar H, Velhal S, Patel V, Bandivdekar A, Degani M, Patravale V. 2019. Tetrahydrocurcumin-loaded vaginal nanomicrobicide for prophylaxis of HIV/AIDS: in silico study, formulation development, and *in vitro* evaluation. *Drug Deliv Transl Res*. 2019 Mar 21. doi: 10.1007/s13346-019-00633-2.

Mishra S, Mishra M, Seth P, Sharma SK. 2011. Tetrahydrocurcumin confers protection against amyloid beta-induced toxicity. *Neuroreport*. 22(1):23-27.

Chapter 3
TETRAHYDROCURCUMIN (THC): THE MAJOR METABOLITE WITH MAJOR BENEFITS

Morales NP, Sirijaroonwong S, Yamanont P, Phisalaphong C. 2015. Electron paramagnetic resonance study of the free radical scavenging capacity of curcumin and its demethoxy and hydrogenated derivatives. *Biol Pharm Bull*. 38(10):1478-1483.

Mukhopadhyay A, Basu N, Ghatak N, Gujral PK. 1982. Anti-inflammatory and irritant activities of curcumin analogues in rats. *Agents Actions*. 12(4):508-515.

Murugan P, Pari L. 2005. Effect of tetrahydrocurcumin on erythromycin estolate-induced lipid peroxidation in rats. *J Basic Clin Physiol Pharmacol*. 16(1):1-15.

Murugan P, Pari L. 2006. Antioxidant effect of tetrahydrocurcumin in streptozotocin–nicotinamide induced diabetic rats. *Life Sci*. 79(18):1720-1728.

Murugan P, Pari L. 2007a. Influence of tetrahydrocurcumin on hepatic and renal functional markers and protein levels in experimental type 2 diabetic rats. *Basic Clin Pharmacol Toxicol*. 101(4):241-245.

Murugan P, Pari L. 2007b. Influence of tetrahydrocurcumin on erythrocyte membrane bound enzymes and antioxidant status in experimental type 2 diabetic rats. *J Ethnopharmacol*. 113(3):479-486.

Murugan P, Pari L. 2007c. Protective role of tetrahydrocurcumin on changes in the fatty acid composition in streptozotocin-nicotinamide induced type 2 diabetic rats. *J Appl Biomed*. 5:31-38.

Murugan P, Pari L, Rao CA. 2008. Effect of tetrahydrocurcumin on insulin receptor status in type 2 diabetic rats: studies on insulin binding to erythrocytes. *J Biosci*. 33(1):63-72.

Muthumani M, Miltonprabu S. 2015. Ameliorative efficacy of tetrahydrocurcumin against arsenic induced oxidative damage, dyslipidemia and hepatic mitochondrial toxicity in rats. *Chem Biol Interact*. 235:95-105.

Naito M, Wu X, Nomura H, Kodama M, Kato Y, Kato Y et al. 2002. The protective effects of tetrahydrocurcumin on oxidative stress in cholesterol-fed rabbits. *J Atheroscler Thromb*. 9(5):243-250.

Nakmareong S, Kukongviriyapan U, Pakdeechote P, Donpunha W, Kukongviriyapan V, Kongyingyoes B et al. 2011. Antioxidant and vascular protective effects of curcumin and tetrahydrocurcumin in rats with L-NAME-induced hypertension. *Naunyn Schmiedebergs Arch Pharmacol*. 383(5):519-529.

Nakmareong S, Kukongviriyapan U, Pakdeechote P, Kukongviriyapan V, Kongyingyoes B, Donpunha W et al. 2012. Tetrahydrocurcumin alleviates hypertension, aortic stiffening and oxidative stress in rats with nitric oxide deficiency. *Hypertens Res*. 35(4):418-425.

Neyrinck AM, Alligier M, Memvanga PB, Nevraumont E, Larondelle Y, Preat V et al. 2013. *Curcuma longa* extract associated with white pepper lessens high fat diet-induced inflammation in subcutaneous adipose tissue. *PLoS One*. 8(11):e81252.

Nikkila EA, Kekki M. 1973. Plasma triglyceride transport kinetics in diabetes mellitus. *Metabolism*. 22(1):1-22.

Novaes JT, Lillico R, Sayre CL, Nagabushnam K, Majeed M, Chen Y et al. 2017. Disposition, metabolism and histone deacetylase and acetyltransferase inhibition activity of tetrahydrocurcumin and other curcuminoids. *Pharmaceutics*. 9(4):45.

Chapter 3
TETRAHYDROCURCUMIN (THC): THE MAJOR METABOLITE WITH MAJOR BENEFITS

Okada K, Wangpoengtrakul C, Tanaka T, Toyokuni S, Uchida K, Osawa T. 2001. Curcumin and especially tetrahydrocurcumin ameliorate oxidative stress-induced renal injury in mice. *J Nutr*. 131(8):2090-2095.

Osawa T, Sugiyama Y, Inayoshi M, Kawakishi S. 1995. Antioxidative activity of tetrahydrocurcuminoids. *Biosci Biotechnol Biochem*. 59(9):1609-1612.

Paglin S, Hollister T, Delohery T, Hackett N, McMahill M, Sphicas E *et al*. 2001. A novel response of cancer cells to radiation involves autophagy and formation of acidic vesicles. *Cancer Res*. 61(2):439-444.

Pan MH, Chen JW, Kong ZL, Wu JC, Ho CT, Lai CS. 2018. Tetrahydrocurcumin attenuates adiposity and hepatic steatosis in high-fat diet induced obese mice. *J Agric Food Chem*. 66 (48): 12685–12695.

Pandit S, Kim HJ, Kim JE, Jeon JG. 2011. Separation of an effective fraction from turmeric against *Streptococcus mutans* biofilms by the comparison of curcuminoid content and anti-acidogenic activity. *Food Chem*. 126(4):1565-1570.

Pari L, Amali DR. 2005. Protective role of tetrahydrocurcumin (THC) an active principle of turmeric on chloroquine induced hepatotoxicity in rats. *J Pharm Pharm Sci*. 8(1):115-123.

Pari L, Karthikesan K. 2009. Protective role of tetrahydrocurcumin and chlorogenic acid on glycoprotein changes in streptozotocin-nicotinamide-induced diabetic rats. *J Pharm Sci & Res*. 1(4):173-180

Pari L, Karthikesan K, Menon VP. 2010. Comparative and combined effect of chlorogenic acid and tetrahydrocurcumin on antioxidant disparities in chemical induced experimental diabetes. *Mol Cell Biochem*. 341(1-2):109-117.

Pari L, Murugan P. 2004. Protective role of tetrahydrocurcumin against erythromycin estolate-induced hepatotoxicity. *Pharmacol Res*. 49(5):481-486.

Pari L, Murugan P. 2005. Effect of tetrahydrocurcumin on blood glucose, plasma insulin and hepatic key enzymes in streptozotocin induced diabetic rats. *J Basic Clin Physiol Pharmacol*. 16(4):257-274.

Pari L, Murugan P. 2006. Tetrahydrocurcumin: effect on chloroquine-mediated oxidative damage in rat kidney. *Basic Clin Pharmacol Toxicol*. 99(5):329-334.

Pari L, Murugan P. 2007a. Antihyperlipidemic effect of curcumin and tetrahydrocurcumin in experimental type 2 diabetic rats. *Ren Fail*. 29(7):881-889.

Pari L, Murugan P. 2007b. Influence of tetrahydrocurcumin on tail tendon collagen contents and its properties in rats with streptozotocin-nicotinamide-induced type 2 diabetes. *Fundam Clin Pharmacol*. 21(6):665-671.

Pari L, Murugan P. 2007c. Tetrahydrocurcumin prevents brain lipid peroxidation in streptozotocin-induced diabetic rats. *J Med Food*. 10(2):323-329.

Pari L, Murugan P. 2007d. Changes in glycoprotein components in streptozotocin--nicotinamide induced type 2 diabetes: influence of tetrahydrocurcumin from *Curcuma longa*. *Plant Foods Hum Nutr*. 62(1):25-29.

Chapter 3
TETRAHYDROCURCUMIN (THC): THE MAJOR METABOLITE WITH MAJOR BENEFITS

Park S, Lee LR, Seo JH, Kang S. 2016. Curcumin and tetrahydrocurcumin both prevent osteoarthritis symptoms and decrease the expressions of pro-inflammatory cytokines in estrogen-deficient rats. *Genes Nutr*. 11(1):2.

Park CS, Jang HJ, Lee JH, Oh MY, Kim HJ. 2018. Tetrahydrocurcumin ameliorates Tacrolimus-induced nephrotoxicity via inhibiting apoptosis. *Transplant Proc*. 50(9):2854-2859.

Peng W, Zhang Y, Yang K, Xiao Y. 2007. Chemical constituents of *Zingiber officinale* (Zingiberaceae). *Yunnan Zhiwu Yanjiu*. 29(1):125-128

Pihlstrom BL, Michalowicz BS, Johnson NW. 2005. Periodontal diseases. *Lancet*. 366(9499):1809-1820.

Plyduang T, Lomlim L, Yuenyongsawad S, Wiwattanapatapee R. 2014. Carboxymethylcellulose–tetrahydrocurcumin conjugates for colon-specific delivery of a novel anti-cancer agent, 4-amino tetrahydrocurcumin. *Eur J Pharm Biopharm*. 88(2):351-360.

Portes E, Gardrat C, Castellan A. 2007. A comparative study on the antioxidant properties of tetrahydrocurcuminoids and curcuminoids. *Tetrahedron*. 63(37):9092-9099.

Prabhu RP, Hegde K, Shabaraya AR, Rao MNA. 2011. Scavenging potential of reactive oxygen species by tetrahydrocurcumin. *J Appl Pharm Sci*. 1(5):114-118.

Prentki M, Nolan CJ. 2006. Islet beta cell failure in type 2 diabetes. *J Clin Invest*.116(7):1802-1812.

Qiu X, Wong G, Audet J, Bello A, Fernando L, Alimonti JB *et al*. 2014. Reversion of advanced Ebola virus disease in nonhuman primates with ZMapp™. *Nature*. 514(7520):47-53.

Rajeswari A, Sabesan M. 2008. Inhibition of monoamine oxidase-B by the polyphenolic compound, curcumin and its metabolite tetrahydrocurcumin, in a model of Parkinson's disease induced by MPTP neurodegeneration in mice. *Inflammopharmacology*. 16(2):96-99.

Ramakrishnan R, Elangovan P, Pari L. 2017. Protective role of tetrahydrocurcumin: an active polyphenolic curcuminoid on cadmium-induced oxidative damage in rats. *Appl Biochem Biotechnol*. 183(1):51-69.

Randino R, Grimaldi M, Persico M, De Santis A, Cini E, Cabri W *et al*. 2016. Investigating the neuroprotective effects of turmeric extract: structural interactions of beta-amyloid peptide with single curcuminoids. *Sci Rep*. 6: 38846.

Ricchi P, Ammirabile M, Spasiano A, Costantini S, Cinque P, Di Matola T *et al*. 2010. Combined chelation therapy in thalassemia major with deferiprone and desferrioxamine: a retrospective study. *Eur J Haematol*. 85(1):36-42.

Robertson RP. 2004. Chronic oxidative stress as a central mechanism for glucose toxicity in pancreatic islet beta cells in diabetes. *J Biol Chem*. 279(41):42351-42354

Sajid R, Ghani, F, Adil, S, Khurshid, M. 2009. Oral iron chelation therapy with deferiprone in patients with Thalassemia Major. *J Pak Med Assoc*. 59(6):388-390.

Sakai Y, Kamiya S. 2003. Method for producing tetrahydrocurcumins. Patent:JP-2003033195-A.

Chapter 3
TETRAHYDROCURCUMIN (THC): THE MAJOR METABOLITE WITH MAJOR BENEFITS

Sales KJ, Katz AA, Davis M, Hinz S, Soeters RP, Hofmeyr MD *et al*. 2001. Cyclooxygenase-2 expression and prostaglandin E2 synthesis are up-regulated in carcinomas of the cervix: a possible autocrine/paracrine regulation of neoplastic cell function via EP2/EP4 receptors. *J Clin Endocrinol Metab*. 86(5):2243-2249.

Samaha HS, Kelloff GJ, Steele V, Rao CV, Reddy BS. 1997. Modulation of apoptosis by sulindac, curcumin, phenylethyl-3-methylcaffeate, and 6-phenylhexyl isothiocyanate: apoptotic index as a biomarker in colon cancer chemoprevention and promotion. *Cancer Res*. 57(7):1301-1305.

Sami Labs Limited. 2003. Indian Institue of Toxicology. The acute oral toxicity (LD50) to the Sprague Dawley rat. Report No. 9340.

Sami Labs Limited. 2009. Compilation report of bioassay of tetrahydrocurcuminoids CG. Report No. 09 222.

Sami Labs Limited. 2010a. Indian Institue of Toxicology. *Salmonella typhimurium* reverse mutation assay with C31962 (Tetrahydrocurcuminoids CG) of Sami Labs Limited., Bangalore. Report No. 10535.

Sami Labs Limited. 2010b. Department of Pharmacy Practive. Al-Ameen College of Pharmacy. Repeated insult patch test on human subjects with RIPT/THC-CG/ C1152 of Sami Labs LTD., Bangalore. Report No. AACP/PP/162.

Sami Labs Limited. 2015. Acute oral toxicity study of tetrahydrocurcuminoids in wistar rats. Report No. VIP1134.

Sami Labs Limited. 2017. A Prospective, open label, two arm clinical study to evaluate the efficacy and safety of C3 Reduct® ODN in the treatment of canker sore and gingivitis.

Sami Labs Limited/ClinWorld Ltd. 2010. A 28-days safety assessment of THC extract. Protocol No. CPL/23/THC/DEC/10.

San Miguel SM, Opperman LA, Allen EP, Zielinski J, Svoboda KK. 2011. Bioactive antioxidant mixtures promote proliferation and migration on human oral fibroblasts. *Arch Oral Biol*. 56(8):812-822.

San Miguel SM, Opperman LA, Allen EP, Zielinski J, Svoboda KK. 2012. Bioactive polyphenol antioxidants protect oral fibroblasts from ROS-inducing agents. *Arch Oral Biol*. 57(12):1657-1667.

San Miguel SM, Opperman LA, Allen EP, Zielinski JE, Svoboda KK. 2013. Antioxidant combinations protect oral fibroblasts against metal-induced toxicity. *Arch Oral Biol*. 58(3):299-310.

Sangartit W, Kukongviriyapan U, Donpunha W, Pakdeechote P, Kukongviriyapan V, Surawattanawan P *et al*. 2014. Tetrahydrocurcumin protects against cadmium-induced hypertension, raised arterial stiffness and vascular remodeling in mice. *PLoS One*. 9(12):e114908.

Sangartit W, Pakdeechote P, Kukongviriyapan V, Donpunha W, Shibahara S, Kukongviriyapan U. 2016. Tetrahydrocurcumin in combination with deferiprone attenuates hypertension, vascular dysfunction, baroreflex dysfunction, and oxidative stress in iron-overloaded mice. *Vascul Pharmacol*. 87:199-208.

Schieffelin JS, Shaffer JG, Goba A, Gbakie M, Gire SK, Colubri A *et al*. 2014. Clinical illness and outcomes in patients with Ebola in Sierra Leone. *N Engl J Med*. 371(22):2092-2100.

Sculley DV, Langley-Evans SC. 2003. Periodontal disease is associated with lower antioxidant capacity in whole saliva and evidence of increased protein oxidation. *Clin Sci(Lond)*. 105(2):167-172.

Scully C, Porter S. 2008. Oral mucosal disease: recurrent aphthous stomatitis. *Br J Oral Maxillofac Surg*. 46(3):198-206.

Sermkaew N, Wiwattanawongsa K, Ketjinda W, Wiwattanapatapee R. 2013. Development, characterization and permeability assessment based on Caco-2 monolayers of self-microemulsifying floating tablets of tetrahydrocurcumin. *AAPS PharmSciTech*. 14(1):321-331.

Sharma K, Sahai M. 2018. Chemical constituents of *Zingiber officinale* rhizome. *J Med Plants Stud*. 6(1):146-149.

Sharma RA, Gescher AJ, Steward WP. 2005. Curcumin: the story so far. *Eur J Cancer*. 41(13):1955-1968.

Shimoda K, Kubota N, Hirano H, Matsumoto M, Hamada H, Hamada H. 2012. Formation of tetrahydrocurcumin by reduction of curcumin with cultured plant cells of *Marchantia polymorpha*. *Nat Prod Commun*. 7(4):529-530.

Somparn P, Phisalaphong C, Nakornchai S, Unchern S, Morales NP. 2007. Comparative antioxidant activities of curcumin and its demethoxy and hydrogenated derivatives. *Biol Pharm Bull*. 30(1):74-78.

Song G, Lu H, Chen F, Wang Y, Fan W, Shao W *et al*. 2018. Tetrahydrocurcumin induced autophagy via suppression of PI3K/Akt/mTOR in non small cell lung carcinoma cells. *Mol Med Rep*. 17(4):5964-5969.

Song KI, Park JY, Lee S, Lee D, Jang HJ, Kim SN *et al*. 2015. Protective effect of tetrahydrocurcumin against cisplatin-induced renal damage: *in vitro* and *in vivo* studies. *Planta Med* 81(4):286-291.

Stebbing J, Filipovic A, Lit LC, Blighe K, Grothey A, Xu Y *et al*. 2013. LMTK3 is implicated in endocrine resistance via multiple signaling pathways. *Oncogene*. 32(28):3371-3380.

Storka A, Vcelar B, Klickovic U, Gouya G, Weisshaar S, Aschauer S *et al*. 2015. Safety, tolerability and pharmacokinetics of liposomal curcumin (Lipocurc™) in healthy humans. *Int J Clin Pharmacol Therapeut*. 53(1): 54-65.

Sugiyama Y, Kawakishi S, Osawa T. 1996. Involvement of the beta-diketone moiety in the antioxidative mechanism of tetrahydrocurcumin. *Biochem Pharmacol*. 52(4):519-525.

Sui Z, Salto R, Li J, Craik C, Ortiz de Montellano PR. 1993. Inhibition of the HIV-1 and HIV-2 proteases by curcumin and curcumin boron complexes. *Bioorg Med Chem*. 1(6):415-422.

Surwase VS, Laddha KS, Kale RV, Hashmi SI, Lokhande SM. 2011. Extraction and isolation of turmerone from turmeric. *EJEAFChe*. 10(5):2173-2179.

Suzuki M, Nakamura T, Iyoki S, Fujiwara A, Watanabe Y, Mohri K *et al*. 2005. Elucidation of anti-allergic activities of curcumin-related compounds with a special reference to their anti-oxidative activities. *Biol Pharm Bull*. 28(8):1438-1443.

Tan A, Wu Y, Wong M, Licollari A, Bolger G, Fanaras JC *et al*. 2016. Use of basic mobile phase to improve chromatography and boost sensitivity for quantifying tetrahydrocurcumin in human plasma by LC–MS/MS.

J Chromatogr B Analyt Technol Biomed Life Sci. 1028:86-93.

Tan S, Calani L, Bresciani L, Dall'asta M, Faccini A, Augustin MA *et al*. 2015. The degradation of curcuminoids in a human faecal fermentation model. *Int J Food Sci Nutr*. 66(7):790-796.

Tan S, Rupasinghe TW, Tull DL, Boughton B, Oliver C, McSweeny C *et al*. 2014. Degradation of curcuminoids by *in vitro* pure culture fermentation. *J Agric Food Chem*. 62(45):11005-11015.

Trivedi MK, Gangwar M, Mondal SC, Jana S. 2017. Protective effects of tetrahydrocurcumin (THC) on fibroblast and melanoma cell lines *in vitro*: it's implication for wound healing. *J Food Sci Technol*. 54(5):1137-1145.

Tsai ML, Tsai SP, Ho CT. 2017. Tetrahydrocurcumin attenuates carbon tetrachloride-induced hepatic fibrogenesis by inhibiting the activation and autophagy of hepatic stellate cells. *J Funct Foods*. 36:418-428.

Tyagi N, Moshal KS, Ovechkin AV, Rodriguez W, Steed M, Henderson B *et al*. 2005. Mitochondrial mechanism of oxidative stress and systemic hypertension in hyperhomocysteinemia. *J Cell Biochem*. 96(4):665-671.

Tyagi N, Ovechkin AV, Lominadze D, Moshal KS, Tyagi SC. 2006. Mitochondrial mechanism of microvascular endothelial cells apoptosis in hyperhomocysteinemia. *J Cell Biochem*. 98(5):1150-1162.

Tyagi N, Qipshidze N, Munjal C, Vacek JC, Metreveli N, Givvimani S *et al*. 2012. Tetrahydrocurcumin ameliorates homocysteinylated cytochrome-c mediated autophagy in hyperhomocysteinemia mice after cerebral ischemia. *J Mol Neurosci*. 47(1):128-138.

Vacek JC, Behera J, George AK, Kamat PK, Kalani A, Tyagi N. 2018. Tetrahydrocurcumin ameliorates homocysteine-mediated mitochondrial remodeling in brain endothelial cells. *J Cell Physiol*. 233(4):3080-3092.

Vogel H, Pelletier J. 1815. Examen chimique de la racine de curmuma. *J de Pharmacie*. I: 289-300.

Wang F, Nguyen M, Qin FX, Tong Q. 2007. SIRT2 deacetylates FOXO3a in response to oxidative stress and caloric restriction. *Aging Cell*. 6(4):505-514.

Wang J, Yu X, Zhang L, Wang L, Peng Z, Chen Y. 2018. The pharmacokinetics and tissue distribution of curcumin and its metabolites in mice. *Biomed Chromatogr*. e4267.

Wang Y, Qin ZH. 2013. Coordination of autophagy with other cellular activities. *Acta Pharmacol Sin*. 34(5):585-594.

Weber WM, Hunsaker LA, Abcouwer SF, Deck LM, Vander Jagt DL. 2005. Anti-oxidant activities of curcumin and related enones. *Bioorg Med Chem*. 13(11):3811-3820.

Wei G, Chen B, Lin Q, Li Y, Luo L, He H *et al*. 2017. Tetrahydrocurcumin provides neuroprotection in experimental traumatic brain injury and the Nrf2 signaling pathway as a potential mechanism. *Neuroimmunomodulation*. 24(6):348-355.

West IC. 2000. Radicals and oxidative stress in diabetes. *Diabet Med*. 17(3):171-180.

Wongeakin N, Sridulyakul P, Jariyapongskul A, Suksamrarn A, Patumraj S. 2009. Effects of curcumin and tetrahydrocurcumin on diabetes induced endothelial dysfunction. *Afr J Biochem Res*. 3(5):259-265.

Wright LE, Frye JB, Gorti, B, Timmermann BN, Funk JL. 2013. Bioactivity of turmeric-derived curcuminoids and related metabolites in breast cancer. *Curr Pharm Des*. 19(34):6218-6225.

Wu JC, Tsai ML, Lai CS, Wang YJ, Ho CT, Pan MH. 2014. Chemopreventative effects of tetrahydrocurcumin on human diseases. *Food Funct*. 5(1):12-17.

Wu JC, Lai CS, Badmaev V, Nagabhushanam K, Ho CT, Pan MH. 2011. Tetrahydrocurcumin, a major metabolite of curcumin, induced autophagic cell death through coordinative modulation of PI3K/Akt-mTOR and MAPK signaling pathways in human leukemia HL-60 cells. *Mol Nutr Food Res*. 55(11):1646-1654.

Xiang L, Nakamura Y, Lim YM, Yamasaki Y, Kurokawa-Nose Y, Maruyama W *et al*. 2011. Tetrahydrocurcumin extends life span and inhibits the oxidative stress response by regulating the FOXO forkhead transcription factor. *Aging (Albany NY)*. 3(11):1098-1109.

Xu S, Touyz RM. 2006. Reactive oxygen species and vascular remodelling in hypertension: still alive. *Can J Cardiol*. 22(11):947-951.

Yodkeeree S, Garbisa S, Limtrakul P. 2008. Tetrahydrocurcumin inhibits HT1080 cell migration and invasion via downregulation of MMPs and uPA. *Acta Pharmacol Sin*. 29(7):853-860.

Yoysungnoen P, Wirachwong P, Changtam C, Suksamrarn A, Patumraj S. 2008. Anti-cancer and anti-angiogenic effects of curcumin and tetrahydrocurcumin on implanted hepatocellular carcinoma in nude mice. *World J Gastroenterol*. 14(13):2003-2009.

Yoysungnoen BB, Bhattarakosol P, Patumraj S, Changtam C. 2015. Effects of tetrahydrocurcumin on hypoxia-inducible factor-1α and vascular endothelial growth factor expression in cervical cancer cell-induced angiogenesis in nude mice. *Biomed Res Int*. 391748.

Yoysungnoen B, Bhattarakosol P, Changtam C, Patumraj S. 2016. Effects of tetrahydrocurcumin on tumor growth and cellular signaling in cervical cancer xenografts in nude mice. *Biomed Res Int*. 2016:1781208.

Zhang J, Ney PA. 2009. Role of BNIP3 and NIX in cell death, autophagy, and mitophagy. *Cell Death Differ*. 16(7):939-946.

Zhang ZB, Luo, DD, Xie JH, Xian YF, Lai ZQ, Liu YH et al. 2018a. Curcumin's metabolites, tetrahydrocurcumin and octahydrocurcumin, possess superior anti-inflammatory effects *in vivo* through suppression of TAK1-NF-κB pathway. *Front Pharmacol*. 9: 1181.

Zhang X, Peng L, Liu A, Ji J, Zhao L, Zhai G. 2018b. The enhanced effect of tetrahydrocurcumin on radiosensitivity of glioma cells. *J Pharm Pharmacol*. 70(6):749-759.

Zhang Y, Kompa AR. 2014. A practical guide to subtotal nephrectomy in the rat with subsequent methodology for assessing renal and cardiac function. *Nephrology (Carlton)*. 19(9):552-561.

Zhang Y, Liu Y, Zou J, Yan L, Du W, Zhang Y *et al*. 2017. Tetrahydrocurcumin induces mesenchymal-epithelial transition and suppresses angiogenesis by targeting HIF-1α and autophagy in human osteosarcoma. *Oncotarget*. 8(53):91134-91149.

Chapter 3
TETRAHYDROCURCUMIN (THC): THE MAJOR METABOLITE WITH MAJOR BENEFITS

Zhao F, Gong Y, Hu Y, Lu M, Wang J, Dong J *et al*. 2015. Curcumin and its major metabolites inhibit the inflammatory response induced by lipopolysaccharide: Translocation of nuclear factor-κB as potential target. *Mol Med Rep*. 11(4):3087-3093.

Zhongfa L, Chiu M, Wang J, Chen W, Yen W, Fan-Havard P *et al*. 2012. Enhancement of curcumin oral absorption and pharmacokinetics of curcuminoids and curcumin metabolites in mice. *Cancer Chemother Pharmacol*. 69(3): 679-689.

Zi D, Zhou ZW, Yang YJ, Huang L, Zhou ZL, He SM, *et al*. 2015. Danusertib induces apoptosis, cell cycle arrest, and autophagy but inhibits epithelial to mesenchymal transition involving pi3k/akt/mtor signaling pathway in human ovarian cancer cells. *Int J Mol Sci*. 16(11):27228-27251.

Chapter 4
Hexahydrocurcumin (HHC)
The Unsung Metabolite of Curcumin

Scope of this Review

This review concentrates on all aspects of HHC including its chemical synthesis, its occurrence in plant kingdom, biosynthesis, biotransformative synthesis by microbes, as a human metabolite, as a product of gut-bacteria metabolism and finally its various pharmacological effects as gleaned through several *in vitro* and *in vivo* studies.

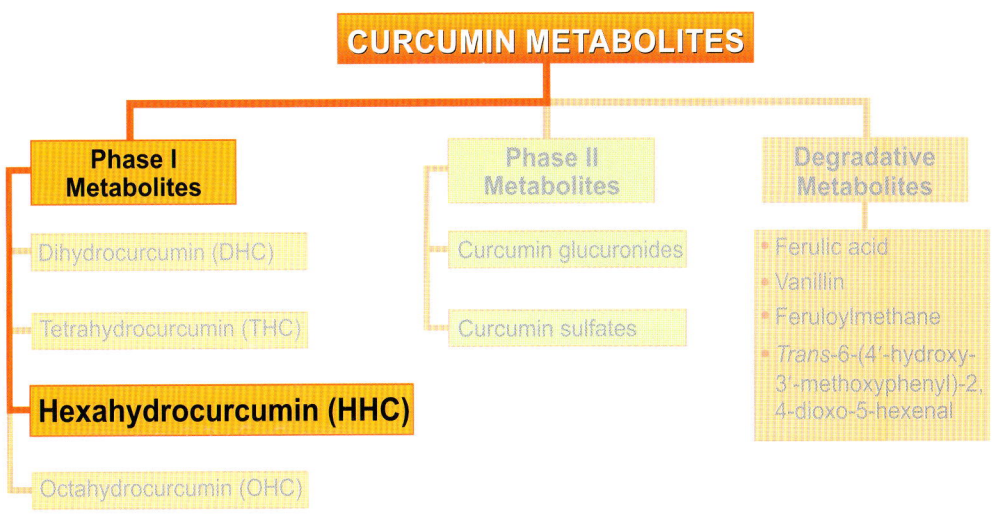

Chapter 4
HEXAHYDROCURCUMIN (HHC): THE UNSUNG METABOLITE OF CURCUMIN

Chapter 4
HEXAHYDROCURCUMIN (HHC): THE UNSUNG METABOLITE OF CURCUMIN

Introduction

The rhizomes of dietary spice turmeric (*C. longa* L.) belong to Zingiberaceae family, are rich in polyphenolic compounds known as curcuminoids, more specifically diarylheptanoids (C6-C7-C6) have been used in traditional medicine and as food additives, especially as a curry spice, preservative, coloring, and flavoring agent in Asian countries such as China and India (Sharma *et al.*, 2005; Shoba *et al.*, 1998). Turmeric contains 2–9% curcuminoids, comprising of curcumin, DMC and BDMC. Despite its perceived poor bioavailability, curcumin has been shown to have potential health benefits that are related to anti-inflammatory (Begum *et al.*, 2008), antioxidant (Aggarwal *et al.*, 2007; Joe *et al.*, 2004) and anticancer (Ireson *et al.*, 2001 & 2002) properties.

Recently, it has been demonstrated that there are other compounds in turmeric that may have pharmacological activities (Aggarwal *et al.*, 2013; Gupta *et al.*, 2013). It is well documented over the years that the phase I metabolism of curcumin **(1)** comprises the reduction of the four double bonds of the heptadiene-3,5-dione structure, such as DHC **(6)**, THC **(7)**, HHC **(8)**, and OHC **(9)** (Fig. 116). Hexahydrocurcumin (HHC) or 5-hydroxy-1,7-bis(4'-hydroxy-3'-methoxyphenyl)-3-heptanone (Fig. 116) is one of the active compounds derived metabolically from its parent compound, curcumin (Dempe *et al.*, 2013; Hoehle *et al.*, 2006; Kuo *et al.*, 2017).

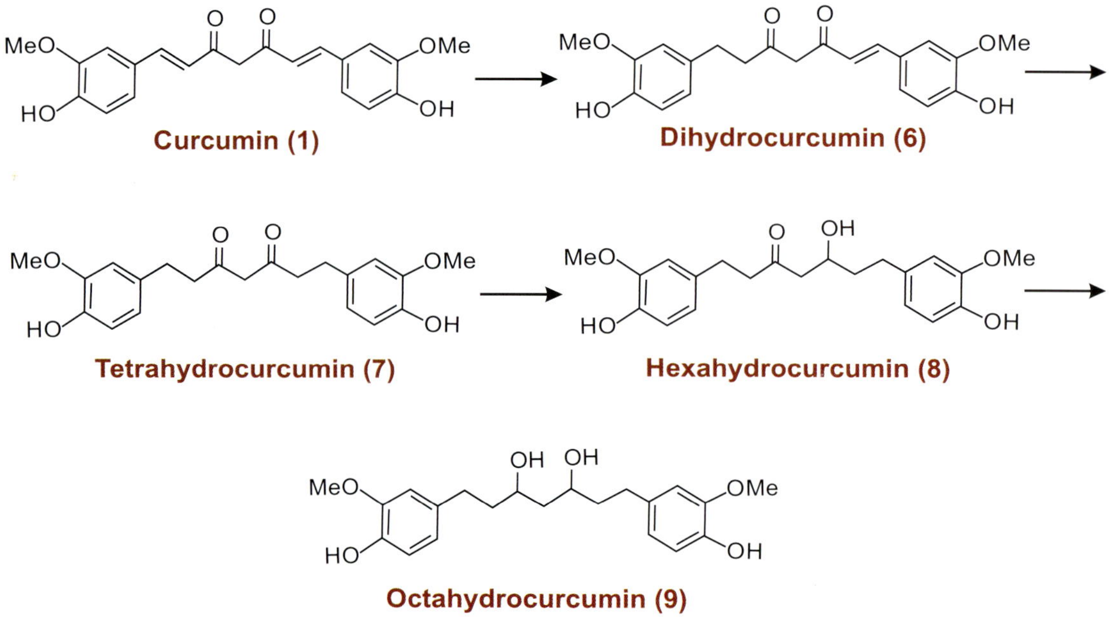

Chapter 4
HEXAHYDROCURCUMIN (HHC): THE UNSUNG METABOLITE OF CURCUMIN

Fig. 116: Reductive metabolites of curcumin in rat liver.
(Adapted from Hoehle *et al.*, 2006)

Studies conducted with precision-cut liver slices from male and female Sprague-Dawley rats showed that THC and HHC are the major reductive metabolites of curcumin observed in most studies, whereas DHC and OHC usually represent minor metabolites or sometimes not detected at all.

Natural Occurrence and Biosynthesis

Hexahydrocurcumin is a naturally occurring compound mainly distributed in the roots and rhizomes of the rhizomatous herbaceous perennial plant genera *Curcuma, Zingiber*, and *Alpinia* of the family Zingiberaceae (Ireson *et al.*, 2001; Lv and She, 2010 & 2012). Isolation of HHC provides an interesting biogenetic linkage between turmeric and ginger, the rhizomes of *Zingiber officinale* Roscoe. Earlier studies on the composition of the non-volatile components or the pungent constituents of ginger have shown the presence of HHC (Connell and McLachlan, 1972; Connell and Sutherland, 1969; Harvey, 1981a & 1981b; Masada *et al.*, 1974; Murata *et al.*, 1972). Kikuzaki *et al.* (1991) isolated HHC from the rhizomes of ginger. Peng *et al.* (2012) isolated HHC from the rhizomes of fresh ginger. Recently, Lin *et al.* (2010) employed n-hexane/chloroform extraction protocol to obtain HHC (0.001%) from the rhizomes of ginger and confirmed by comparison with literature values. All the above reports clearly support the presence of HHC in natural plants of dietary importance.

Interestingly, HHC occurs naturally in either of the two enantiomeric forms and also as a racemic mixture. In *Z. officinale*, it occurs in the "*S*" form (Chen *et al.*, 2009; Kikuzaki *et al.*, 1991) whereas "*R*" form occurs in *Alpinia officinarum* (Itokawa *et al.*, 1985) (Fig. 117). However, HHC is reported to occur as a racemic form in another edible *Curcuma* species, namely *Curcuma xanthorriza* (Uehara *et al.*, 1987). Thus, all stereoisomeric forms of HHC (**8A** & **8B**) seem to occur naturally in the plant kingdom.

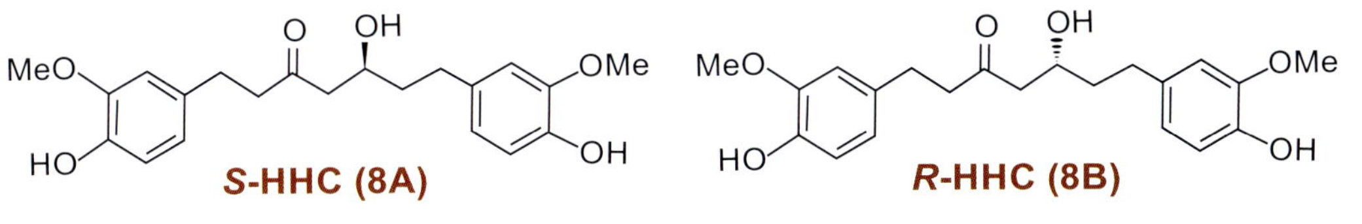

Fig. 117: HHC occurs naturally in either of the two enantiomeric forms, *S*-HHC (**8A**) and *R*-HHC (**8B**). (Adapted from Chen *et al.*, 2009; Itokawa *et al.*, 1985; Kikuzaki *et al.*, 1991)

Chapter 4
HEXAHYDROCURCUMIN (HHC): THE UNSUNG METABOLITE OF CURCUMIN

The "*S*" form was reported to have positive specific rotation, $[\alpha]_D$ value of $+9^0$ in chloroform solvent, whereas "*R*" form isolated from *Alpinia* had a rotation of -10^0. It was further observed that the signs of the cotton effect in the n-π* transition near 300 nm were further supportive of these assignments of configurations. It may be noted that assignment of "*S*" configuration of HHC in *Zingiber* species is further in line with the "*S*" configuration reported for gingerols (Connell and McLachlan, 1972; Murata *et al.*, 1972; Raghuveer and Govindarajan, 1979).

The stereochemical course of metabolic reduction of curcumin to HHC in any animal species has never been reported. However, it has been shown (Li *et al.*, 2012) that the curcumin (**1**), through a series of metabolic steps in rats, gives rise to both forms (**23** & **24**) as racemic mixture (Fig. 118). Hence it is presumed that in mammalian systems HHC metabolite might be scalemic/racemic in nature since non-discriminatory reductive enzyme systems or enzymes of opposite enantio-specificities would appear to be present.

Recently, Jia *et al.* (2017) employed a three-step strategy to identify curcuminoids in turmeric samples: a) the combination of various skeletons and aryl groups, b) by extracting the corresponding precursor ions in positive and negative modes to make sure whether they exist in the sample or not, and c) characterizing the detected compounds by their specific product ions and retention times. To identify the curcuminoids in turmeric samples the authors used a single UHPLC-QTOF-MS/MS platform. By this

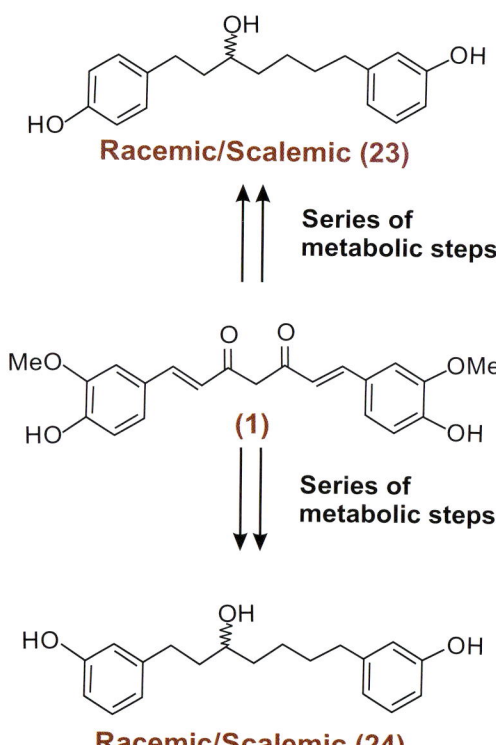

Fig. 118: Scheme showing the metabolic steps in rats that gives rise to both the forms of (**23**) and (**24**) as racemic mixture.
(Adapted from Li *et al.*, 2012)

approach, 101 chromatographic peaks (12 curcuminoids exhibited keto-enol tautomerism and 89 curcuminoids including 16 novel ones) were detected and identified in turmeric extracts based on a previous study about the fragmentation patterns of known curcuminoids (Jiang *et al.*, 2006).

Harvey (1981a) investigated the compounds present in ginger and identified HHC as its *tris*-silylated derivative. Also identified the dehydrated HHC as well as desmethyl-HHC analog. Later Li *et al.* (2012) demonstrated that DMC **(2)** is metabolized to both the positional isomers of the corresponding hexahydro derivatives (**25** & **26**) (Fig. 119).

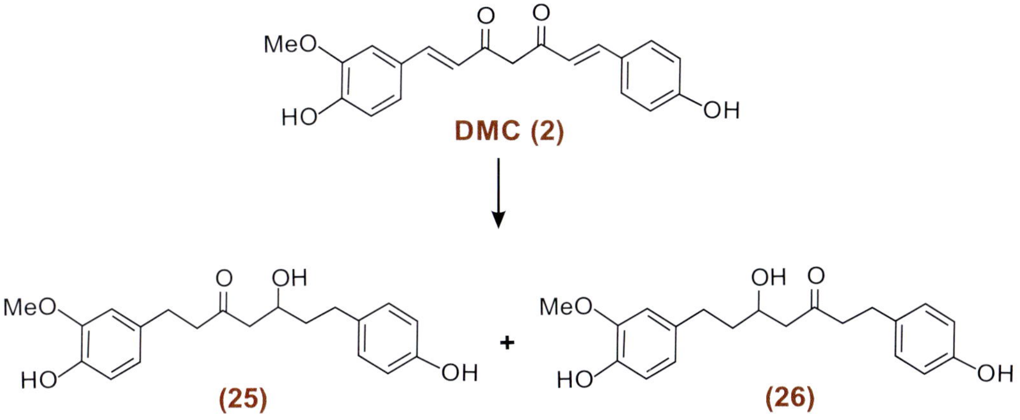

HH-DMCs

Fig. 119: Naturally occurring hexahydro-DMCs.
(Adapted from Li *et al.*, 2012)

Cellular & Mammalian Metabolism of Curcumin & HHC

In studies involving animals and human subjects, researchers have identified numerous metabolites of curcumin which include hydrogenated (dihydro, tetrahydro, hexahydro, and octahydro metabolites), desmethyl, glucuronide, and sulfate metabolites (Holder et al., 1978; Ireson et al., 2002). Biotransformation of curcumin has been characterized by the structures of its metabolites, including HHC in the suspensions of human and rat hepatocytes in comparison with that in rats *in vivo* after intravenous or oral administration of curcumin in rats. The HPLC assay and mass spectrometric techniques were used to detect the curcumin metabolites. The curcumin biotransformation produces, HHC and OHC which were identified in small amounts in rat plasma. However, the major metabolites of curcumin in suspensions of human or rat hepatocytes were identified as HHC and OHC. These findings clearly support the possibility that the metabolite was generated from curcumin via HHC (Ireson et al., 2001).

Earlier studies conducted using *in vitro* models of hepatic and intestinal cells, subcellular fractions and clinical studies in cancer patients indicated the biosynthesis of phase I metabolites of curcumin (Cheng et al., 2001; Garcea et al., 2004; Hoehle et al., 2006; Holder et al., 1978; Ireson et al., 2001 & 2002; Pan et al., 1999; Sharma et al., 2005). It is well documented that the phase I metabolism of curcumin comprises the reduction of the four double bonds of the heptadiene-3,5-dione structure. **Both THC and HHC are the major metabolites observed in most studies, whereas DHC and OHC usually represent minor metabolites.** The enzyme responsible for the bio-reduction of curcuminoids have been found to reside in the cytosol of liver and intestine and that include alcohol dehydrogenase. It was also established that incubation of curcuminoids with liver slices from rat resulted in the reduction of curcumin to DHC, THC, HHC, and OHC (Fig. 116), and consequently, these metabolites were glucuronidated resulting in tetrahydro, hexahydro, and octahydro forms being mainly present as glucuronides or conjugated with sulfate (Hoehle et al., 2006).

HEXAHYDROCURCUMIN (HHC): THE UNSUNG METABOLITE OF CURCUMIN

In addition, studies conducted by Hoehle *et al.* (2006) with precision-cut liver slices from male and female Sprague-Dawley rats showed that the major reductive metabolite of curcumin was HHC. The HPLC profile of the phase I metabolite of curcumin extracted from the incubation medium of male rat liver slice after enzymatic hydrolysis showed two peaks, which upon GC-MS analysis showed the GC retention time and mass spectrum as same as for authentic HHC (Hoehle *et al.*, 2006) (Fig. 120). Among the reductive metabolites, HHC was found to be more stable (Hoehle *et al.*, 2006). Earlier studies have reported that about 60% of the given dose of curcumin (400 mg) was absorbed both in the stomach and small intestine, while the unabsorbed curcumin was largely found in the large intestine (Ravindranath and Chandrasekhara, 1980). Wang *et al.* (1997) have shown that the stability of curcumin varied in different physiological matrices. Curcumin degraded rapidly both in phosphate buffer and serum-free medium after 37 °C incubation for 1 h. In a medium containing 10% fetal calf serum and in human blood, less than 20% of curcumin decomposed within 1 h. However, it was reported that more than 50% of curcumin still remained after incubation for 8 h. Hexahydrocurcumin

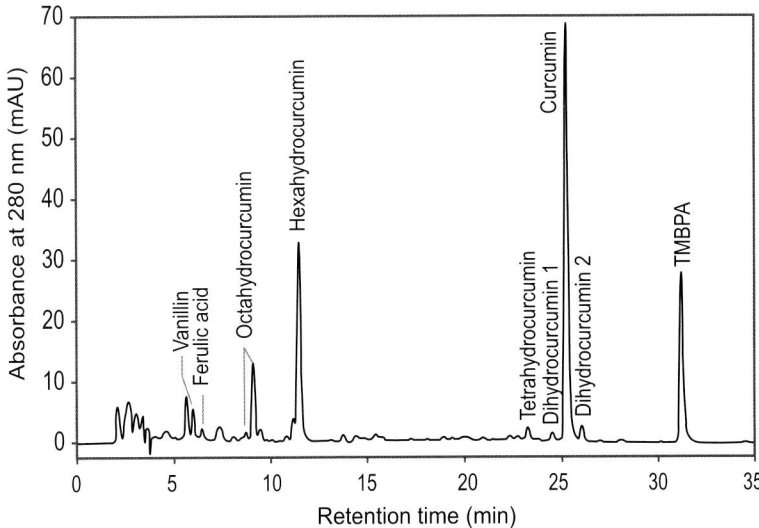

Fig. 120: HPLC profile of the phase I metabolites of curcumin extracted from the medium of a 24 h incubation of 200 μM curcumin with the slice of a male Sprague-Dawley rat liver after conjugate hydrolysis with β-glucuronidase/arylsulfatase from *H. pomatia*. 3,5,3′,5′-Tetramethyl-bisphenol A (TMBPA), internal standard. (Adapted from Hoehle *et al.*, 2006)

has been found as a major curcumin metabolite in mice and humans (Hoehle *et al.*, 2006; Holder *et al.*, 1978; Ireson *et al.*, 2001 & 2002; Pan *et al.*, 1999).

Recently, Li *et al.* (2012) isolated new as well as known metabolites of curcuminoids in rat feces and urine after oral administration of curcumin by gavage and suggested possible pathways for their production. The structures of fourteen phase I reductive metabolites derived from curcuminoids were identified by ESI-MS and NMR spectroscopy and clearly confirmed by using chiral column chromatography (Fig. 121).

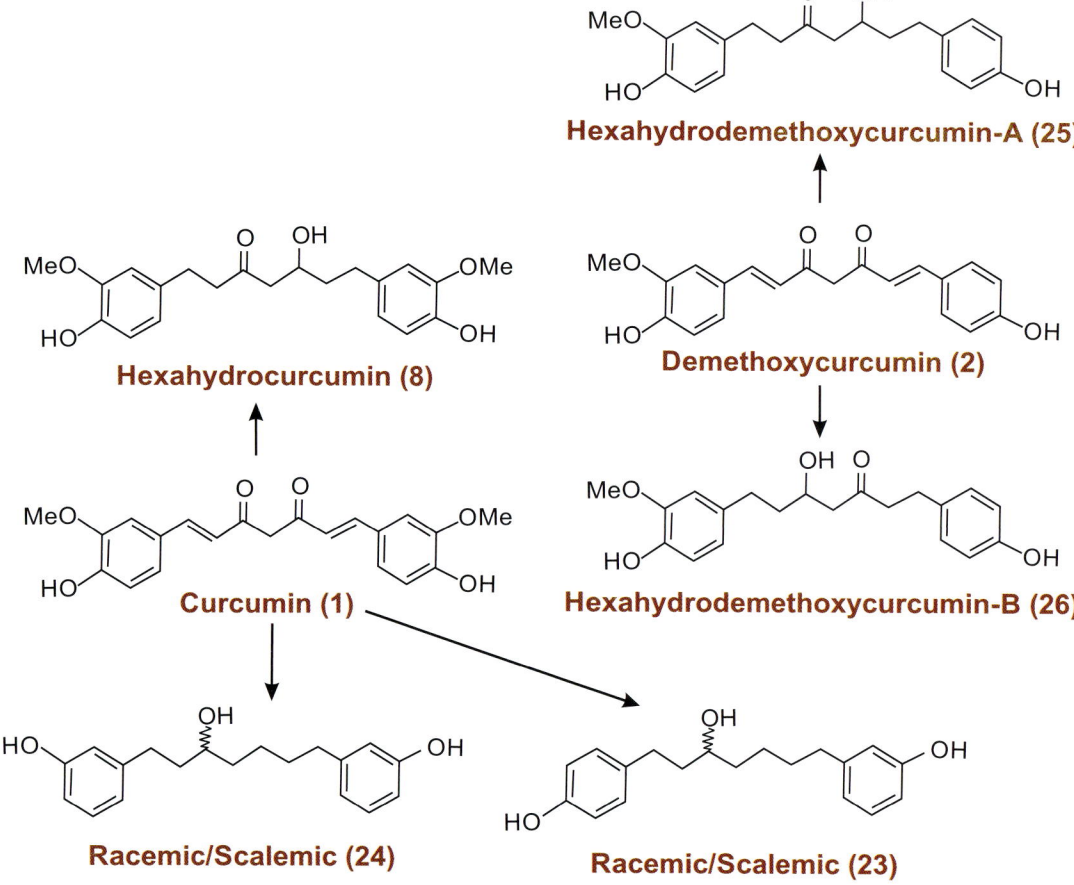

Fig. 121: Structures of curcuminoids metabolites identified in rat feces and urine after oral administration of curcumin by gavage. (Adapted from Li *et al.*, 2012)

Interestingly, it has been reported that the newly identified metabolites, namely 3-hydroxy-[1-(4-hydroxyphenyl)-7-(3-hydroxyphenyl)] heptane **(23)**, and 3-hydroxy-1,7-bis(3-hydroxyphenyl) heptane **(24)** occurred as pairs of enantiomers. Similarly, the known metabolites, such as hexahydrodemethoxycurcumin-A **(25)** and hexahydrodemethoxycurcumin-B **(26)** were also shown to occur in pairs of enantiomers. We speculate that in the mammalian system, the metabolite HHC is composed of both the enantiomers of HHC, namely (S)- and (R)-hexahydrocurcuminoids (Fig. 117) (Murata *et al.*, 1972; Kikuzaki *et al.*, 1991; Itokawa *et al.*, 1985; Uehara *et al.*, 1987). Also, metabolism changes the structure not only on the aliphatic chain, but also on the substituent groups in the benzene rings. These findings are important for understanding the metabolism of curcuminoids in rats and provide useful information and reference for further metabolic investigations on curcuminoids in humans.

It is important to mention here that HHC was found as a stable curcumin metabolite in mice and humans (Holder *et al.*, 1978; Ireson *et al.*, 2001 & 2002). In this context, Holder *et al.* (1978) reported that although some curcumin was found in bile after intravenous administration of 50 mg/kg [3H]-Curcumin in rats, most of the radioactivity in the bile was present in glucuronide conjugates of THC and HHC. The orally administered curcumin was metabolized into curcumin glucuronides and curcumin sulfates by conjugation, whereas THC, HHC, and DHC are formed by reduction after intraperitoneal administration of curcumin (Srivastava *et al.*, 2017).

Chapter 4
HEXAHYDROCURCUMIN (HHC): THE UNSUNG METABOLITE OF CURCUMIN

Preparation of HHC by Hydrogenation

Earlier, Sompran *et al.* (2007) reported the synthesis of HHC through the catalytic hydrogenation reaction of curcumin in alcohol solvent over a period of five hours with palladium on charcoal and other synthesized metabolites were confirmed using MS and NMR spectra (Deters *et al.*, 2008; Roughley and Whiting, 1973). The scheme on the conversion of curcumin to THC, HHC and OHC is shown in Fig. 122.

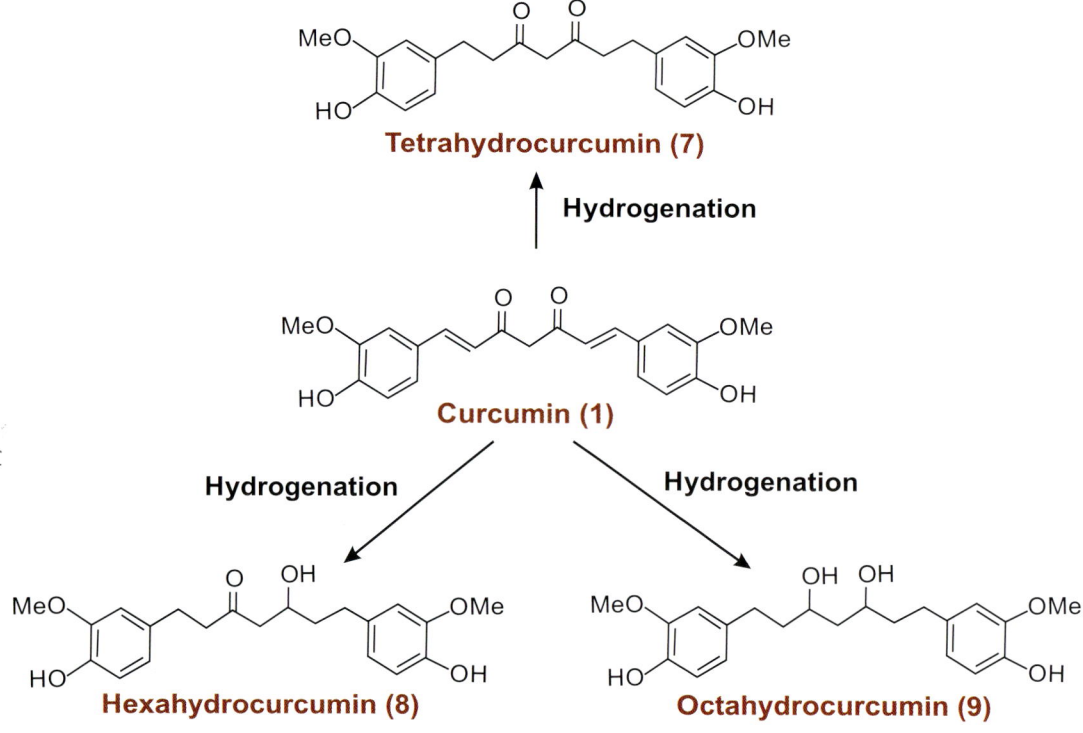

Fig. 122: Conversion of curcumin to THC, HHC and OHC by hydrogenation.

Earlier, Uehara *et al.* (1987) synthesized HHC **(8)** by hydrogenation of curcumin **(1)**. Similarly, Changtam *et al.* (2010) synthesized HHC **(8)** from curcumin by catalytic hydrogenation reaction in ethanol for 5 h, with palladium on charcoal as the catalyst. Hexahydrocurcumin was isolated from the mixture of THC **(7)** and OHC **(9)** by using silica gel column chromatography.

Microbial Biotransformation of Curcumin to HHC

Many approaches have been used to study microbial transformation of curcumin to understand the effect of the intestinal bacteria on curcumin metabolism. With an effort to provide clarification on the curcumin metabolism, studies have focused on curcumin-converting microorganisms and functional analyses of the curcumin-converting enzymes and genes. In this context, Hassaninasab *et al.* (2011) for the first time, identified an NADPH-dependent reductase, an enzyme found in *E. coli* isolated from human feces, that was capable of promoting a cascade reduction of curcumin. Interestingly, Zhang *et al.* (2013) used a novel yeast strain *Pichia kudriavzevii* ZJPH0802 from a soil sample for converting curcumin to its derivatives, namely HHC and THC. Similarly, Herath *et al.* (2007) reported that curcumin fermentation with the microorganism *Pichia anomala* (ATCC 20170) yielded four major metabolites including HHC, and two minor metabolites. It has been reported that the structures of major metabolites, including HHC, were established on the basis of spectroscopic data.

Recently, Younis *et al.* (2016) isolated eight metabolites by microbial transformation, namely THC **(7)**, HHC **(8)**, OHC **(9)**, demethoxyhexahydrocurcumin (DMHHC) **(26)**, demethoxyoctahydrocurcumin (DMOHC) **(27)**, vanillin **(13)**, bisdemethylcurcumin or didesmethylcurcumin (DDMC) **(5)**, and curcumin-4-O-β-D-glucoside **(28)** (Fig. 123) from curcumin **(1)**. Microbial transformation of curcumin **(1)** was carried out after screening for more than forty strains of fungi of different classes. After screening, *Alternaria alternata* AUMC 4685, *Cunninghamella blackesleeana* NRRL 1369, *Cunninghamella elegans* NRRL 2310 and *Penicillium brevicompactum* AUMC 2751 were found to be the most efficient microorganisms for maximum biotransformation of curcumin into several metabolites. The chemical structures of these metabolites were established by using physical and spectroscopic techniques, including melting points, UV, IR, ^{1}H-NMR, ^{13}C-NMR and ESI-MS. It has been reported that HHC exhibited more potent cytotoxic effect than curcumin with respect to antimicrobial activity.

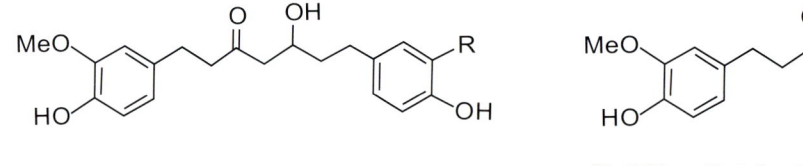

Fig. 123: Chemical structures of curcumin and its isolated metabolites.
(Adapted from Younis *et al.*, 2016)

Gut Microbiota Influence the Fate of Curcumin to Produce HHC in the Colon

Earlier studies show that orally administered curcumin was absorbed from the alimentary tract and present in the general blood circulation after largely being metabolized to the various forms of curcumin metabolites, including HHC (Asai and Miyazawa, 2000; Ireson *et al.*, 2001). It has been suggested that intestinal tract plays a critical role in the metabolic disposition of curcumin. The human large intestine hosts a highly complex microbial ecosystem containing ~10^{14} bacterial cells comprising approximately 1000 distinct species (Fava and Danese, 2011; Tuohy *et al.*, 2012). These gut microbiota can transform polyphenolic compounds by ring cleavage, reduction, decarboxylation, demethylation and dihydroxylation, thereby allowing the absorption of low molecular weight metabolites (Aura, 2008). The human GI microbiota consisting of the majority of bacteria, a few archaea, known as the microbiome, viruses, fungi, and other uni- and multicellular eukaryotes, are exclusively concentrated in the colon (Lepczynska *et al.*, 2017). An important function of gut microbiota is its conversion of dietary plant substances into bioactive molecules (Carmody and Turnbaugh, 2014). The biotransformation of turmeric curcuminoids, namely curcumin, DMC, and BDMC by human gut microbiota is known to produce a series of reduced curcumin metabolites. It has been reported that HHC, the phase I reductive metabolite of curcumin was isolated and identified in feces and urine after oral administration in male Wistar rats (Zeng *et al.*, 2007). Tan *et al.* (2014) also reported that a series of reduced curcumin metabolites are produced by intestinal bacteria, such as *E. coli* and *E. fergusonii*. However, metabolic fate of curcumin in the GI is yet to be fully elucidated.

Recently Li *et al.* (2017), for the first time, established the metabolic fate of curcumin in the GI-tract of mice by administering curcumin in the diet for 6 weeks.

The authors reported that curcumin was metabolized (Phase I) in the GI tract to produce three metabolic products, namely THC, HHC and OHC. Subsequently, curcumin and the phase I metabolites were further metabolized to yield their corresponding conjugated phase II metabolites. It was shown that the above mentioned metabolic processes of curcumin occurred in the stomach but only to a minimal extent compared to the small intestine. It has been reported that the phase I metabolites of curcumin, namely THC and HHC, were detected only in the cecum and colon. On the other hand, phase II metabolites of curcumin (i.e., conjugated forms of curcumin) were found in the small intestine, suggesting gut microbiota plays a role in the deconjugation of phase II metabolites to convert them back to the respective phase I metabolites in the cecum and colon. In addition, it was shown that during the anaerobic fermentation, phase II metabolites (isolated from the small intestine of a curcumin-fed mouse) were deconjugated to yield phase I metabolites by mouse and human fecal bacteria. Furthermore, curcumin could be transformed to yield THC, HHC and OHC by fecal bacteria, and fission metabolites such as ferulic acid.

In order to further establish the potential role of gut microbiota in the biotransformation process of curcumin, Li *et al.*, (2017) treated curcumin-fed mice with dextran sulfate sodium (DSS), an agent capable of altering gut microbiota, in the drinking water. DSS-mediated alteration of microbiota has established already via next-generation sequencing of fecal microbiota. Mice treated without DSS served as controls. Analyses of colonic content by LC/MS showed that DSS-treated mice exhibited a totally different profile of curcumin metabolites in the colon. It was reported that much higher levels of phase II metabolites and less of fission metabolites of curcumin were observed in DSS treated mice than the control mice. Overall, the study revealed that the composition of gut microbiota plays a significant role in the biotransformation of curcumin in the colon, thereby, having a significant influence on the health benefits of dietary curcumin (Li et al., 2017).

Pharmacological Significance

Antimicrobial Activity

Recently, Younis *et al.* (2016) reported the antibacterial and antifungal activities of curcumin and its isolated metabolites, assessed using agar well diffusion method. It has been reported that curcumin and its metabolites, including HHC showed antimicrobial activity against *Staphylococcus aureus*, *Escherichia coli*, *Candida albicans*, and *Aspergillus niger* at various levels. Interestingly, it was found that HHC showed the highest antimicrobial activity compared to curcumin, or THC or OHC. The antibacterial and antifungal activities of curcumin are already known (Ali, 2017; Moghadamtousi *et al.*, 2014; Mohammed and Habil, 2015). In an earlier study, Chattopadhyay *et al.* (2004) reported that curcumin extract exhibited antibacterial activity against a broad range of microbes, especially against Gram-positive strains and multiple antibiotic resistant bacteria. The results of Younis *et al.* (2016), also correlate with Shahi *et al.* (2000) who reported that curcumin exhibited potent growth inhibitory effect against Gram positive (*S. aureus* and *S. mutans*), Gram negative bacteria (*E. coli* and *P. aeruginosa*) and pathogenic yeast *C. albicans*. Therefore, the data from the available studies suggests that HHC possesses higher antimicrobial activity than that of curcumin. *Candida albicans* is an opportunistic fungal pathogen, which ranks as the fourth leading cause of nosocomial infectious diseases in humans (Chauhan *et al.*, 2006). Similarly, *A. niger*, appeared to be a secondary invader and caused lung damage by the production of oxalic acid (Metzger *et al.*, 1984). Earlier, it has been reported that HHC exhibited moderate activity against both *A. niger* and *C. albicans* (Singh and Jain, 2012).

Anthelmintic and Larvicidal Activities

Earlier studies have shown the efficacy of *Z. officinale* to destroy *Dirofilaria immitis* (Datta and Sukul, 1987), *Anisakis larvae* (Goto *et al.*, 1990), *Schistosoma mansoni* (Adewunmi *et al.*, 1990; Sanderson *et al.*, 2002), and gastrointestinal nematodes (Iqbal *et al.*, 2006). In this context, some components of ginger (e.g., [6]-gingerol, [10]-shogaol, [10]-gingerol, [6]-shogaol) and HHC were found to exert an anthelmintic effect against some parasitic species both *in vitro* and *in vivo* (Lin *et al.*, 2010 & 2014).

Lin *et al.* (2010) investigated the larvicidal effect or ability to halt spontaneous movement of the parasite *Angiostrongylus cantonensis* by [10]-shogaol, [6]-gingerol, [10]-gingerol, [6]-shogaol and HHC at various concentrations from 24 to 72 h. The findings revealed that these compounds were shown to have a larvicidal effect. However, as shown in Figs. 124A & 124B, [10]-gingerol has a maximum larvicidal effect and loss of spontaneous parasite movements when compared to HHC (Lin *et al.*, 2010). Synthesis of newer analogues of HHC could help to overcome this limitation to exert beneficial larvicidal effect.

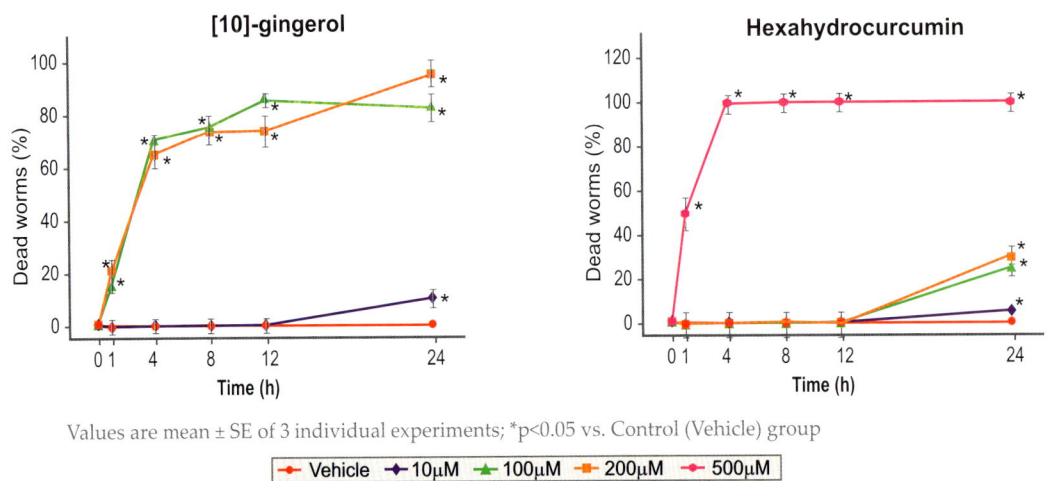

Values are mean ± SE of 3 individual experiments; *$p<0.05$ vs. Control (Vehicle) group

Fig. 124A: Time course and dose-dependent effect of [10]-gingerol and HHC on the larvicidal activity. (Adapted from Lin *et al.*, 2010)

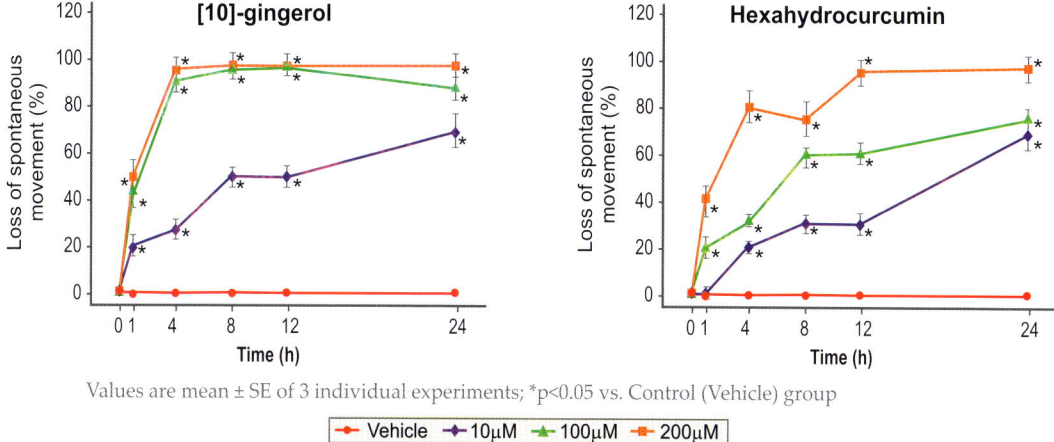

Fig. 124B: Time course and dose-dependent effect of [10]-gingerol and HHC on the loss of spontaneous movements. (Adapted from Lin *et al.*, 2010)

Antioxidant Potential

Hydrogenated derivatives of curcumin, THC, HHC and OHC exhibit strong antioxidant activity compared to curcumin (Li F *et al.*, 2012; Somparn *et al.*, 2007). It has been indicated that the antioxidant activity of HHC and OHC were found to be equal and reported that one molecule of THC, HHC or OHC can trap more than 3 molecules of peroxyl radicals (Somparn *et al.*, 2007) as shown in Table 15.

Another study by Li *et al.* (2012) reported that HHC, and 1-dehydro-[6]-gingerdione exhibit comparable potencies in scavenging DPPH radical with inhibition exceeding 58%, significantly stronger than [6]-shogaol and [6]-dehydroshogaol at the same time-point ($p < 0.05$). However, through comparison of the IC_{50} values, Morales *et al.* (2015) showed that curcumin had comparable scavenging activity as the reference antioxidant, trolox. All other derivatives, except BDMC, showed significantly higher efficacy compared to curcumin and trolox. The relative rank order of the DPPH scavenging potency of curcumin and its derivatives is as follows: OHC > DMC ≥ THC ≥ HHC > Curcumin = Trolox >> BDMC.

Table 15: Antioxidant activities of curcumin and its derivatives on the rate of AAPH-induced oxidation of linoleic acid. (Adapted from Somparn et al., 2007)

Antioxidant	R_{inh}/R_o [a]	Antioxidant activity (min/μM) [b]	n [c]
Curcumin	0.09 ± 0.01*	46.2 ± 8.1*	2.7
DMC	0.26 ± 0.02*, **	20.3 ± 2.8**	2.0
BDMC	0.30 ± 0.01*, **	10.0 ± 1.2**	1.4
THC	0.13 ± 0.01*, **	69.3 ± 6.6*, **	3.4
HHC	0.20 ± 0.03*, **, †	30.8 ± 3.3*, **, †	3.8
OHC	0.19 ± 0.02*, **, †	40.3 ± 8.3*, †	3.1
Trolox	0.51 ± 0.03	16.0 ± 1.2	2.0

Values are mean ± SD of 3 independent experiments; *$p<0.05$ vs. Trolox; **$p<0.05$ vs. Curcumin; †$p<0.05$ vs. THC.
[a] The initial rates of oxidation in the presence of 3 μM antioxidant (except BDMC 12 μM) compared to the control.
[b] Slope of the plot between inhibition time (T_{inh}) vs. antioxidant concentrations.
[c] n represents the stoichiometric number of peroxyl radicals trapped per molecule of antioxidant.
R_{inh}: Initial Oxidation Rate; R_o: Absence of Antioxidant; T_{inh}: Inhibition Time.

Anti-inflammatory Potential

Evidence from recent studies have suggested that HHC isolated from ginger extract showed phase II enzymes induction and anti-inflammatory activity in a LPS-stimulated macrophage (RAW 264.7) bioassay (Li et al., 2012).

Inhibition of phospholipase A2 (PLA2)

The enzyme phospholipase A2 is responsible for the hydrolysis of membrane phospholipids that release arachidonic acid, which serves as a substrate for pro-inflammatory mediators, such as prostaglandins and leukotrienes (Kudo and Murakami, 2002). The binding of the substrate to PLA2 occurs through a well-formed hydrophobic channel. Blocking the hydrophobic channel is an effective way to inhibit PLA2. Computational molecular docking studies indicated that HHC fits better than curcumin at the active site of phospholipase 2, the main enzyme in the arachidonic acid cascade (Dileep *et al.*, 2011).

Inhibition of COX-2 Expression

Hexahydrocurcumin possesses strong anti-inflammatory and anti-carcinogenesis potencies against the formation of COX-2-derived PGE_2 and down regulating the expression of COX-2, an important enzyme in carcinogenesis (Lee *et al.*, 2005; Srimuangwong *et al.*, 2012a & 2012b). Hexahydrocurcumin was reported to have a reduced ability to inhibit COX-2 expression compared to curcumin in a few studies (Ireson *et al.*, 2001). Srimuangwong *et al.* (2012a & 2012b) demonstrated that HHC is a selective COX-2 inhibitor. It has been shown that HHC downregulated COX-2 expression without altering the level of COX-1, a protective enzyme.

Inhibition of NF-κB, iNOS and COX-2 Expression

Zhao *et al.* (2015) investigated the effect of curcumin and its metabolites (THC, HHC, and OHC) on the expression of inducible NO synthase (iNOS), COX-2 and activated NF-κB. It has been reported that LPS- mediated upregulation of iNOS and COX-2, as well as NF-κB activation in RAW 264.7 cells were significantly inhibited by curcumin and its three metabolites. However, it was shown that curcumin was more potent than its three metabolites, of which THC was observed to be pharmacologically most active (Zhao *et al.*, 2015).

In another study using LPS-stimulated macrophage, Lee *et al.* (2005) also showed that HHC has a potent activity against COX-2 derived PGE_2 formation with an IC_{50} value of 0.7 µM (Lee *et al.*, 2005). Pan *et al.* (1999) also evaluated the inhibitory effects of curcumin and its metabolites, THC, HHC, and OHC, on the iNOS in RAW 264.7 cells activated with LPS. The result showed that HHC is less effective in reducing 130-kDa protein and 4.5-kb mRNA levels of iNOS in LPS-activated macrophages compared to curcumin.

Effect on Nitric oxide

Nitric oxide (NO) plays an important role in inflammation and in multiple stages of carcinogenesis (Pan *et al.*, 1999). A study by Morales *et al.* (2015) reported that hydrogenated derivatives, HHC and OHC, had the lowest scavenging capacity for NO. It is suggested that the structure of the heptanedione linkage is important for NO scavenging activity, as loss of the double bond in this structure markedly reduced the activity as is the case for HHC and OHC (Morales *et al.*, 2015; Pan *et al.*, 1999).

Modulation of Cytokines

The overproduction of NO was potently inhibited by curcumin and its three metabolites. While curcumin and THC significantly inhibited the release of major cytokines, including TNF-α and IL-6, the other two metabolites, HHC and OHC, did not substantially influence cytokine release (Zhao *et al.*, 2015).

Anti-allergic Activity

Degranulation is a characteristic feature of activated mast cells or basophils upon the stimulation of cross-linking antigens (Yamada *et al.*, 1982). Measurements of inhibitory capacity on the release of β-hexosaminidase have been used commonly as a reliable parameter to predict possible anti-allergic activities of either natural or synthetic compounds (Beaven and Metzger, 1993). Chen *et al.* (2009) evaluated anti-allergic potency of five pure phenolic compounds (HHC, [6]-dehydrogingerdione, [10]-gingerol, [6]-gingerol, and [6]-shogaol) isolated from the rhizomes of *Z. officinale*. Rat basophilic leukemia (RBL-2H3) cells were incubated with all the above compounds at various concentrations and the release of β-hexosaminidase was measured kinetically and compared to that from untreated cells. All phenolic compounds at 120 µM exhibited similar inhibitory capacities and kinetics. They showed a moderate initial inhibition (60-70%) at the lowest concentration (1 µM) and reached their highest degree of inhibition at 100 and 200 µM concentrations. However, it has been reported that among all the compounds tested, HHC demonstrated the most potent inhibitory effect (Fig. 125), suggesting that HHC isolated from the rhizomes of *Z. officinale* has significant anti-allergic potency (Chen *et al.*, 2009).

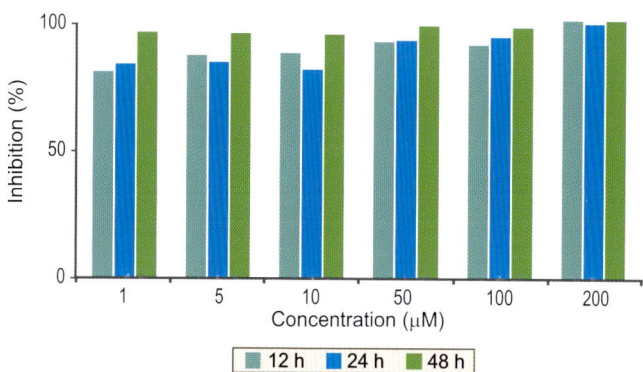

Fig. 125: Time-course inhibitory effects of different concentrations of HHC on β-hexosaminidase release from antigen-stimulated RBL-2H3 (rat basophilic leukemia) cells.
(Adapted from Chen *et al.*, 2009)

Immunomodulatory Activity

Lymphocytes and monocytes represent the innate and adaptive arms of immune response. Monocytes differentiate into tissue macrophages and dendritic cells and function as phagocytic and antigen presenting cells, while lymphocytes get activated in an antigen dependent manner. Peripheral blood mononuclear cells (PBMCs) are used to investigate immune modulatory effects of food bioactive compounds (Kleiveland, 2015). An earlier study evaluated the effect of various curcuminoids and curcumin derivatives (curcumin, isocurcumin, bisdesmethoxycurcumin, diacetylcurcumin, THC, HHC, and OHC as well as vanillin, ferulic acid and dihydroferulic acid) on OKT3 (mouse anti-human CD3 antibody)-

induced proliferation of human PBMC, and established first structure–activity relationships. Additionally, the radical scavenging activities of these curcuminoids were also determined by using a chemical assay to show a possible relationship to their immunosuppressive effects. It was also shown that curcumin inhibited OKT3-induced proliferation of human PBMC in a dose-dependent manner with an IC$_{50}$ value of 2.8 μM (Deters *et al.*, 2008).

The key findings from the above study indicated that the immunosuppressive effect of THC, HHC, and OHC was much higher than that of ferulic acid, dihydroferulic acid, and vanillin and the substances with the strongest effect on scavenging radicals were THC, HHC, and OHC with IC$_{50}$ values of 10.0, 11.7, and 12.3 μM, respectively (Deters *et al.*, 2008). Based on the above findings it was inferred that the curcuminoid-induced inhibition of OKT3-induced PBMC proliferation may not be mediated by the radical scavenging activity. It is suggested that other mechanisms could be responsible for the immunosuppressive effect of the curcuminoids such as inhibition of CD28 costimulatory pathway (Ranjan *et al.*, 1998) or modulation of the transcription factors c-Jun N-terminal kinase (JNK) and NF-κB (Chen and Tan, 1998; Singh and Aggarwal, 1995), and that need further studies specifically with HHC.

Neuroprotective Potential

Alzheimer's disease (AD) is a progressive neurodegenerative disorder and the most common cause of dementia in adults. The deposition of senile plaques composed by fibrillar aggregates of amyloid β-peptide (Aβ) is generally agreed as a characteristic hallmark of the pathology and is considered fundamental in disease pathogenesis (Hardy and Selkoe, 2002). Studies show that the main components of the plaques are the peptides Aβ (1-40) and Aβ (1-42), which occur as fibrillar aggregates in equilibrium with soluble oligomers and random coil or α-helical monomers (Iversen *et al.*, 1995). The turmeric phytocomplex is therapeutic despite the unfavorable pharmacokinetic properties. Curcumin alone and its metabolites such as THC, HHC and OHC are biologically active (Ireson *et al.*, 2001; Pan *et al.*, 1999) and interact with the helical form of Aβ and prevent the formation of membrane-disrupting aggregates (Randino *et al.*, 2016).

In the context of the neuroprotective effects of HHC, Quitschke *et al.* (2013) used amyloid protein precursor (APP)$_{swe}$, PS1dE9 mice model to assess the effect of curcuminoids on the potential for plaque prevention. For the study on plaque prevention, female APP$_{swe}$, PS1dE9 transgenic mice were given intravenous injections of serum-solubilized curcumin via the tail vein once per week starting at 4 months of age for a period of 8 months. The results indicated that although weekly long-term injections did not result in a significant reduction in plaque load, intravenous injection of curcuminoids at higher concentrations and at a biweekly frequency between the ages of 11 and 12 months reduced the plaque load to approximately 70% of the control value. Both HHC and OHC, were detected in plasma and brain. However, HHC was the main reduction metabolite detected in the brain, with peak concentration reaching approximately 40 nmol/g at five minutes after injection. It is, therefore, suggested that inhibition of plaque formation and plaque resolution depends on a more frequent administration of curcuminoids (Quitschke *et al.*, 2013).

A most recent study investigated whether HHC, through its antioxidant and anti-inflammatory activities, reduces apoptosis following cerebral I/R to attenuate brain damage and improves the outcome in a rat stroke model (Wicha *et al.*, 2017). For this purpose, the rats with cerebral I/R were treated with HHC (10, 20 and 40 mg/kg). Sham-operated and vehicle-treated rats served as controls. The rats were tested for neurological deficits and the pathology of the brain after 24 h. The findings showed that HHC treatment, at all doses, significantly reduced the neurological deficit scores and the infarct volume in rats compared to vehicle control (Fig. 126).

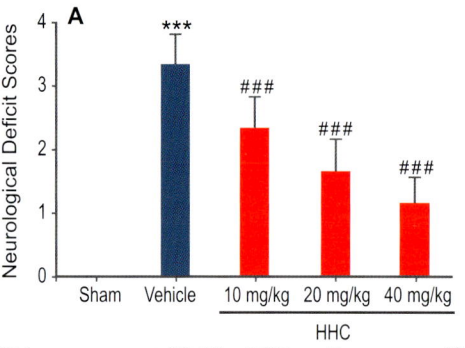
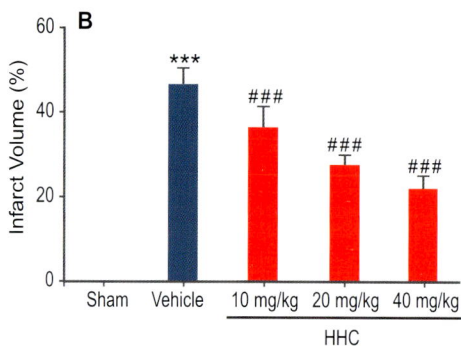

Values are mean ± SD; ***p<0.001 vs. Sham group; ###p<0.001 vs. Vehicle group.

Fig. 126: Impact of HHC on the neurological deficit and brain infarction after cerebral I/R in rats.
Dose-dependent effect of HHC on the initiation of the reperfusion.
(A) HHC effect on the neurological deficit scores after cerebral I/R.
(B) HHC effect on the percentage of infarct volume after I/R in different groups.
(Adapted from Wicha *et al.*, 2017)

The authors reported that HHC treatment markedly reduced the oxidative stress and inflammation, by decreasing the levels of MDA and NO with the reduction in expression of NF-κB (p65) and COX-2 in the I/R rats. In addition, HHC was also shown to enhance the expression of Nrf2 (nucleus) protein, heme oxygenase-1 (HO-1), the antioxidative enzymes, and the superoxide dismutase (SOD) activity in the I/R rats. In addition, HHC treatment also significantly decreased Bax and cleaved caspase-3 and increased Bcl-XL, with a decrease in the apoptotic neuronal cells. The authors concluded that the antioxidant properties of HHC may play an important role in improving functional outcomes and may offer significant neuroprotection against I/R damage (Wicha *et al.*, 2017).

Cardioprotective Potential

Anti-atherosclerotic Activity

It is widely known that inflammation and oxidative stress contribute to atherogenesis and consistently earlier studies also have shown the anti-atherogenic effect of curcumin in animal models of atherosclerosis (Olszanecki et al., 2005). In a long-term study by Shin et al. (2011) the effect of curcumin in lowering plasma and hepatic cholesterol levels and reducing early atherosclerotic lesion was comparable to lovastatin (Shin et al., 2011). Moreover, ginger extract has also been shown to reduce aortic lesions by 44% in mouse models of atherosclerosis (Fuhrman et al., 2000). Based on these studies, it is relevant to infer that HHC from ginger or as a metabolite of curcumin may play a potential role against the pathogenesis of atherosclerosis.

Anti-angiogenic Activity

Corneal neovascularization is an abnormal formation of new blood vessels in a previously avascular cornea which is usually caused by infections, traumatic or inflammatory events at the corneal surface. To understand the effect of HHC on corneal neovascularization, Kuo et al. (2018) studied the effect of HHC on the expression of basic fibroblast growth factor (bFGF), and vascular endothelial growth factor (VEGF) that are associated with neovascularization. In this study, a subconjunctival injection of HHC at a dose of 1 µg for 60 days successfully inhibited corneal neovascularization in male Sprague-Dawley rats compared with the control. Inhibition of corneal neovascularization was also associated with the reduced expression of the protein for bFGF and VEGF (evident from Western blot analysis for the respective proteins), however, the effect induced by HHC was insignificant or reduced after 60 days. In this study, the authors report that there was no inhibition of normal limbal vessels (Kuo et al., 2018).

Anti-platelet Aggregation Activity

Platelet aggregation plays an important role in thrombosis and haemostasis. The first step in platelet response to vascular injury is irreversible attachment to the altered surfaces followed by platelet aggregation. Curcumin exerts its potent anti-platelet activity through the inhibition of COX activity and the blockade of calcium signaling (Shah et al., 1999). Consistently, a recent study showed that treatment of human platelet-rich plasma with HHC resulted in an inhibitory effect on platelet aggregation, suggesting the potential of this compound as an anti-platelet aggregation agent in humans (Dong et al., 2012).

Vasorelaxant Effect

Hyperhomocysteinemia (Hhcy), a powerful independent risk factor for various cardiovascular disease, has been shown to induce endothelial dysfunction due to a decrease in bioavailable NO and increased vascular oxidant stress (Abahji et al., 2007). Endothelium-dependent vasorelaxations are impaired in animals and human with Hhcy (Tep-Areenan and Suksamrarn, 2012; Williams and Schalinske, 2010). A study by Moohammadaree et al. (2015) demonstrated the vasorelaxant effect of HHC in isolated rat aortic rings, and provided insights into the mechanism of action, by recording the isometric tension of the aortic rings using the organ bath system. Hexahydrocurcumin at a dose of 1 nM to 1 mM relaxed the endothelium-intact aortic rings precontracted with phenylephrine (PE) and potassium chloride (KCl) in a concentration-dependent manner in both endothelium-intact and endothelium-denuded arteries. In Ca^{2+}-free Krebs solution, HHC significantly inhibited the $CaCl_2$-induced contraction in high K^+ depolarized rings and suppressed the transient contraction induced by PE and caffeine in a concentration-dependent manner (Figs. 127A & 127B). These results suggest that the vasorelaxant effect of HHC is mediated by the endothelium-independent pathway, probably because of the inhibition of extracellular Ca^{2+} influx through voltage-operated Ca^{2+} channels and receptor-operated Ca^{2+} channels, the inhibition of Ca^{2+} mobilization from intracellular stores, as well as inhibition of PKC-mediated Ca^{2+}-independent contraction. Moreover, HHC produces vasorelaxant effects probably by stimulating the β-adrenergic receptor (Moohammadaree et al., 2015).

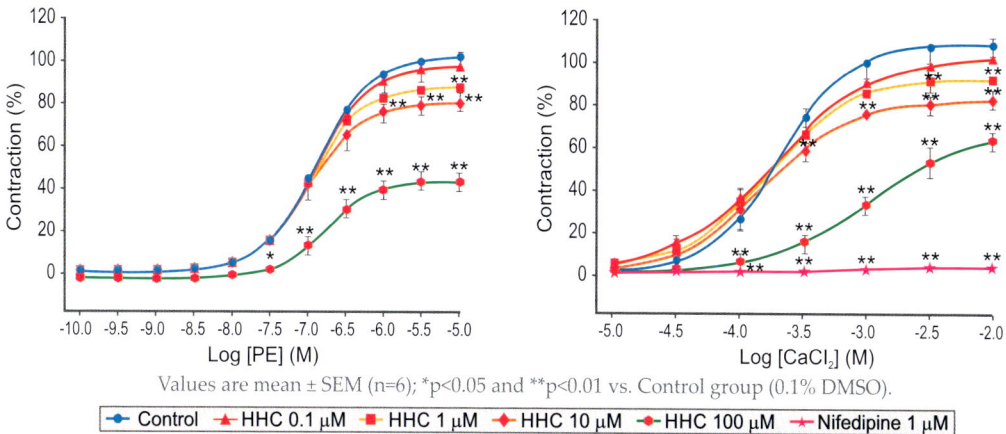

Fig. 127A: The dose-dependent inhibitory effects of HHC on the vascular contraction induced by cumulative 0.1 nM to 10 μM of phenylephrine (PE) in endothelium-intact rat aortic rings.
(Adapted from Moohammadaree *et al.*, 2015)

Fig. 127B: The dose-dependent effect of HHC and nifedipine on $CaCl_2$-induced contractile response in endothelium-denuded rings. The cumulative-concentration curves were determined in Ca^{2+}-free Krebs solution after intracellular and extracellular Ca^{2+} depletion. The $CaCl_2$-contractile effect was dependent on the Ca^{2+} influx via the VOCC, induced by KCl (80 mM). (Adapted from Moohammadaree *et al.*, 2015)

Secondly, a critical factor in excitation-contraction coupling in smooth muscle contraction was shown to be the accumulation of intracellular Ca^{2+} concentration through an influx of extracellular Ca^{2+} via Ca^{2+} channels as well as Ca^{2+} release from intracellular stores (Jackson *et al.*, 2000). Therefore, Moohammadaree *et al.*, (2015) determined whether the vasorelaxant ability of HHC may responsible for the modulation of the intracellular Ca^{2+} ion level in the smooth muscle cells (SMC). Their finding indicated that the vasodilator effect of HHC might be by acting as the blockade of both the receptor-operated Ca^{2+} channels (ROCC) and the voltage-operated Ca^{2+} channels (VOCC) and relaxed the aortic rings precontracted with either PE or KCl.

In addition, as shown in Fig. 128A, HHC was also observed to relax phorbal-12-myristate-13-acetate (PMA) (an activator of protein kinase C) precontracted aortic rings in a concentration-dependent manner with EC_{50} values equivalent to 93.36 ± 1.03 μM. Also, pre-incubation with propranolol (a β-adrenergic receptor blocker) significantly attenuated HHC-induced vasorelaxation (Figs. 128A & 128B) (Moohammadaree et al., 2015).

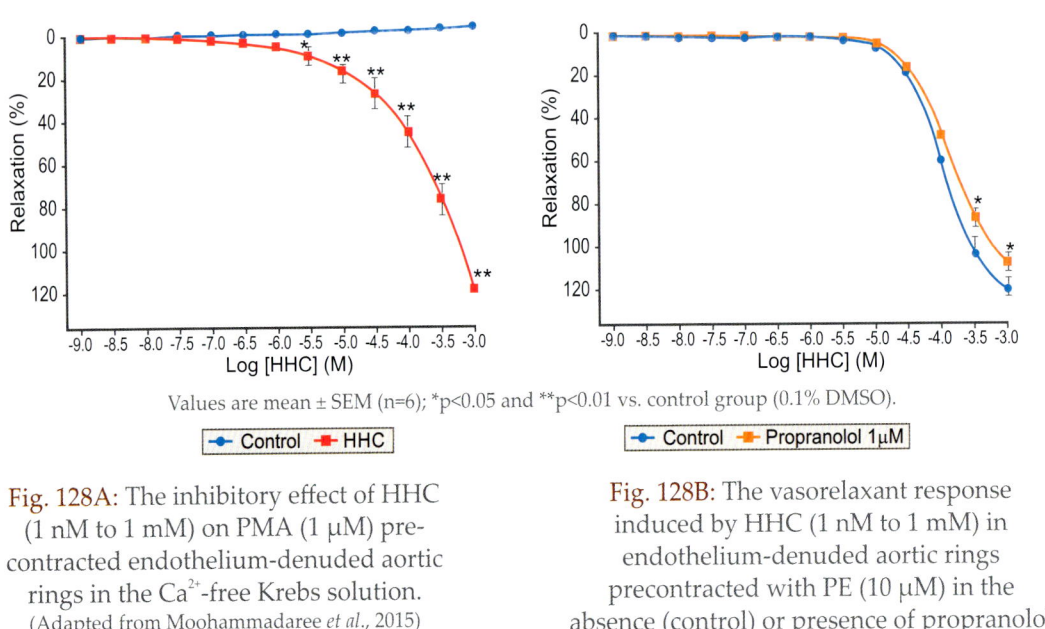

Fig. 128A: The inhibitory effect of HHC (1 nM to 1 mM) on PMA (1 μM) pre-contracted endothelium-denuded aortic rings in the Ca^{2+}-free Krebs solution.
(Adapted from Moohammadaree et al., 2015)

Fig. 128B: The vasorelaxant response induced by HHC (1 nM to 1 mM) in endothelium-denuded aortic rings precontracted with PE (10 μM) in the absence (control) or presence of propranolol (a nonselective β-receptor antagonist, 1 μM).
(Adapted from Moohammadaree et al., 2015)

In summary, the study provides key evidence that HHC contributes to the relaxation of aortic rings in rats through an endothelium-independent mechanism. Involvement of HHC on vasorelaxation is based on four mechanisms, namely

A) Activation through β-adrenoceptors
B) Inhibition of extracellular Ca^{2+} influx via the ROCC and the VOCC
C) Inhibition of Ca^{2+} mobilization from intracellular stores
D) Inhibition of protein kinase C (PKC) mediated Ca^{2+}-independent contraction

(Moohammadaree et al., 2015).

Anticancer Activity

The anticancer activity of HHC and other related health benefits are primarily attributed to its function as an antioxidant, anti-inflammatory and capable of inducing cytotoxic effects against cancer proliferation. In this section, we will highlight those aspects based on the information available from several study reports and literature. Earlier studies have revealed that curcumin metabolites have antioxidant, anti-inflammatory and anticancer activities. Most importantly, HHC also exhibits stronger antioxidant activity than curcumin (Li *et al.*, 2012; Somparn *et al.*, 2007). As a primary mechanism(s) of anticancer activity in colon cancer models, HHC was found to inhibit COX-2 expression effectively compared to curcumin (Ireson *et al.*, 2002). Prostaglandin E_2 (PGE_2) is a major product of COX-2 enzymes implicated in colorectal carcinogenesis and has been shown to stimulate the growth of human colorectal carcinoma cells (Shao *et al.*, 2003). Hexahydrocurcumin was also found to inhibit the biosynthesis of PGE_2 in LPS-stimulated macrophages (Li *et al.*, 2012). In addition, HHC was shown to decrease the level of phorbol ester-induced PGE_2 production in human colonic epithelial cells (HCECs), but weakly inhibits COX-2 protein (Du *et al.*, 2006). On the other hand, Srimuangwong *et al.* (2012b) have shown that HHC could be a selective COX-2 inhibitor at the mRNA level. This finding was further supported by the observation that HHC significantly down-regulates COX-2 mRNA expression compared to the control (control: 100.05% ± 0.03% vs. HHC: 61.01% ± 0.35%, $p<0.05$) but does not alter COX-1 mRNA.

Cytotoxic Effect on Colon Cancer Cells

Studies on the cytotoxicity of HHC and its effect on cell cycle in human colorectal cancer cells SW480 revealed that HHC extracted from *Z. officinale*, is cytotoxic to colorectal cells (Srimuangwong *et al.*, 2012b). Treatment of SW480 with HHC (100 µM) resulted in a massive accumulation of the cells in the G1/G0 phase of the cell cycle, suggesting that the cytotoxic effect of HHC may prove useful in cancer prevention (Chen *et al.*, 2011). In addition, Srimuangwong *et al.* (2012b) also showed that HHC significantly decreased the cell viability of human colon cancer cells (HT-29) compared to the control.

Inhibitory Effect on COX-2 Protein Expression in Colon Cancer Cells

In a combination study, it was shown that HHC with 5-Fluorouracil (5-FU) at a low dose significantly reduced the cell viability to a greater degree than monotherapy, indicating their synergistic effect against the growth of HT-29 colon cancer cells. In addition, treatment of 5-FU at a concentration of 5 μmol/L in combination with HHC (25 μmol/L) significantly down-regulated COX-2 mRNA expression in HT-29 colon cancer cells compared to the effects of 5-FU or HHC alone (HHC + 5-FU: 31.93% ± 5.69%, 5-FU: 100.66% ± 4.52% respectively) (Srimuangwong et al., 2012b) (Fig.129). These findings also suggest that the synergistic effect of 5-FU and HHC on HT-29 human colon cancer cell growth inhibition is comparable to that of curcumin and 5-FU combination treatment of the same colon cancer cells (Du et al., 2006).

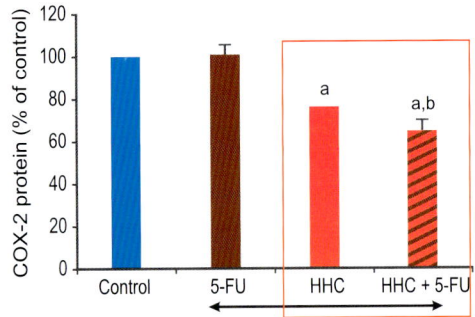

Values are expressed as percentage of control (Mean ± SE)
[a]p<0.05 vs. Control group; [b]p<0.05 vs. 5-FU or HHC monotherapy (n =3);

Fig. 129: Effect of 5-fluorouracil (5-FU) in combination with HHC on COX-2 protein expression in colon cancer (HT-29) cells.
(Adapted from Srimuangwong et al., 2012b)

Synergistic Effect of HHC with 5-Fluorouracil (5-FU) on Colon Cancer

Using a methylating agent 1,2-dimethylhydrazine (DMH)-induced colon cancer in male Wistar rats, Srimuangwong *et al.* (2012a) have demonstrated the effects of HHC alone and in combination with 5-FU on colon crypts. Compound 5-FU is widely used in the treatment of cancer, including colon cancer. Hexahydrocurcumin at an oral dose of 50 mg/kg, for 16 weeks reduced aberrant crypt foci (ACF) that are indicative of early changes in the colon before colorectal polyp formation. This study also showed down regulation of COX-2 expression in Wistar rats. A combination of HHC with 5-FU exhibited a synergistic effect in decreasing ACF formation significantly (Table 16). The synergistic effect of using 5-FU, a conventional chemotherapy drug, in combination with HHC has been demonstrated to have enhanced cell growth inhibition and down-regulation of COX-2 mRNA in colon cancer cells provides evidence that these two compounds in combination may have an enormous potential for the treatment of human colon cancer (Srimuangwong *et al.*, 2012b).

Table 16: HHC or 5-FU alone and their combination of dimethylhydrazine-exposed aberrant crypt foci formation in rats.
(Adapted from Srimuangwong *et al.*, 2012a)

Groups	Total ACF	Large ACF
Vehicle	1558.20 ± 17.37	262.20 ± 10.18
5-Fluorouracil	1231.20 ± 25.62[a]	111.00 ± 7.88[a]
Curcumin	1284.20 ± 25.47[a]	178.00 ± 7.33[a]
Hexahydrocurcumin	1086.80 ± 53.47[a]	186.60 ± 21.51[a]
5-Fluorouracil + Curcumin	880.20 ± 13.67[a,b,c]	122.00 ± 5.94[a]
5-Fluorouracil + Hexahydrocurcumin	665.80 ± 16.64[a,b,d]	119.00 ± 17.92[a,d]

Value are mean ± SE; [a]$p<0.01$ vs. Vehicle group; [b]$p<0.01$ vs. 5-Fluorouracil monotherapy; [c]$p<0.01$ vs. Curcumin monotherapy; [d]$p<0.01$ vs. Hexahydrocurcumin monotherapy; ACF: Aberrant Crypt Foci.

In summary, findings from the above studies suggest that HHC can inhibit the initiation and promotion of colorectal carcinogenesis, which is very much like the property of parent compound, curcumin (Shpitz et al., 2006). Also, HHC in combination with 5-FU exerted a synergistic effect in reducing the total number of ACFs higher than the treatment with either HHC or 5-FU alone. Furthermore, HHC also enhanced the inhibitory effects of 5-FU on HT-29 human colon cancer cell growth and downregulated the expression of COX-2 at the mRNA and protein levels (Srimuangwong et al., 2012a). Therefore, it is plausible to state that HHC augments the chemotherapeutic effects of 5-FU against the initiation of colorectal carcinogenesis.

Conclusion

Based on recent studies on HHC as presented in the appropriate sections, we believe that there is compelling evidence to investigate further on the health benefits of HHC. The potential pharmacotherapeutic activities of HHC are summarized in Fig. 130. Most importantly, the available data presented on the overall bioactivity profile of a major reductive metabolite HHC clearly reveals its multiple health benefits. It is also evident that HHC occurs naturally in plants such as turmeric and ginger highlighting the importance of the dietary source of HHC. This review provides information on HHC as a single reductive metabolite that possesses strong antioxidant, anti-inflammatory, anti-allergic, anthelmintic/larvicidal and cardioprotective effects at very low doses that could be achieved through regular dietary supplements.

Chapter 4
HEXAHYDROCURCUMIN (HHC): THE UNSUNG METABOLITE OF CURCUMIN

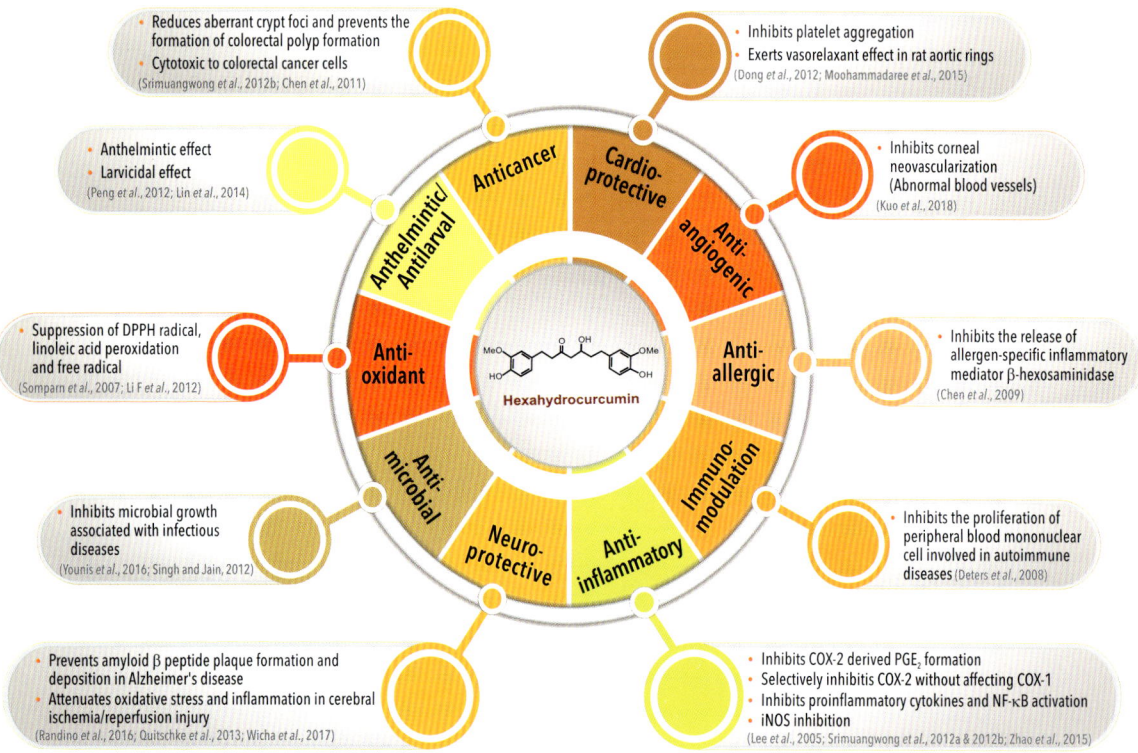

Fig. 130: Schematic representation on pharmacotherapeutic activities of HHC.

References

Abahji TN, Nill L, Ide N, Keller C, Hoffmann U, Weiss N. 2007. Acute hyperhomocysteinemia induces microvascular and macrovascular endothelial dysfunction. *Arch Med Res*. 38 (4):411-416.

Adewunmi CO, Oguntimein BO, Furu P. 1990. Molluscicidal and antischistosomal activities of *Zingiber officinale*. *Planta Med*. 56 (04):374-376.

Aggarwal BB, Sundaram C, Malani N, Ichikawa H. 2007. Curcumin: the Indian solid gold. *Adv Exp Med Biol*. 595: 1-75.

Aggarwal BB, Yuan W, Li S, Gupta SC. 2013. Curcumin-free turmeric exhibits anti-inflammatory and anticancer activities: Identification of novel components of turmeric. *Mol Nutr Food Res*. 57 (9):1529-1542.

Ali N. 2017. *In vitro* studies of antimicrobial activity of (*Curcuma longa* L.) rhizomes against *Helicobacter pylori*. *Iraq Med. J*. 1 (1):7-9.

Asai A, Miyazawa T. 2000. Occurrence of orally administered curcuminoid as glucuronide and glucuronide/sulfate conjugates in rat plasma. *Life Sci*. 67 (23):2785-2793.

Aura AM. 2008. Microbial metabolism of dietary phenolic compounds in the colon. *Phytochem Rev*. 7 (3):407-429.

Beaven MA, Metzger H. 1993. Signal transduction by Fc receptors: the Fc epsilon RI case. *Immunol Today*. 14 (5):222-226.

Begum AN, Jones MR, Lim GP, Morihara T, Kim P, Heath DD. 2008. Curcumin structure-function, bioavailability, and efficacy in models of neuroinflammation and Alzheimer's disease. *J Pharmacol Exp Ther*. 326 (1):196-208.

Carmody RN, Turnbaugh PJ. 2014. Host-microbial interactions in the metabolism of therapeutic and diet-derived xenobiotics. *J Clin Invest*. 124 (10):4173-4181.

Changtam C, de Koning HP, Ibrahim H, Sajid MS, Gould MK, Suksamrarn A. 2010. Curcuminoid analogs with potent activity against *Trypanosoma* and *Leishmania* species. *Eur J Med Chem*. 45 (3):941-956.

Chattopadhyay I, Biswas K, Bandyopadhyay U, Banerjee RK. 2004. Turmeric and curcumin: Biological actions and medicinal applications. *Curr Sci*. 87:44-53.

Chauhan N, Latge JP, Calderone R. 2006. Signalling and oxidant adaptation in *Candida albicans* and *Aspergillus fumigatus*. *Nat Rev Microbiol*. 4 (6):435-444.

Chapter 4
HEXAHYDROCURCUMIN (HHC): THE UNSUNG METABOLITE OF CURCUMIN

Chen BH, Wu PY, Chen KM, Fu TF, Wang HM, Chen CY. 2009. Antiallergic potential on RBL-2H3 cells of some phenolic constituents of *Zingiber officinale* (ginger). *J Nat Prod*. 72 (5):950-953.

Chen CY, Yang WL, Kuo SY. 2011. Cytotoxic activity and cell cycle analysis of hexahydrocurcumin on SW 480 human colorectal cancer cells. *Nat Prod Commun*. 6 (11):1671-1672.

Chen YR, Tan TH. 1998. Inhibition of the c-Jun N-terminal kinase (JNK) signaling pathway by curcumin. *Oncogene*. 17 (2):173-178.

Cheng AL, Hsu CH, Lin JK, Hsu MM, Ho YF, Shen TS *et al*. 2001. Phase I clinical trial of curcumin, a chemopreventive agent, in patients with high-risk or pre-malignant lesions. *Anticancer Res*. 21 (4B):2895-2900.

Connell D, McLachlan R. 1972. Natural pungent compounds: IV. Examination of the gingerols, shogaols, paradols and related compounds by thin-layer and gas chromatography. *J Chromatogr A*. 67 (1):29-35.

Connell D, Sutherland M. 1969. A re-examination of gingerol, shogaol, and zingerone, the pungent principles of ginger (*Zingiber officinale* Roscoe). *Aust J Chem*. 22 (5):1033-1043.

Datta A, Sukul NC. 1987. Antifilarial effect of *Zingiber officinale* on *Dirofilaria immitis*. *J Helminthol*. 61 (3):268-270.

Dempe JS, Scheerle RK, Pfeiffer E, Metzler M. 2013. Metabolism and permeability of curcumin in cultured Caco-2 cells. *Mol Nutr Food Res*. 57 (9):1543-1549.

Deters M, Knochenwefel H, Lindhorst D, Koal T, Meyer HH, Hansel W *et al*. 2008. Different curcuminoids inhibit T-lymphocyte proliferation independently of their radical scavenging activities. *Pharm Res*. 25 (8):1822-1827.

Dileep KV, Tintu I, Sadasivan C. 2011. Molecular docking studies of curcumin analogs with phospholipase A2. *Interdiscip Sci*. 3 (3):189-197.

Dong HP, Yang RC, Chunag IC, Huang LJ, Li HT, Chen HL *et al*. 2012. Inhibitory effect of hexahydrocurcumin on human platelet aggregation. *Nat Prod Commun*. 7(7):883-884.

Du B, Jiang L, Xia Q, Zhong L. 2006. Synergistic inhibitory effects of curcumin and 5-fluorouracil on the growth of the human colon cancer cell line HT-29. *Chemotherapy*. 52 (1):23-28.

Fava F, Danese S. 2011. Intestinal microbiota in inflammatory bowel disease: friend of foe? *World J Gastroenterol*. 17 (5):557-566.

Fuhrman B, Rosenblat M, Hayek T, Coleman R, Aviram M. 2000. Ginger extract consumption reduces plasma cholesterol, inhibits LDL oxidation and attenuates development of atherosclerosis in atherosclerotic, apolipoprotein E-deficient mice. *J Nutri*. 130 (5):1124-1131.

Garcea G, Jones DJ, Singh R, Dennison AR, Farmer PB, Sharma RA *et al*. 2004. Detection of curcumin and its metabolites in hepatic tissue and portal blood of patients following oral administration. *Br J Cancer*. 90 (5):1011-1015.

Goto C, Kasuya S, Koga K, Ohtomo H, Kagei N. 1990. Lethal efficacy of extract from *Zingiber officinale* (traditional Chinese medicine) or [6]-shogaol and [6]-gingerol in Anisakis larvae *in vitro*. *Parasitol Res*. 76 (8):653-656.

Gupta SC, Sung B, Kim JH, Prasad S, Li S, Aggarwal BB. 2013. Multitargeting by turmeric, the golden spice: From kitchen to clinic. *Mol Nutr Food Res*. 57 (9):1510-1528.

Hardy J, Selkoe DJ. 2002. The amyloid hypothesis of Alzheimer's disease: progress and problems on the road to therapeutics. *Science*. 297 (5580):353-356.

Harvey D. 1981a. Gas chromatographic and mass spectrometric studies of ginger constituents: Identification of gingerdiones and new hexahydrocurcumin analogues. *J Chromatogr A*. 212 (1):75-84.

Harvey D. 1981b. The mass spectra of the trimethylsilyl derivatives of ginger constituents. *Biological Mass Spectrometry*. 8 (11):546-552.

Hassaninasab A, Hashimoto Y, Tomita-Yokotani K, Kobayashi M. 2011. Discovery of the curcumin metabolic pathway involving a unique enzyme in an intestinal microorganism. *Proc Natl Acad Sci USA*.108 (16):6615-6620.

Herath W, Ferreira D, Khan IA. 2007. Microbial metabolism. Part 7: Curcumin. *Nat Prod Res*. 21 (5):444-450.

Hoehle SI, Pfeiffer E, Solyom AM, Metzler M. 2006. Metabolism of curcuminoids in tissue slices and subcellular fractions from rat liver. *J Agric Food Chem*. 54 (3): 756-764.

Holder GM, Plummer JL, Ryan AJ. 1978. The metabolism and excretion of curcumin (1,7-bis-(4-hydroxy-3-methoxyphenyl)-1,6-heptadiene-3,5-dione) in the rat. *Xenobiotica*. 8 (12):761-768.

Iqbal Z, Lateef M, Akhtar MS, Ghayur MN, Gilani AH. 2006. *In vivo* anthelmintic activity of ginger against gastrointestinal nematodes of sheep. *J Ethnopharmacol*. 106 (2):285-287.

Ireson CR, Jones DJ, Orr S, Coughtrie MW, Boocock DJ, Williams ML *et al*. 2002. Metabolism of the cancer chemopreventive agent curcumin in human and rat intestine. *Cancer Epidemiol Biomarkers Prev*. 11 (1):105-111.

Ireson C, Orr S, Jones DJ, Verschoyle R, Lim CK, Luo JL *et al*. 2001. Characterization of metabolites of the chemopreventive agent curcumin in human and rat hepatocytes and in the rat *in vivo*, and evaluation of their ability to inhibit phorbol ester-induced prostaglandin E2 production. *Cancer Res*. 61 (3):1058-1064.

Itokawa H, Morita H, Midorikawa I, Aiyama R, Morita M. 1985. Diarylheptanoids from the rhizome of *Alpinia officinarum* Hance. *Chem Pharm Bull*. 33 (11):4889-4893.

Iversen LL, Mortishire-Smith RJ, Pollack SJ, Shearman MS. 1995. The toxicity *in vitro* of beta-amyloid protein. *Biochem J*. 311 (Pt 1):1-16.

Jackson WF. 2000. Ion channels and vascular tone. *Hypertension*. 35 (1 Pt 2):173-178.

Jia S, Du Z, Song C, Jin S, Zhang Y, Feng Y *et al*. 2017. Identification and characterization of curcuminoids in turmeric using ultra-high performance liquid chromatography-quadrupole time of flight tandem mass spectrometry. *J Chromatogr A*. 1521:110-122.

Jiang H, Timmermann BN, Gang DR. 2006. Use of liquid chromatography-electrospray ionization tandem mass spectrometry to identify diarylheptanoids in turmeric (*Curcuma longa* L.) rhizome. *J Chromatogr A*. 1111 (1):21-31.

Joe B, Vijaykumar M, Lokesh BR. 2004. Biological properties of curcumin-cellular and molecular mechanisms of action. *Crit Rev Food Sci Nutr*. 44 (2):97-111.

Chapter 4
HEXAHYDROCURCUMIN (HHC): THE UNSUNG METABOLITE OF CURCUMIN

Kikuzaki H, Usuguchi J, Nakatani N. 1991. Constituents of Zingiberaceae. I. diarylheptanoids from the rhizomes of ginger (*Zingiber officinale* Roscoe). *Chem Pharm Bull*. 39 (1):120-122.

Kleiveland CR. 2015. Peripheral blood mononuclear cells. In the impact of food bioactives on health, *Springer*. pp 161-167.

Kudo I, Murakami M. 2002. Phospholipase A2 enzymes. *Prostaglandins Other Lipid Mediat*. 68:3-58.

Kuo CN, Chen CH, Chen SN, Huang JC, Lai LJ, Lai CH et al. 2018. Anti-angiogenic effect of hexahydrocurcumin in rat corneal neovascularization. *Int Ophthalmol*. 38(2):747-756.

Lee SL, Huang WJ, Lin WW, Lee SS, Chen CH. 2005. Preparation and anti-inflammatory activities of diarylheptanoid and diarylheptylamine analogs. *Bioorg Med Chem*. 13 (22):6175-6181.

Lepczynska M, Bialkowska J, Dzika E, Piskorz-Ogorek K, Korycinska J. 2017. Blastocystis: how do specific diets and human gut microbiota affect its development and pathogenicity? *Eur J Clin Microbiol Infect Dis*.1-10.

Li F, Nitteranon V, Tang X, Liang J, Zhang G, Parkin KL et al. 2012. In vitro antioxidant and anti-inflammatory activities of 1-dehydro-[6]-gingerdione, 6-shogaol, 6-dehydroshogaol and hexahydrocurcumin. *Food Chem*. 135 (2):332-337.

Li J, Liu Y, Wei JQ, Wang K, Chen LX, Yao XS et al. 2012. Isolation and identification of phase 1 metabolites of curcuminoids in rats. *Planta Med*. 78 (12):1351-1356.

Li Z, Sun Y, Song M, Li F, Xiao H. 2017. Gut microbiota dictate metabolic fate of curcumin in the colon. *FASEB J*. 31 (1 Supplement):646.12-646.12

Lin RJ, Chen CY, Chung LY, Yen CM. 2010. Larvicidal activities of ginger (*Zingiber officinale*) against *Angiostrongylus cantonensis*. *Acta Trop*. 115 (1):69-76.

Lin RJ, Chen CY, Lu CM, Ma YH, Chung LY, Wang JJ et al. 2014. Anthelmintic constituents from ginger (*Zingiber officinale*) against *Hymenolepis nana*. *Acta Trop*. 140:50-60.

Lv H, She G. 2012. Naturally occuring diarylheptanoids-A supplementary version. *Rec Nat Pro*. 6 (4):321-333.

Lv H, She G. 2010. Naturally occurring diarylheptanoids. *Nat Prod Commun*. 5 (10):1687-1708.

Masada Y, Inoue T, Hashimoto K, Fujioka M, Uchino C. 1974. Studies on the constituents of ginger (*Zingiber officinale* Roscoe) by GC-MS (author's transl). *Yakugaku zasshi: Journal of the Pharmaceutical Society of Japan*. 94 (6):735-738.

Metzger JB, Garagusi VF, Kerwin DM. 1984. Pulmonary oxalosis caused by *Aspergillus niger*. *Am Rev Respir Dis*.129 (3):501-502.

Moghadamtousi ZS, Kadir AH, Hassandarvish P, Tajik H, Abubakar S, Zandi K. 2014. A review on antibacterial, antiviral, and antifungal activity of curcumin. *BioMed Res Int*. 2014:186864.

Mohammed NA, Habil NY. 2015. Evaluation of antimicrobial activity of curcumin against two oral bacteria. *ACIS, Special Issue: Artifical nano sensory system 3(2)*: 18-21.

Moohammadaree A, Changtam C, Wicha P, Suksamrarn A, Tocharus J, Tocharus C. 2015. Mechanisms of vasorelaxation induced by hexahydrocurcumin in isolated rat thoracic aorta. *Phytother Res*. 29 (11):1806-1813.

Morales NP, Sirijaroonwong S, Yamanont P, Phisalaphong C. 2015. Electron paramagnetic resonance study of the free radical scavenging capacity of curcumin and its demethoxy and hydrogenated derivatives. *Biol Pharm Bull*. 38 (10):1478-1483.

Murata T, Shinohara M, Miyamoto M. 1972. Isolation of hexahydrocurcumin, dihydrogingerol and two additional pungent principles from ginger. *Chem Pharm Bull*. 20 (10):2291-2292.

Olszanecki R, Jawien J, Gajda M, Mateuszuk L, Gebska A, Korabiowska M *et al*. 2005. Effect of curcumin on atherosclerosis in apoE/LDLR-double knockout mice. *J Physiol Pharmacol*. 56 (4):627-635.

Pan MH, Huang TM, Lin JK. 1999. Biotransformation of curcumin through reduction and glucuronidation in mice. *Drug Metab Dispos*. 27 (4):486-494.

Peng F, Tao Q, Wu X, Dou H, Spencer S, Mang C *et al*. 2012. Cytotoxic, cytoprotective and antioxidant effects of isolated phenolic compounds from fresh ginger. *Fitoterapia*. 83 (3):568-585.

Quitschke WW, Steinhauff N, Rooney J. 2013. The effect of cyclodextrin-solubilized curcuminoids on amyloid plaques in Alzheimer transgenic mice: brain uptake and metabolism after intravenous and subcutaneous injection. *Alzheimer's Res Ther*. 5 (2):16.

Raghuveer K, Govindarajan V. 1979. Evaluation of spices and oleoresins vii. gas chromatographic examination of gingerol, shogaol and related compounds in ginger. *J Food Qual*. 2 (1):41-54.

Randino R, Grimaldi M, Persico M, De Santis A, Cini E, Cabri W *et al*. 2016. Investigating the neuroprotective effects of turmeric extract: Structural interactions of beta-Amyloid peptide with single curcuminoids. *Sci Rep*. 6:38846.

Ranjan D, Johnston TD, Wu G, Elliott L, Bondada S, Nagabhushan M. 1998. Curcumin blocks cyclosporine A-resistant CD28 costimulatory pathway of human T-cell proliferation. *J Surg Res*. 77 (2):174-178.

Ravindranath V, Chandrasekhara N. 1980. Absorption and tissue distribution of curcumin in rats. *Toxicology*. 16 (3):259-265.

Roughley PJ, Whiting DA. 1973. Experiments in the biosynthesis of curcumin. *J Chem Soc Perkin Trans* 1. 2379-2388.

Sanderson L, Bartlett A, Whitfield PJ. 2002. *In vitro* and *in vivo* studies on the bioactivity of a ginger (*Zingiber officinale*) extract towards adult schistosomes and their egg production. *J Helminthol*. 76 (3):241-247.

Shah BH, Nawaz Z, Pertani SA, Roomi A, Mahmood H, Saeed SA *et al*. 1999. Inhibitory effect of curcumin, a food spice from turmeric, on platelet-activating factor- and arachidonic acid-mediated platelet aggregation through inhibition of thromboxane formation and Ca^{2+} signaling. *Biochem Pharmacol*. 58 (7):1167-1172.

Shahi SK, Shukla AC, Bajaj AK, Banerjee U, Rimek D, Midgely G *et al*. 2000. Broad spectrum herbal therapy against superficial fungal infections. *Skin Pharmacol Appl Skin Physiol*. 13(1):60-64.

Shao J, Lee SB, Guo H, Evers BM, Sheng H. 2003. Prostaglandin E2 stimulates the growth of colon cancer cells via induction of amphiregulin. *Cancer Res*. 63 (17):5218-5223.

Sharma RA, Gescher AJ, Steward WP. 2005. Curcumin: the story so far. *Eur J Cancer*. 41 (13):1955-1968.

Shin SK, Ha TY, McGregor RA, Choi MS. 2011. Long-term curcumin administration protects against atherosclerosis via hepatic regulation of lipoprotein cholesterol metabolism. *Mol Nutr Food Res*. 55 (12):1829-1840.

Shoba G, Joy D, Joseph T, Majeed M, Rajendran R, Srinivas PS.1998. Influence of piperine on the pharmacokinetics of curcumin in animals and human volunteers. *Planta Med*. 64 (4):353-356.

Shpitz B, Giladi N, Sagiv E, Lev-Ari S, Liberman E, Kazanov D *et al*. 2006. Celecoxib and curcumin additively inhibit the growth of colorectal cancer in a rat model. *Digestion*. 74 (3-4):140-144.

Singh RP, Jain DA. 2012. Antimicrobial Activity of hydrogenated derivatives of curcumin. *J Pharm Res*. 5 (7):3650-3653.

Singh S, Aggarwal BB. 1995. Activation of transcription factor NF-κB is suppressed by curcumin (diferuloylmethane). *J Biol Chem*. 270 (42):24995-25000.

Somparn P, Phisalaphong C, Nakornchai S, Unchern S, Morales NP. 2007. Comparative antioxidant activities of curcumin and its demethoxy and hydrogenated derivatives. *Biol Pharm Bull*. 30 (1):74-78.

Srimuangwong K, Tocharus C, Tocharus J, Suksamrarn A, Chintana PY. 2012a. Effects of hexahydrocurcumin in combination with 5-fluorouracil on dimethylhydrazine-induced colon cancer in rats. *World J Gastroenterol*. 18 (47):6951-6959.

Srimuangwong K, Tocharus C, Yoysungnoen Chintana P, Suksamrarn A, Tocharus J. 2012b. Hexahydrocurcumin enhances inhibitory effect of 5-fluorouracil on HT-29 human colon cancer cells. *World J Gastroenterol*. 18 (19):2383-2389.

Srivastava AK, Singh D, Roy BK. 2017. Structural interactions of curcumin biotransformed molecules with the N-terminal residues of cytotoxic-associated gene a protein provide insights into suppression of oncogenic activities. *Interdiscip Sci*. 9 (1):116-129.

Tan S, Rupasinghe TW, Tull DL, Boughton B, Oliver C, McSweeny C *et al*. 2014. Degradation of curcuminoids by *in vitro* pure culture fermentation. *J Agric Food Chem*. 62 (45):11005-11015.

Tep-Areenan P, Suksamrarn S. 2012. Mechanisms of vasorelaxation to gamma-mangostin in the rat aorta. *J Med Assoc Thai*. 95 Suppl 12:S63-8.

Tuohy KM, Conterno L, Gasperotti M, Viola R. 2012. Up-regulating the human intestinal microbiome using whole plant foods, polyphenols, and/or fiber. *J Agric Food Chem*. 60 (36):8776-8782.

Uehara SI, Yasuda I, Akiyama K, Morita H, Takeya K, Itokawa H. 1987. Diarylheptanoids from the rhizomes of *Curcuma xanthorrhiza* and *Alpinia officinarum*. *Chem Pharm Bull*. 35 (8):3298-3304.

Wang YJ, Pan MH, Cheng AL, Lin LI, Ho YS, Hsieh CY *et al*. 1997. Stability of curcumin in buffer solutions and characterization of its degradation products. *J Pharm Biomed Anal*. 15 (12):1867-1876.

Wicha P, Tocharus J, Janyou A, Jittiwat J, Changtam C, Suksamrarn A *et al*. 2017. Hexahydrocurcumin protects against cerebral ischemia/reperfusion injury, attenuates inflammation, and improves antioxidant defenses in a rat stroke model. *PloS One*. 12 (12):e0189211.

Williams KT, Schalinske KL. 2010. Homocysteine metabolism and its relation to health and disease. *Biofactors*. 36 (1):19-24.

Yamada H, Damiano V, Tsang A, Meranze D, Glasgow J, Abrams W *et al*. 1982. Neurtrophil degranulation in cadmium-chloride-induced acute lung inflammation. *Am J Pathol*. 109 (2):145-156

Younis AM, Ibrahim ARS, Ibrahim SM, AboulSoud KA, Kabbash AM. 2016. Microbial transformation of curcumin and evaluation of the biological activities of the isolated metabolites. *J Pharm Sci & Res*. 8 (10):1169-1178.

Zeng Y, Qiu F, Takahashi K, Liang J, Qu G, Yao X. 2007. New sesquiterpenes and calebin derivatives from *Curcuma longa*. *Chem Pharm Bull*. 55 (6):940-943.

Zhang W, Huang J, Wo X, Wang P. 2013. Microbial transformation of curcumin to its derivatives with a novel *Pichia kudriavzevii* ZJPH0802 strain. *Appl Biochem Biotechnol*.170 (5):1026-1037.

Zhao F, Gong Y, Hu Y, Lu M, Wang J, Dong J *et al*. 2015. Curcumin and its major metabolites inhibit the inflammatory response induced by lipopolysaccharide: Translocation of nuclear factor-κB as potential target. *Mol Med Rep*. 11 (4):3087-3093.

Chapter 5

Octahydrocurcumin (OHC)
The Final Reductive Metabolite of Curcumin

Scope of this Review

Curcumin, an important polyphenolic compound derived from *Curcuma longa* (turmeric), is well known for its pharmacological activities. The focus of this review is to enlighten the pharmacological properties of OHC.

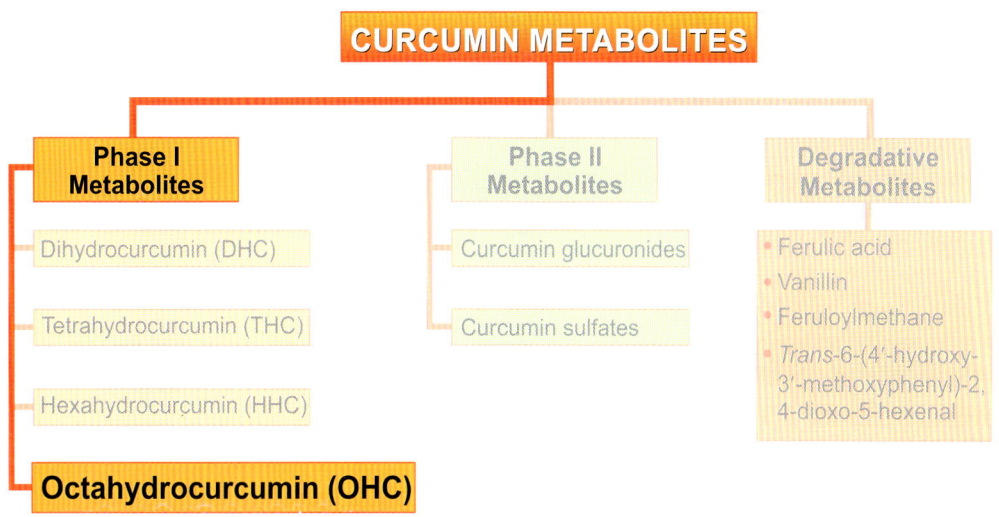

Chapter 5
OCTAHYDROCURCUMIN (OHC): THE FINAL REDUCTIVE METABOLITE OF CURCUMIN

Chapter 5
OCTAHYDROCURCUMIN (OHC): THE FINAL REDUCTIVE METABOLITE OF CURCUMIN

Introduction

Curcumin undergoes rapid metabolism primarily by reduction followed by conjugation after oral administration (Schneider *et al.*, 2015). Consecutive reduction of the double bonds in the heptadienedione chain results in the formation of several-reduced forms including THC, HHC, and OHC in the liver as well as intestinal mucosa by phase I metabolism, in which the hexahydro product is a major metabolite and much smaller amounts of the products are OHC, THC, and DHC (Ireson *et al.*, 2002). Octahydrocurcumin, also known as hexahydrocurcuminol or 1,7-bis(4'-hydroxy-3'-methoxyphenyl)-heptane-3,5-diol is the final reductive metabolite of curcumin.

Natural Occurrence

Uehara *et al.* (1987) isolated OHC along with other diarylheptanoids from rhizomes of *C. xanthorrhiza* of the family Zingiberaceae. In an earlier study, OHC has been isolated from *Z. officinale* (Kikuzaki *et al.*, 1991) and *A. officinarum*. In a recent study, Jia *et al.* also identified OHC during characterization of curcuminoids in turmeric using UHPLC-QTOF-MS/MS (Jia *et al.*, 2017).

Preparation of OHC by Hydrogenation

Octahydrocurcumin is derived from HHC by hydrogenation or by reduction with sodium borohydride (Hoehle *et al.*, 2006). Somparn *et al.* reported the synthesis of OHC via a two steps process (Somparn *et al.*, 2007). First, curcumin was converted to THC by hydrogenation with palladium-carbon (Pd/C) as the catalyst (Roughley and Whiting, 1973), and then HHC and OHC were synthesized from THC by reduction with sodium borohydride (Venkateswarlu *et al.*, 2001). Recently, Moohammadaree *et al.* have synthesized HHC, THC and OHC through the catalytic hydrogenation reaction of curcumin in alcohol solvent over a period of five hours with palladium on charcoal. Octahydrocurcumin was obtained in 11% yield from the mixture after purification over silica gel column chromatography (Moohammadaree *et al.*, 2015).

Biotransformation - In vivo

Earlier reports indicate that the enzyme responsible for the bioreduction of curcuminoids have been found to reside in the cytosol of liver and intestine and that include alcohol dehydrogenase (Hoehle *et al.*, 2006). Curcumin and its reduced metabolites appear to be easily conjugated *in vivo* and *in vitro*. After systemic absorption, alcohol dehydrogenase reduces curcumin to THC and HHC in the liver, whereas formation of DHC and OHC required an unidentified microsomal enzyme (Schneider *et al.*, 2015), citing the previous publications (Hoehle *et al.*, 2006; Ireson *et al.*, 2001 & 2002).

However, Ireson *et al.* reported that the candidate enzyme responsible for the final reduction step, the generation of OHC from HHC in microsomes is cytochrome P450 reductase, but suggested that it has to be experimentally confirmed (Ireson *et al.*, 2002).

Two phases of curcumin metabolism in the liver and intestine of rats and humans, and in the plasma of mice, have been reported; phase I metabolism comprises the reduction of the four double bonds of the heptadiene-3,5-dione structure: namely, curcumin **(1)** → DHC **(6)** → THC **(7)** → HHC **(8)** → OHC **(9)** (Fig. 131). During phase II, curcumin and its reduced metabolites are conjugated as a monoglucuronide, a monosulfate and a mixed sulfate/glucuronide (Hoehle *et al.*, 2006; Ireson *et al.*, 2001 & 2002; Pan *et al.*, 1999).

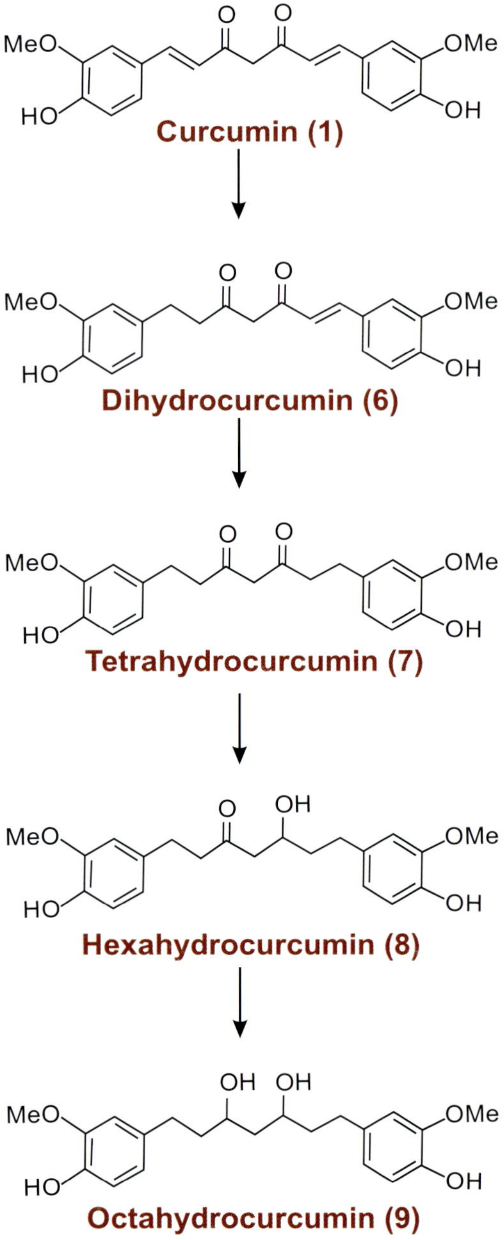

Chapter 5
OCTAHYDROCURCUMIN (OHC): THE FINAL REDUCTIVE METABOLITE OF CURCUMIN

Fig. 131: Chemical structures of reductive metabolites of curcumin in rat liver.
(Adapted from Hoehle *et al.*, 2006)

Chapter 5
OCTAHYDROCURCUMIN (OHC): THE FINAL REDUCTIVE METABOLITE OF CURCUMIN

Microbial Transformation of Curcumin to OHC

Biotransformation is the modification of a definite compound to a distinct product with structural similarity, using biological catalysts including microorganisms like fungi, bacteria and even cell-free systems. In this context, Maehara *et al*. investigated the microbial conversion of curcumin by using endophytic fungi, especially by *Diaporthe sp* (CLO-13) associated with the rhizome of *C. longa* and identified the existence of (3*S*, 5*S*) form of OHC **(21)**, *meso*-OHC **(22)**, along with compounds **(19)** and **(20)** (Figs. 132 & 133) (Maehara *et al*., 2011).

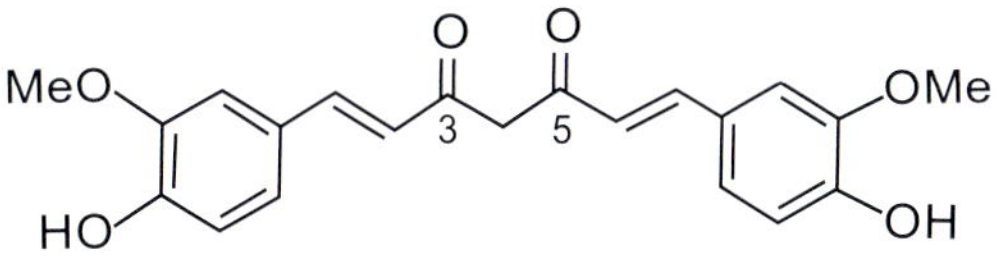

Curcumin (1)

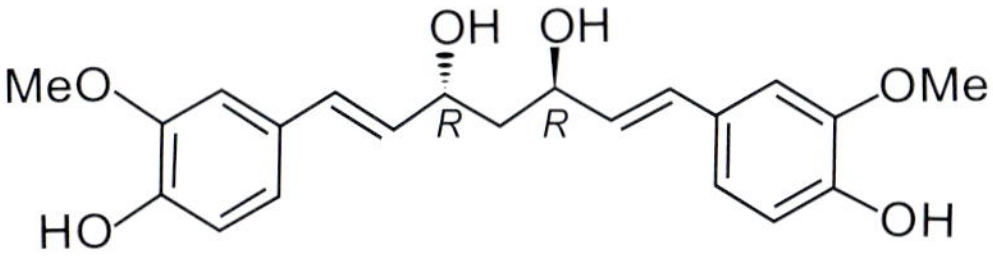

(3*R*,5*R*)-tetrahydrocurcumin (19)

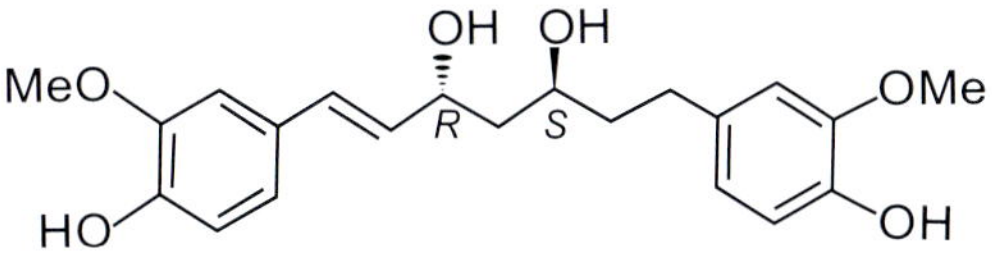

Neohexahydrocurcumin (20)

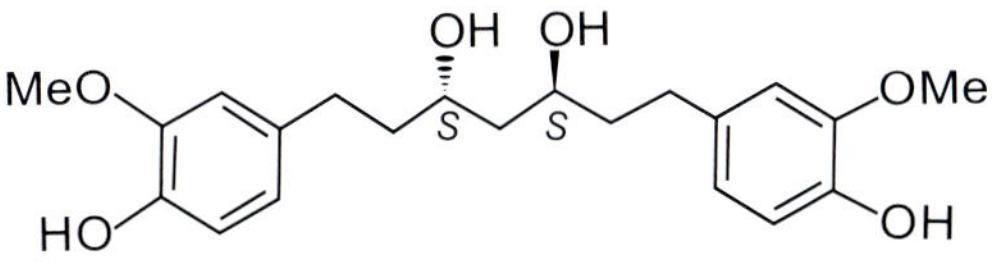

(3*S*,5*S*)-octahydrocurcumin (21)

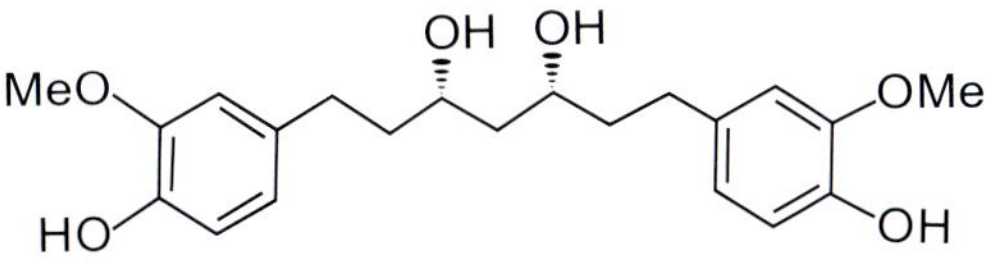

***Meso*-octahydrocurcumin (22)**

Fig. 132: Chemical structures of curcumin and its microbial conversion products.
(Adapted from Maehara *et al*., 2011)

OCTAHYDROCURCUMIN (OHC): THE FINAL REDUCTIVE METABOLITE OF CURCUMIN

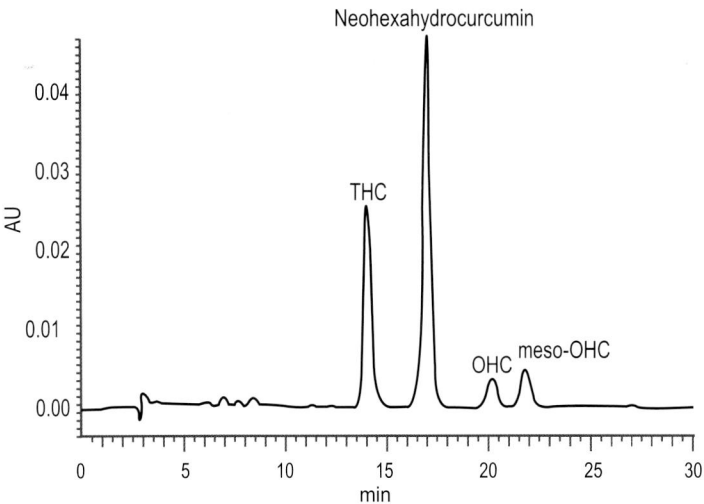

Fig. 133: HPLC profile of microbial conversion products [2 days after adding curcumin]. (Adapted from Maehara *et al.*, 2011)

Studies conducted by Younis *et al.* on biotransformation of curcumin using the fungal strain *Alternaria alternate* confirmed the presence of OHC. In this study, curcumin was fermented for two weeks and extracted with ethyl acetate. The ethyl acetate layer was evaporated and the product was further purified over column chromatography to obtain HHC and OHC in pure form (Younis *et al.*, 2016).

Biotransformation of Curcumin to OHC by Gut Microbiota

In a recent study, Li *et al.* fed a diet containing curcumin (0.05% w/w) to male CD-1 mice for 5 weeks and showed that curcumin has undergone phase I metabolism in the small intestine to yield HHC and OHC, its two major metabolites. It was reported that during the Phase II metabolism, curcumin, HHC and OHC were converted to their respective conjugates namely, glucuronides and sulfates in the small intestine. However, curcumin, HHC and OHC were also found to exist as non-conjugated forms in the cecum perhaps may be due to the action of gut microbiota. These findings suggest that gut microbiota in the cecum and colon plays an important role in the deconjugation process of the phase II metabolites that converts them back again to their respective phase I metabolites (Li *et al.*, 2017).

Pharmacological Significance

Antioxidant Potential

Inhibition of peroxidation

Curcumin, the main chemical constituent of turmeric rhizome, is well-known for its potent antioxidant effect. However, Maehara *et al.* reported that the curcumin converted products showed antioxidant activity by inhibiting the peroxidation of microsomal and mitochondrial lipids prepared from rat liver (Table 17) (Maehara *et al.*, 2011).

Table 17: Effect of OHC on mitochondrial and microsomal lipid peroxidation.
(Adapted from Maehara et al., 2011)

	IC$_{50}$ (μg/mL)	
	Mitochondria	Microsome
Curcumin	8.9	30.1
THC	6.8	7.0
Neo-HHC	8.9	12.5
OHC	13.4	27.6
Meso-OHC	13.5	28.1

Lower the IC$_{50}$ value, better the activity

It has been shown that the degree of inhibition of lipid peroxidation based on the IC$_{50}$ values in rat mitochondria was in the order of THC > Curcumin > OHC. The results indicate that OHC inhibited peroxidation of microsomes compared to curcumin (8.9 μg/mL) at a higher IC$_{50}$ value of 13.4 μg/mL.

DPPH radical scavenging

Antioxidant properties of individual curcuminoids (Curcumin, DMC and BDMC), and hydrogenated derivatives, namely THC, HHC, and OHC were assessed using DPPH radical assay. Curcumin and its derivatives, including OHC have comparable potencies in scavenging DPPH radical antioxidant activities than trolox. Based on the IC$_{50}$ values, the scavenging activity of OHC was found to be significant (23.6 μM) and comparable to those of HHC (21.6 μM) and curcumin (35.1 μM) (Somparn et al., 2007).

However, in a recent study, Morales et al. showed that while curcumin had comparable radical scavenging activity as the reference antioxidant trolox, the hydrogenated derivatives of curcumin including OHC showed significantly higher DPPH scavenging efficacy compared to curcumin (Table 18). The relative rank order of the DPPH scavenging potency of curcumin and its derivatives based on the IC$_{50}$ values is as follows: OHC > DMC ≥ THC ≥ HHC > Curcumin = Trolox >> BDMC (Morales et al., 2015).

Table 18: The IC_{50} and scavenging capacity values of DPPH by curcumin and its derivatives.
(Adapted from Morales *et al.*, 2015)

	DPPH	
	IC_{50} (μM)	Scavenging capacity (mol/mol test compound)
Curcumin	38.4 ± 1.4	3.4
DMC	20.9 ± 1.6	3.1
BDMC	85.6 ± 6.0	1.7
THC	20.7 ± 2.1	4.1
HHC	23.4 ± 1.7	3.7
OHC	14.7 ± 1.9	3.8
Trolox	39.3 ± 2.1	1.7

Values are mean ± SD of three independent experiments.

Lower the IC_{50} value, better the activity

Earlier, Deters *et al.* reported that the DPPH radical scavenging activities of dihydroferulic acid, ferulic acid and curcumin were in the middle range with IC_{50} values of 19.5, 37 and 40 μM respectively. The lowest effects as radical scavengers were observed in experiments with vanillin, isocurcumin, diacetylcurcumin and BDMC with IC_{50} values higher than 100 μM. Based on these results, the authors concluded that reduction of the 1,6-heptadiene structure (THC, HHC, and OHC) increases the radical scavenging effects of curcumin (Deters *et al.*, 2008).

In summary, reduced metabolites of curcumin exhibited stronger DPPH scavenging activity compared to curcumin.

Effect on AAPH-induced red blood cell hemolysis

Somparn *et al.* studied the effects of curcumin and its metabolites on AAPH-induced hemolysis in red blood cells and compared their effects with trolox, a standard antioxidant. Curcumin and its metabolites have been shown to exert significant protective effects by reducing the red blood cell hemolysis induced by AAPH. It was observed that the order of inhibitory activity was as follows: OHC > THC = HHC > Trolox > Curcumin = DMC (Somparn *et al.*, 2007).

Inhibition of AAPH-induced linoleic acid oxidation

Curcumin and its metabolites THC, HHC, and OHC at 3 µM concentration decreased the rate of conjugated diene formation during linoleic acid oxidation about 2 to 6 fold more potently than trolox, a standard derivative of vitamin E with antioxidant properties. Further analysis using AAPH-induced linoleic oxidation model showed that the antioxidant activity of OHC was significant (40.3 ± 8.3) and comparable to curcumin and HHC (46.2 ± 8.1 and 30.8 ± 3.3 respectively) (Table 19) (Somparn *et al.*, 2007).

Table 19: Antioxidant activities of curcumin and its derivatives on the rate of AAPH-induced oxidation of linoleic acid. (Adapted from Somparn *et al.*, 2007)

Antioxidant	R_{inh}/R_o [a]	Antioxidant activity (min/µM) [b]	n [c]
Curcumin	0.09 ± 0.01*	46.2 ± 8.1*	2.7
DMC	0.26 ± 0.02*,**	20.3 ± 2.8**	2.0
BDMC	0.30 ± 0.01*,**	10.0 ± 1.2**	1.4
THC	0.13 ± 0.01*,**	69.3 ± 6.6*,**	3.4
HHC	0.20 ± 0.03*,**,†	30.8 ± 3.3*,**,†	3.8
OHC	0.19 ± 0.02*,**,†	40.3 ± 8.3*,†	3.1
Trolox	0.51 ± 0.03	16.0 ± 1.2	2.0

Values are mean ± SD of 3 independent experiments; *p<0.05 vs. Trolox; **p<0.05 vs. Curcumin; †p<0.05 vs. THC.
[a] The initial rates of oxidation in the presence of 3 µM antioxidant (except BDMC 12 µM) compared to the control.
[b] Slope of the plot between inhibition time (T_{inh}) vs. Antioxidant concentrations.
[c] n represents the stoichiometric number of peroxyl radicals trapped per molecule of antioxidant.
R_{inh}: Initial Oxidation Rate; R_o: Absence of Antioxidant; T_{inh}: Inhibition Time

Anti-inflammatory Potential

Effect on Nitric oxide (NO)

Zhao *et al*. compared the anti-inflammatory activity of curcumin and its three metabolites THC, HHC and OHC with varying concentrations ranging from 3.125 to 25 µM, in LPS-stimulated RAW 264.7 macrophage cells. The results of the study showed that overproduction of LPS-induced NO was significantly inhibited by curcumin and its metabolites in a dose-dependent manner. In addition, the inhibitory effect of OHC on the LPS- induced NO overproduction was significant at 25 µM (Fig. 134) (Zhao *et al*., 2015).

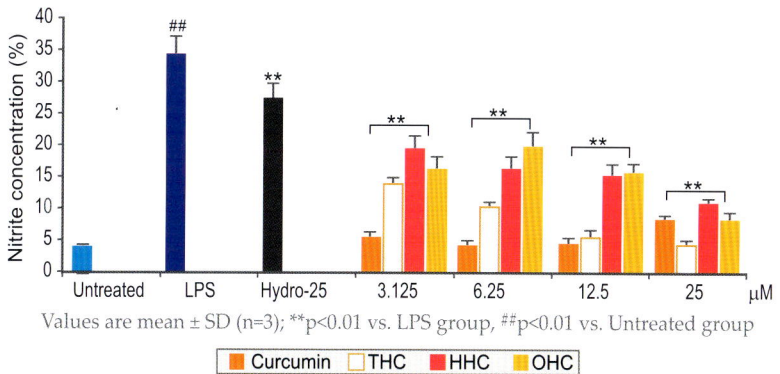

Fig. 134: Dose-dependent effects of curcumin and its metabolites on nitrite concentration in RAW 264.7 cells. (Adapted from Zhao *et al*., 2015)

Effect on iNOS and COX-2

Zhao *et al*. investigated the inhibitory effects of curcumin and its metabolites on iNOS, and cyclooxygenase 2 (COX-2) in RAW 264.7 cells. It has been shown that curcumin and its three metabolites were able to inhibit LPS-induced up regulation of iNOS and COX-2 expression. At the same time, curcumin was found to exert more potent effect on LPS-stimulated RAW 264.7 cells. Among the three metabolites of curcumin, OHC showed moderate inhibition on the iNOS and COX-2 expression (Fig. 135) (Zhao *et al*., 2015).

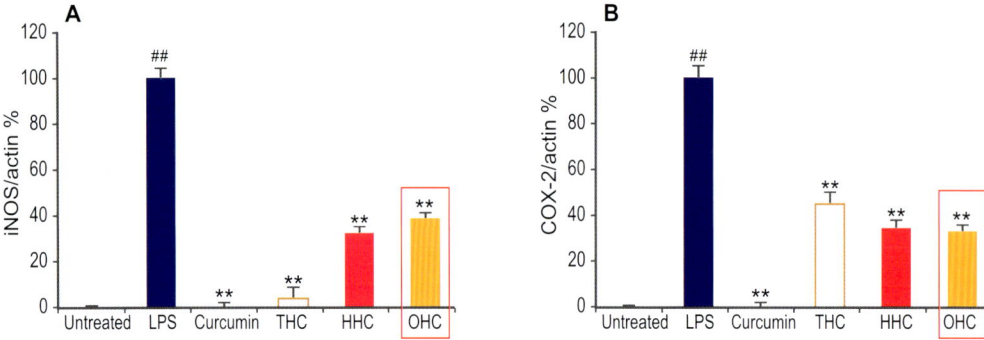

Values are mean ± SD (n=3); **$p<0.01$ vs. LPS group, ##$p<0.01$ vs. Untreated group

Fig. 135: Effect of curcumin and its metabolites on inhibition of iNOS (A) and COX-2 (B) expression in LPS-induced RAW 264.7 cells. (Adapted from Zhao *et al.*, 2015)

Earlier, using similar *in vitro* models, Pan *et al.* investigated the inhibitory effects of curcumin and its metabolites, THC, HHC, and OHC, on the induction of NO synthase (iNOS) in RAW 264.7 cells that are pre-activated with LPS (Pan *et al.*, 1999). Western blotting and Northern blotting analyses demonstrated that curcumin strongly reduced the protein and mRNA levels of iNOS in LPS-activated macrophages compared to its metabolites, THC, HHC, and OHC.

Effect on IκB kinases

The anti-inflammatory effect of curcumin and its metabolite OHC was measured by examining the activities on NF-κB. As presented in Figs. 136A & 136B, when compared with the effect of curcumin on cytoplasmic IκB-α protein and the nuclear protein p65, OHC was found to be more effective, suggesting a potential role of OHC on anti-inflammatory activities.

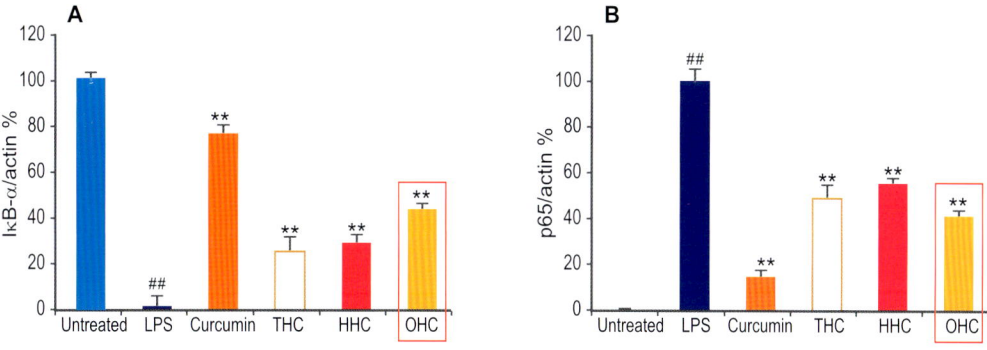

Values are mean ± SD(n=3); **p<0.01 vs. LPS only group, ##p<0.01 vs. Untreated group.

Fig. 136: Densitometric analysis of cytoplasmic IκB-α (A) and nuclear p65 protein (B) expression. β-actin was used as an internal control. (Adapted from Zhao et al., 2015)

In a similar study, earlier Pan *et al.* reported that curcumin inhibits IκB kinase 1 (IKK1) and IκB kinase 2 (IKK2) activities induced by LPS. However, THC, HHC, and OHC were less active against IκB kinase 1 (IKK1) and IκB kinase 2 (IKK2) activities (Pan et al., 1999).

Effect and mechanisms of OHC under inflammatory conditions

Recently, Zhang *et al.* (2018a) compared the *in vivo* anti-inflammatory effects of OHC and curcumin using three common inflammatory animal models, namely

a) Xylene-induced ear edema in mice

b) The vascular permeability assay using acetic acid-induced murine model

c) Carrageen-induced paw edema, a non-immune and an acute inflammatory model

The results indicated that OHC in a dose-dependent manner suppressed the formation of ear edema induced by xylene (Fig. 137A), inhibited the Evans blue dye leakage in peritoneal cavity elicited by acetic acid (Fig. 137B) and reduced paw edema provoked by carrageenan (Fig. 137C).

Chapter 5
OCTAHYDROCURCUMIN (OHC): THE FINAL REDUCTIVE METABOLITE OF CURCUMIN

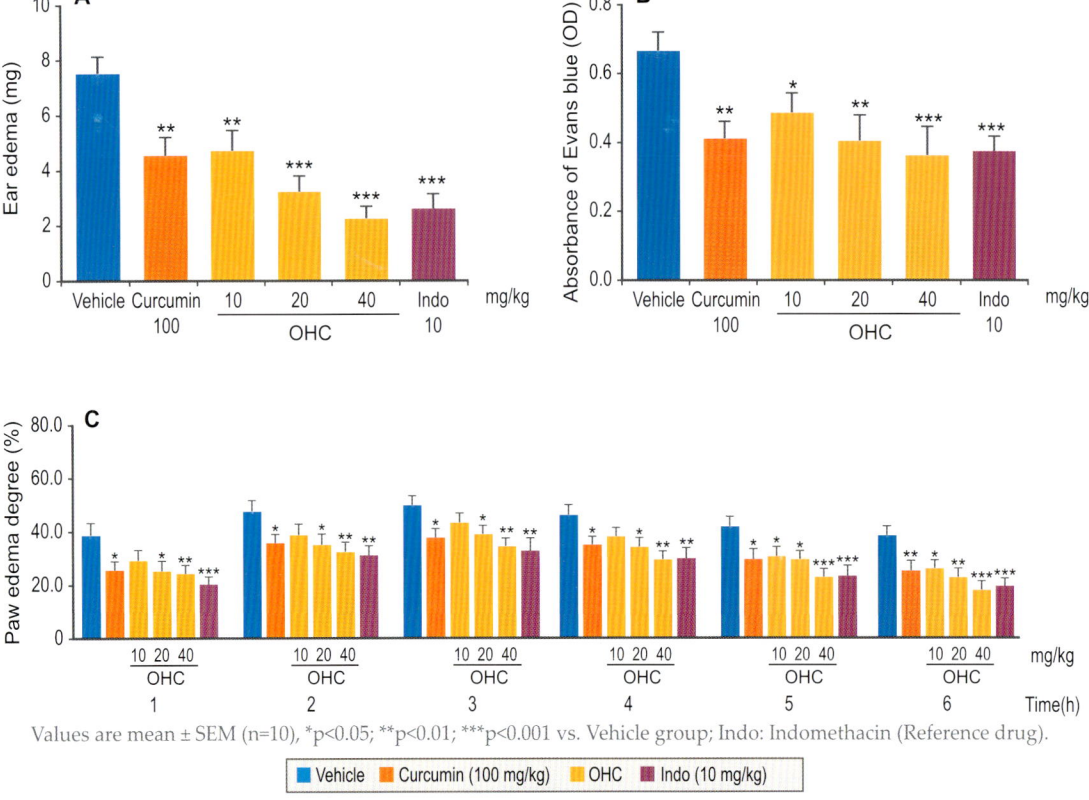

Fig. 137: Effect of OHC on xylene-induced ear edema (A), acetic-acid-induced vascular permeability (B) and carrageenan-induced paw edema (C) in mice.
(Adapted from Zhang *et al.*, 2018a)

The results revealed that OHC has an excellent safety profile with LD_{50} value greater than 10,000 mg/kg surpassing that of curcumin. Also, OHC was shown to suppress IL-1β, IL-6, TNF-α and PGE2 at the tissue level, suggesting its ability to alleviate acute inflammation by inhibiting pro-inflammatory mediators. In addition, OHC significantly inhibited COX-2 expression without affecting COX-1. Importantly, by inhibiting the levels of pro-inflammatory mediators and suppressing the expression of COX-2, OHC was shown to be more effective than curcumin. Based on the results it was indicated that OHC might possess a superior COX-2 selective inhibitory effect than curcumin.

The authors (Zhang *et al.*, 2018a) suggested that the difference in the *in vivo* anti-inflammatory activities of OHC and curcumin may be due to their structural differences. Hydrogenation at conjugated double bonds of the pentadiene and β-diketone of curcumin and its conversion to OHC could be attributed to a significant increase in the anti-inflammatory effects in carrageenan-induced mouse paw edema. It was also shown that suppression of NF-κB pathways through the inactivation of TAK1, inhibition of COX-2 and other mediators of inflammation are responsible for the potent anti-inflammatory effects of OHC. It was concluded that OHC mediates more pronounced anti-inflammatory effects than curcumin, suggesting that OHC might be one of the important bioactive anti-inflammatory metabolites of curcumin *in vivo*, and a promising new chemical entity for further development of potent anti-inflammatory therapeutics.

Immunosuppressive Effect

Deters *et al.* investigated the inhibitory effects of THC, HHC, OHC and curcumin using mouse anti-human CD3 antibody (OKT3)-induced proliferation of human peripheral blood mononuclear cell (PBMC). It was found that the immunosuppressive effect of OHC was lower than that of curcumin. The authors suggest that the number of carbon atoms of the 1,6-heptadiene-3,5-dione structure was more important for the inhibitory effect (Deters *et al.*, 2008), however a synergistic effect of OHC and curcumin could enhance the total immunosuppressive effects.

Hepatoprotective Potential

Acetaminophen (APAP) overdose is a leading cause of drug-induced hepatotoxicity that accounts for more than 40% of acute liver failure in the United States, Great Britain and Europe (Lee, 2017). Hepatotoxicity due to APAP overdose is associated with oxidative stress. In a recent study, Luo *et al.* (2019) investigated the potential mechanisms of OHC against APAP-induced hepatotoxicity in comparison with curcumin using male Kunming mice. Findings of this study showed that pretreatment of mice with OHC (100 mg/kg bw) substantially attenuated liver histopathological changes (Fig. 138) and enhanced liver function by decreasing the serum levels of alanine transaminase (ALT) and aspartate aminotransferase (AST) in a dose-dependent manner (Figs. 139A & 139B).

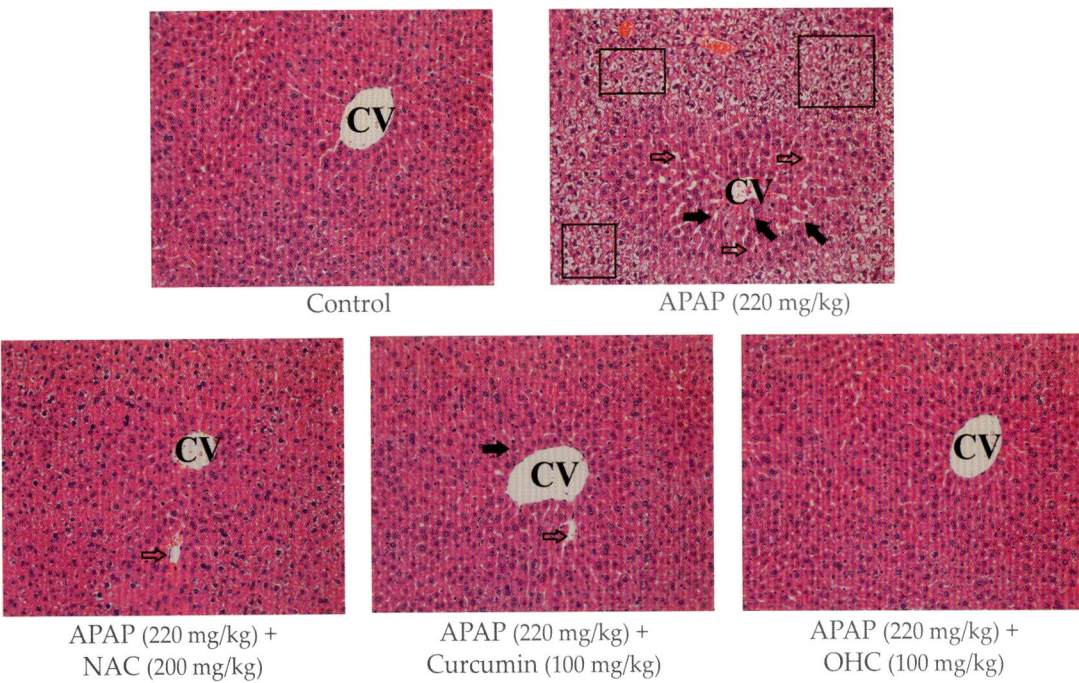

CV: Central vessel; Solid arrows: Inflammatory cell infiltration; Open arrow: Sinusoidal dilation; Rectangle: Vacuolation; The scale indicates 50 μm; APAP: Acetaminophen; NAC: N-acetyl cysteine.

Fig. 138: Effects of OHC and curcumin on the liver histological alternations (original magnification × 100). (Adapted from Luo *et al.*, 2019)

Chapter 5
OCTAHYDROCURCUMIN (OHC): THE FINAL REDUCTIVE METABOLITE OF CURCUMIN

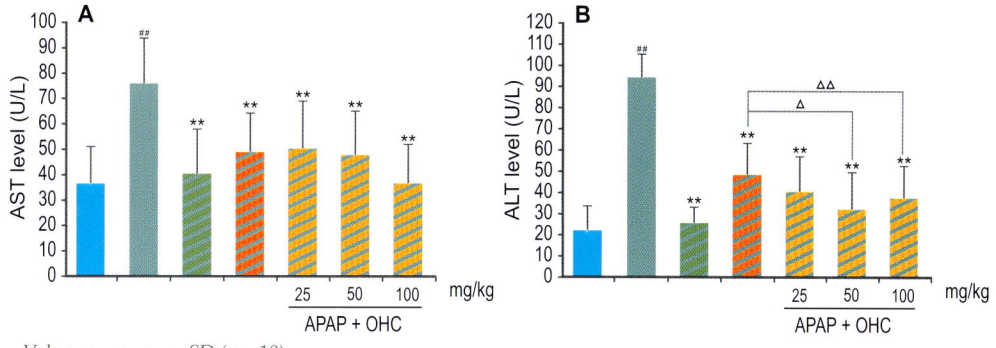

Values are mean ± SD (n = 10).
##p<0.01 vs. Control group; **p<0.01 vs. APAP-treated group; Δp< 0.05, ΔΔp< 0.01 vs. Curcumin group;
APAP: Acetaminophen; NAC: N-acetyl cysteine; AST: Aspartate transaminase; ALT: Alanine transaminase.

Fig. 139: Effects of OHC and curcumin on the levels of AST (A) and ALT (B) in serum.
(Adapted from Luo *et al.*, 2019)

Besides, OHC significantly restored the hepatic antioxidant status by reducing the level of malondialdehyde (MDA) and ROS. Furthermore, OHC as an antioxidant increased the levels of GSH, SOD, CAT and T-AOC (total antioxidant capacity). In addition, OHC markedly suppressed the activity and expressions of CYP2E1 at the mRNA level by 2-fold. Moreover, OHC activated the Keap1-Nrf2 pathway and enormously enhanced the translational activation of Nrf2-targeted genes against oxidative stress, via inhibiting the expression of Keap1 and blocking the interaction between Keap1 and Nrf2. Particularly, OHC exerted superior hepatoprotective and antioxidant activities compared to curcumin.

Anticancer Activity

Attempts have been made to investigate the anti-tumor effect and underlying mechanism of OHC, a hydrogenated metabolite of curcumin in comparison with curcumin, the parent compound, in a mouse hepatoma 22 (H22) cells-induced ascites tumor mice model (Zhang *et al.*, 2018b). It has been reported that treatment with OHC (5, 10 and 20 mg/kg) exerted a dose-dependent decrease on the mortality of mice compared to the mice in the vehicle (tumor control), implying that OHC might possess effective anti-hepatocellular carcinoma (HCC) effect. It was also observed that OHC significantly decreased the body weight of the tumor-bearing mice (Fig. 140A), abdominal circumference, volume of ascites and cancer cell viability as compared to the vehicle control. Importantly, OHC (20 mg/kg) treatment significantly enhanced the survival rate of mice similar to cyclophosphamide (CTX), a reference drug, treated group than that of the curcumin (100 mg/kg) as shown in Fig. 140B, suggesting that OHC might be more effective than curcumin in suppressing the H22-induced ascites tumor in mice.

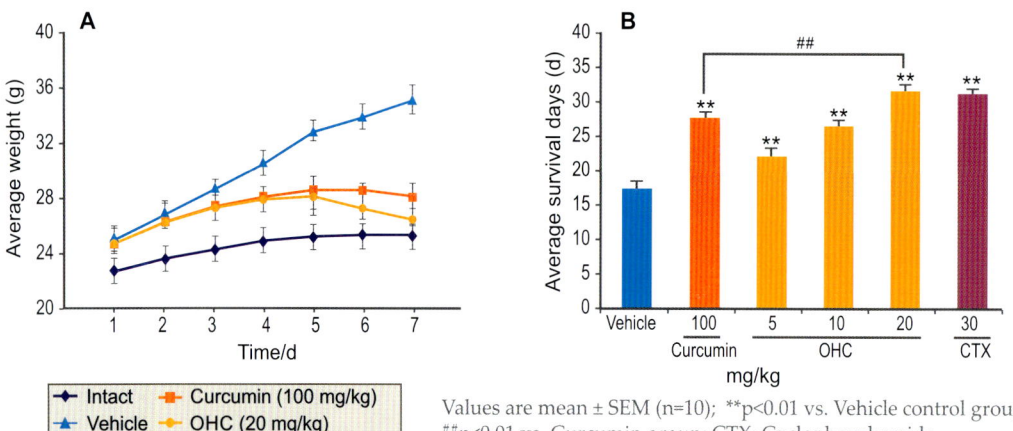

Fig. 140: Effects of OHC on the survival rate, body weight in ascites tumor-bearing mice. (A) The change in body weight (B) The average survival days of CTX, curcumin and OHC in tumor-bearing mice. (Adapted from Zhang *et al.*, 2018b)

The overall findings suggest that OHC had a relatively wide margin of safety at a dose ranging from 5 to 20 mg/kg, and exhibited superior effect compared to curcumin in suppressing the tumor growth, including body weight of the tumor-bearing mice, abdominal circumference, ascites volume and cancer cells viability.

Mechanistically, it has been reported that OHC significantly induced H22 cells apoptosis by upregulating the p53 expression, an important pro-apoptotic protein that plays a major role in cancer development and progression to activate the mitochondrial pathway by interacting with the Bcl-2 family protein (Purvis *et al.*, 2012; Yang *et al.*, 2013) and downregulating the MDM2 expression, a negative regulator of p53 (Haupt *et al.*, 1997). In addition, OHC also remarkably decreased the Bcl-2 and Bcl-xl protein expressions, and increased the Bax and Bad expressions in ascitic cells. Importantly, OHC substantially induced the release of cytochrome c, caspase-3, caspase-9 and the cleavage of PARP to induce H22 cells apoptosis. Thus, OHC was more effective in suppressing H22-induced HCC through activation of the mitochondrial apoptosis pathway and thus be a promising anti-HCC agent (Zhang *et al.*, 2018b).

Conclusion

The summary of this review emphasizes the fact that while curcumin is well known for its pharmacological activities, some specific activities of octahydrocurcumin are also equally important contributing to the total health benefits of curcumin. The existing body of evidence suggests that octahydrocurcumin is a very safe material possessing superior antioxidant properties while sharing anti-inflammatory activity of curcumin.

Chapter 5
OCTAHYDROCURCUMIN (OHC): THE FINAL REDUCTIVE METABOLITE OF CURCUMIN

References

Deters M, Knochenwefel H, Lindhorst D, Koal T, Meyer HH, Hansel W *et al*. 2008. Different curcuminoids inhibit T-lymphocyte proliferation independently of their radical scavenging activities. *Pharm Res*. 25(8):1822-1827.

Haupt Y, Maya R, Kazaz A, Oren M. 1997. Mdm2 promotes the rapid degradation of p53. *Nature*. 387(6630): 296-299.

Hoehle SI, Pfeiffer E, Solyom AM, Metzler M. 2006. Metabolism of curcuminoids in tissue slices and subcellular fractions from rat liver. *J Agric Food Chem*. 54(3):756-764.

Ireson C, Orr S, Jones DJ, Verschoyle R, Lim CK, Luo JL *et al*. 2001. Characterization of metabolites of the chemopreventive agent curcumin in human and rat hepatocytes and in the rat *in vivo*, and evaluation of their ability to inhibit phorbol ester-induced prostaglandin E2 production. *Cancer Res*. 61(3):1058-1064.

Ireson CR, Jones DJ, Orr S, Coughtrie MW, Boocock DJ, Williams ML *et al*. 2002. Metabolism of the cancer chemopreventive agent curcumin in human and rat intestine. *Cancer Epidemiol Biomarkers Prev*. 11(1):105-111.

Jia S, Du Z, Song C, Jin S, Zhang Y, Feng Y *et al*. 2017. Identification and characterization of curcuminoids in turmeric using ultra-high performance liquid chromatography-quadrupole time of flight tandem mass spectrometry. *J Chromatogr A*. 1521:110-122.

Kikuzaki, H, Kobayashi, M, Nakatani, N. 1991. Constituents of Zingiberaceae. Part 4. Diarylheptanoids from rhizomes of *Zingiber officinale*. *Phytochemistry*. 30(11):3647-3651.

Lee WM. 2017. Acetaminophen (APAP) hepatotoxicity-Isn't it time for APAP to go away? *J Hepatol*. 67(6): 1324-1331.

Li Z, Sun Y, Song M, Li F, Xiao H. 2017. Gut microbiota dictate metabolic fate of curcumin in the colon. *The FASEB J*. 31(1 Supplement):646.612-646.612.

Luo DD, Chen JF, Liu JJ, Xie JH, Zhang ZB, Gu JY *et al*. 2019. Tetrahydrocurcumin and octahydrocurcumin, the primary and final hydrogenated metabolites of curcumin, possess superior hepatic-protective effect against acetaminophen-induced liver injury: Role of CYP2E1 and Keap1-Nrf2 pathway. *Food Chem Toxicol*. 123:349-362.

Maehara S, Ikeda M, Haraguchi H, Kitamura C, Nagoe T, Ohashi K *et al*. 2011. Microbial conversion of curcumin into colorless hydroderivatives by the endophytic fungus *Diaporthe* sp. associated with *Curcuma longa*. *Chem Pharm Bull*. 59(8):1042-1044.

Chapter 5
OCTAHYDROCURCUMIN (OHC): THE FINAL REDUCTIVE METABOLITE OF CURCUMIN

Moohammadaree A, Changtam C, Wicha P, Suksamrarn A, Tocharus J, Tocharus C. 2015. Mechanisms of vasorelaxation induced by hexahydrocurcumin in isolated rat thoracic aorta. *Phytother Res*. 29(11):1806-1813.

Morales NP, Sirijaroonwong S, Yamanont P, Phisalaphong C. 2015. Electron paramagnetic resonance study of the free radical scavenging capacity of curcumin and its demethoxy and hydrogenated derivatives. *Biol Pharm Bull*. 38(10):1478-1483.

Pan MH, Huang TM, Lin JK. 1999. Biotransformation of curcumin through reduction and glucuronidation in mice. *Drug Metab Dispos*. 27(4):486-494.

Purvis JE, Karhohs KW, Mock C, Batchelor E, Loewer A, Lahav G. 2012. p53 dynamics control cell fate. *Science*. 336(6087):1440-1444.

Roughley PJ, Whiting DA. 1973. Experiments in the biosynthesis of curcumin. *J Chem Soc Perkin Trans*.1:2379-2388.

Schneider C, Gordon ON, Edwards RL, Luis PB. 2015. Degradation of curcumin: from mechanism to biological implications. *J Agric Food Chem*. 63(35):7606-7614.

Somparn P, Phisalaphong C, Nakornchai S, Unchern S, Morales NP. 2007. Comparative antioxidant activities of curcumin and its demethoxy and hydrogenated derivatives. *Biol Pharm Bull*. 30(1):74-78.

Uehara SI, Yasuda I, Akiyama K, Morita H, Takeya K, Itokawa H. 1987. Diarylheptanoids from the rhizomes of *Curcuma xanthorrhiza* and *Alpinia officinarum*. *Chem Pharm Bull*. 35(8):3298-3304.

Venkateswarlu S, Ramachandra MS, Rambabu M, Subbaraju GV. 2001. Synthesis of gingerenone-A and hirsutenone. *Indian J Chem. B*; 40:495-497.

Yang Y, Xia T, Li N, Zhang J, Yang Y, Cong W *et al*. 2013. Combined effects of p53 and MDM2 polymorphisms on susceptibility and surgical prognosis in hepatitis B virus-related hepatocellular carcinoma. *Protein Cell*. 4(1):71-81.

Younis AM, Ibrahim ARS, Ibrahim SM, AboulSoud KA, Kabbash AM. 2016. Microbial transformation of curcumin and evaluation of the biological activities of the isolated metabolites. *J Pharm Sci & Res*. 8(10):1169-1178.

Zhang ZB, Luo, DD, Xie JH, Xian YF, Lai ZQ, Liu YH *et al*. 2018a. Curcumin's metabolites, tetrahydrocurcumin and octahydrocurcumin, possess superior anti-inflammatory effects *in vivo* through suppression of TAK1-NF-κB pathway. *Front Pharmacol*. 9:1181.

Zhang Z, Luo D, Xie J, Lin G, Zhou J, Liu W *et al*. 2018b. Octahydrocurcumin, a final hydrogenated metabolite of curcumin, possesses superior anti-tumor activity through induction of cellular apoptosis. *Food Funct*. 9(4):2005-2014.

Zhao F, Gong Y, Hu Y, Lu M, Wang J, Dong J *et al*. 2015. Curcumin and its major metabolites inhibit the inflammatory response induced by lipopolysaccharide: Translocation of nuclear factor-κB as potential target. *Mol Med Rep*. 11(4):3087-3093.

Epilogue

Curcuminoids are one of the dominant dietary supplements enjoying the confidence of the populace. While the health benefits of curcuminoids are indisputable, their mechanism of action presents an interesting mystery especially given that they are not soluble in water and hence perceived to be poorly bioavailable in the body. While various theories had been proposed and concerted efforts had been expended to increase the bioavailability of curcuminoids, the importance of curcuminoid metabolites has been relegated to the background. The preceding chapters bring out the various pharmacological actions of the reductive metabolites of curcumin in great detail. Thus, it stands to reason that these reductive metabolites of curcuminoids jointly work with curcumin in conferring the health benefits.

Sabinsa's curcuminoids product, Curcumin C3 Complex®, has been the most studied product in the world. With a large number of clinical and preclinical studies supporting its premier position, Sabinsa's Curcumin C3 Complex® is the leading product in the market. With the importance of the reductive metabolites of curcuminoids being recognized more and more, Sabinsa introduced C3 Reduct®, a product based on curcumin metabolites, Tetrahydrocurcuminoids, which is gaining increasing importance as attested by numerous studies and increasing utility. The GRAS status of C3 Reduct® should further expand the horizon of its usage pattern. It appears clear that a bright future awaits the reductive metabolites of curcuminoids.

It is fit to state that the reductive metabolites of curcuminoids are now finally emerging from the long shadow of curcumin and proffer themselves as potential nutrients.

Glossary

5-FU
5-Fluorouracil: A drug commonly used in the treatment of cancer.

8-OHdG
8-Hydroxy-2'-deoxyguanosine: The most representative product of oxidative modifications of DNA, urinary 8-OHdG and potentially the best non-invasive biomarker of oxidative damage to DNA.

A549 cells
A widely utilized human lung cancer cells to study a variety of molecular characteristics for human tumors in culture.

AAPH
2,2'-Azobis (2-amidinopropane) dihydrochloride: A water-soluble, heat-labile azo compound which undergoes thermal decomposition to produce carbon-centred free radicals, and is used in the study of lipid peroxidation and the characterization of antioxidants.

ABTS
2,2'-Azino-bis(3-ethylbenzothiazoline-6-sulphonic acid): A chemical compound used for kinetic studies of specific enzymes. It is commonly used in the enzyme-linked immunosorbent assay (ELISA) procedures for the measurement of antioxidant activity.

ACC
Acetyl-CoA carboxylase: A biotin-dependent enzyme that catalyzes the irreversible carboxylation of acetyl-CoA to produce malonyl-CoA.

AD
Alzheimer's disease: A progressive form of dementia that interferes with memory, thinking, and behavior.

ACF
Aberrant crypt foci: Clusters of abnormal tube-like glands in the lining of the colon and rectum that aid in early detection of colorectal cancer.

AGEs
Advanced glycation end products: They are proteins or lipids and get glycated during exposer to sugar. They are harmful on accumulation in the body and could cause several complication including diabetes and aging.

Akt
A serine/threonine-specific protein kinase that plays a key role in multiple cellular processes such as glucose metabolism, apoptosis, cell proliferation, transcription and cell migration.

ALP
Alkaline phosphatase: An enzyme found in several tissues throughout the body. The highest concentrations of ALP are present in the cells that comprise bone and the liver. Elevated levels of ALP in the blood are most commonly caused by liver disease or bone disorders.

ALT
Alanine aminotransferase: Also known as serum glutamic-pyruvic transaminase (SGPT), an enzyme found mostly in the cells of the liver and kidney. It is used for diagnosing the liver damage.

AMES Test
A method for evaluating mutagenic effects of implant device, chemicals, and drug utilizing bacteria to detect carcinogens and mutagens.

GLOSSARY

AMPK
5' Adenosine monophosphate-activated protein kinase: An enzyme that plays a role in cellular energy homeostasis.

APP$_{swe}$
The "Swedish" mutation of the amyloid precursor protein dissociates components of object-location memory in aged Tg2576 mice.

APAP
Acetaminophen, also called N-acetyl para-aminophenol or paracetamol: One of the most widely used over-the-counter non-opioid analgesic and antipyretic agents to treat pain and fever.

AST
Aspartate transaminase or aspartate aminotransferase, also known as AspAT/ASAT/AAT or (serum) glutamic oxaloacetic transaminase (GOT, SGOT): An important enzyme in amino acid metabolism, and is used for diagnosing liver disorder.

ASVD
Arteriosclerotic vascular disease: It is closely related to the medical condition atherosclerosis. It encompasses coronary heart disease, cerebrovascular disease, and peripheral arterial disease and also responsible for the majority of cases of CVD in both developing and developed countries.

ATCC
American Type Culture Collection: A nonprofit organization which collects, stores, and distributes standard reference microorganisms, cell lines and other materials for research and development.

AUC
Area under curve: The definite integral in a plot of drug concentration in blood plasma vs. time.

Aβ
Amyloid-beta peptide: A peptide derived from amyloid precursor protein (APP) and forms the amyloid plaques which are markers of Alzheimer's disease in the brain and are believed to be the culprit in initiating the pathological cascade of the disease.

BALB/c
A nude mouse developed through crosses and back-crosses between BALB/cABom-nu and BALB/cAnNCrj-nu at Charles River Laboratories.

BAX
Bcl-2-associated X protein: Acts as anti- or pro-apoptotic regulator that are involved in a wide variety of cellular activities.

Bcl-2 and Bcl-xL
B cell lymphoma: Regulator proteins that induce to inhibit apoptosis or programmed cell death.

BDMC
Bisdemethoxycurcumin: A natural demethoxy derivative of curcumin.

bFGF
Basic fibroblast growth factor: A potent angiogenic factor and endothelial cell mitogen.

Biotransformation
A process of chemical modification made by an organism on a chemical compound. Bio-transformation also means chemical alteration of chemicals such as nutrients, amino acids, toxins, and drugs in the body. It is also needed to render non-polar compounds polar so that they are not reabsorbed in renal tubules and are excreted.

BMI
Body Mass Index: A measure of body fat based on height and weight that applies to adult men and women.

GLOSSARY

BUN
Blood Urea Nitrogen: A medical test that measures the amount of urea nitrogen present in blood.

CaSki cells
Cervical cancer cells: A model system used to study cancer biology.

CAT
Catalase: An antioxidant enzyme present in all aerobic organisms. It catalyzes the decomposition of hydrogen peroxide to water and oxygen. It protects cells from oxidative damage by reactive oxygen species.

CCl_4
Carbon tetrachloride: An organic solvent most commonly used as hepatotoxic agent for the induction of liver injuries in experimental animals.

Cd
Cadmium is a natural element found in tiny amounts in air, water, soil, and food. Exposure to cadmium occurs mostly in workplaces where cadmium products are made. Occupational exposure to various cadmium compounds is associated with an increased risk of lung cancer.

CD-1 mice
The original group of Swiss mice that served as progenitors of this stock consisted of two male and seven female albino mice derived from a non-inbred stock. Generally used for genetics, toxicology, pharmacology, and aging research.

$CDCl_3$
Chloroform-d (deuterochloroform): A deuterated solvent useful in NMR-based research and analyses.

CGA
Chlorogenic acid: A natural phenolic compound, widely found in fruits, vegetables (apples, pears, carrots, tomatoes, and sweet potatoes), coffee and tea.

CHC
Curcumin with polyvinylpyrrolidone (PVP) and natural antioxidants: A specific mixture used for a particular study.

CIPN
Chemotherapy-induced peripheral neuropathy: Chemotherapeutic drugs used to treat cancer can damage peripheral nerves that are away from the brain and spinal cord. It is a progressive, enduring, and often irreversible condition featuring pain, numbness, tingling and sensitivity to cold in the hands and feet (sometimes progressing to the arms and legs) that afflicts between 30% and 40% of patients undergoing chemotherapy.

CKD
Chronic kidney disease: A type of kidney disease in which there is gradual loss of kidney function over a period of months or years, and it may be caused by diabetes, high blood pressure and other disorders.

CLL
Chronic lymphocytic leukemia: A most common blood and bone marrow disease in adults that usually gets worse slowly.

CMC
Carboxymethyl cellulose: A food grade water-soluble polymer obtained from cellulose used as thickener and stabilizer.

COX-1
Cyclooxygenase-1: A constitutively expressed form (normal for homeostasis) of enzyme that acts to speed up the production of certain chemical messengers, called prostaglandins which is responsible for inflammation, pain and fever.

GLOSSARY

COX-2
Cyclooxygenase-2: An enzyme primarily responsible for inflammation and pain.

CPR
Cytochrome P450 reductase: A membrane-bound protein that catalyzes electron transfer from NADPH to all known microsomal cytochromes P450.

CQ
Chloroquine: A medication used to prevent and to treat malaria.

CTX
Cyclophosphamide (aka Cytoxan): A common chemotherapeutic agent that has immuno-modulatory effects in addition to its direct cytotoxic activity.

CurA
An *Escherichia coli* gene that catalyzes the NADPH-dependent, sequential reduction of curcumin, first to the stable intermediate dihydrocurcumin and then to tetrahydrocurcumin.

Curcumin
A bright yellow chemical substance and the principal curcuminoid of turmeric (*Curcuma longa*), a member of the ginger family, Zingiberaceae. It is used as an herbal supplement, cosmetics ingredient, food flavoring, and food coloring.

CuZn SOD
Copper-zinc superoxide dismutase: An abundant copper- and zinc-containing protein present in the cytosol, nucleus, peroxisomes, and mitochondrial intermembrane space of human cells. Primarily it acts as an antioxidant enzyme, lowering the steady-state concentration of superoxide, but when mutated, it can also cause disease.

CYP2E1
Cytochrome P450 2E1: A member of the cytochrome P450 mixed-function oxidase system that carry out oxidative metabolism of many endogenous and foreign chemicals.

CYP4A
Cytochrome P450 4A - One of eighteen subfamilies in the CYP4 family and presently consists of twenty individual forms in nine different mammalian species and is responsible for the metabolism of arachidonic acid to its omega-hydroxy product dichloro fluorescein diacetate - a quantitative method for oxidative stress assessment of nanoparticle-treated cells.

DCFH-DA
Dichloro-dihydro-fluorescein diacetate assay: A quantitative method for oxidative stress assessment of nanoparticle-treated cell.

DDMC
Didesmethylcurcumin: A metabolite formed by microbial transformation of curcumin.

DFA
Dihydroferulic acid: One of the minor degradation products of curcumin.

DHC
Dihydrocurcumin: A naturally occurring molecule present in the plants of dietary importance and also one of the phase I reductive metabolites of curcumin.

DMC
Demethoxycurcumin: A natural demethoxy derivative of curcumin.

DMHHC
Demethoxyhexahydrocurcumin: A metabolite formed by microbial transformation of curcuminoids.

GLOSSARY

DMOHC
Demethoxyoctahydrocurcumin: A metabolite formed by microbial transformation of curcuminoids.

DMRT
Duncan's Multiple Range test: A post hoc test to measure specific differences between pairs of means.

DOPAL
3,4-Dihydroxyphenylacetaldehyde: An endogenous catecholaldehyde produced by enzymatic oxidative deamination of dopamine, a toxic agent to catecholaminergic neurons.

DOPG
1,2-Dioleoyl-sn-glycero-3-[phospho-rac-(1-glycerol)]: A lipid that has significant influence on multidrug transport.

DPPH
1,1 diphenyl-2-picrylhydrazyl: A colored compound widely used in quantitative assay in biochemistry to evaluate the properties of chemical constituents for scavenging free radicals.

DRAM
Damage regulated autophagy modulator: A p53 target gene encoding a lysosomal protein that induces autophagy, a process that degrades cytosolic proteins and organelles.

DSS
Dextran sulfate sodium: A sulfated polysaccharide with variable molecular weights. Administration of DSS causes human ulcerative colitis-like pathologies due to its toxicity to colonic epithelial cells, which results in compromised mucosal barrier function.

EBOV
Ebola virus: Discovered in 1976. Belongs to the family Filoviridae, causes hemorrhagic fever that could lead to death in a few days.

EC_{50}
Half maximal (50%) effective concentration: Refers to the concentration of a drug, antibody or toxicant which induces a response halfway between the baseline and maximum after a specified exposure time. It is commonly used as a measure of a drug's potency.

ECM
Extra cellular matrix: The non-cellular component present within all tissues and organs and provides not only essential physical scaffolding for the cellular constituents but also initiates crucial biochemical and biomechanical cues that are required for tissue morphogenesis, differentiation and homeostasis.

EGFR
Epidermal growth factor receptor: A transmembrane receptor protein in humans.

EMT
Epithelial-mesenchymal transition: A process whereby epithelial cells are transformed into mesenchymal cells.

eNOS
Endothelial nitric oxide synthase: A dimeric enzyme that is likely to be uncoupled in pro-oxidant states, thus changing its functional activity, giving rise to superoxide formation instead of NO. eNOS has a protective function in the cardiovascular system, which is attributed to NO production.

ERK
Extracellular signal regulated kinase: A specific subtype of mitogen-activated protein kinase (MAPK) that have been extensively linked to regulation of synaptic plasticity and memory formation in many systems.

GLOSSARY

Erα
Estrogen receptor-α: A key transcription factor in breast cancer believed to promote proliferation of breast cancer cells by binding to proximal promoters of key oncogenes.

FA
Ferulic acid: A naturally occurring molecule present in leaves and seeds of most plants and also one of the minor degradation products of curcumin.

FDA
U.S. Food and Drug Administration: An agency within the U.S. Department of Health and Human Services (HHS) that oversees the manufacturing and distribution of food, pharmaceuticals, medical devices, tobacco and other consumer products and veterinary medicine.

Fe-NTA
Ferric nitrilotriacetate: A potent nephrotoxic agent that induces acute and subacute renal proximal tubular necrosis by catalyzing the decomposition of hydrogen peroxide–derived production of hydroxyl radicals, which are known to cause lipid peroxidation and DNA damage.

FFAs
Free fatty acids: Fatty acids produced from triglycerides (TGs) by hydrolytic reactions in any of the steps of the process.

FK506
Tacrolimus also known as fujimycin: A potent immunosuppressive agent with significant nephrotoxic properties.

FOXO
Forkhead box class O family member proteins: Transcription factors essential regulators of cellular homeostasis, including glucose and lipid metabolism, oxidative stress response and redox signaling, cell cycle progression, and apoptosis.

FRAP
Ferric ion reducing antioxidant power: An antioxidant capacity assay that uses trolox as a standard.

G6PD
Glucose-6-phosphate dehydrogenase: The rate-limiting enzyme that determines the production of reduced nicotinamide adenine dinucleotide phosphate (NADPH) and ribose-5-phosphate (R5P) from the pentose phosphate cycle.

GI
Gastrointestinal: An organ system within humans and other animals which take in food, digests it to extract and absorb energy and nutrients, and expels the remaining waste as feces.

GOT
Glutamic-oxaloacetic transaminase: A pyridoxal phosphate-dependent enzyme which exists in cytoplasmic and mitochondrial forms, GOT1 and GOT2, respectively. It plays a role in amino acid metabolism and the urea and tricarboxylic acid cycle.

GPT
Glutamic pyruvic transaminase: Also known as alanine aminotransaminase (ALT), plays a key role in the intermediary metabolism of glucose and amino acids.

Gpx
Glutathione peroxidase: A cytosolic enzyme that catalyzes the reduction of hydrogen peroxide to water and oxygen as well as catalyzing the reduction of peroxide radicals to alcohols and oxygen.

GLOSSARY

GPX-1
Glutathione peroxidase 1: An intracellular antioxidant enzyme that reduces hydrogen peroxide to water to limit its harmful effects.

GRASP65
Golgi reassembly and stacking protein 65: A peripheral golgi protein localized to a *cis*-golgi protein implicated in diverse aspects of protein transport and structure related to the golgi complex, including the stacking of the golgi stack and/or the linking of mammalian golgi stacks into the golgi ribbon.

GRASPs
Golgi reassembly and stacking proteins: Required for polysaccharide secretion and virulence in *Cryptococcus neoformans*.

GSH
Reduced glutathione: A reduced form of glutathione, a potent antioxidant in plants, animals, bacteria and fungi.

GST
Glutathione-S-transferase: Belongs to a family of Phase II detoxification enzymes that have the primary role to detoxify xenobiotics by catalyzing the conjugation of the reduced form of glutathione (GSH).

H22 cells
Hepatoma cell line: Derived from murine hepatic carcinoma cells.

H4IIE cells
Rat hepatoma cells: A bioassay tool to assess the potential toxicity of dioxin-like chemicals.

Hb
Hemoglobin: The iron-containing oxygen-transport metalloprotein in the red blood cells (erythrocytes) of almost all vertebrates (the exception being the fish family Channichthyidae) as well as the tissues of some invertebrates.

HCC
Hepatocellular carcinoma: The most common type of primary liver cancer occured predominantly in patients with underlying chronic liver disease.

HCEC cells
Human colonic 2 epithelial cells: A valuable cell-line for studying colon stem cell biology, differentiation and pathogenesis.

Hcy
Homocysteine: A non-proteinogenic α-amino acid and a homologue of the amino acid cysteine. Its elevation in the blood causes increased oxidative stress and generation of excessive free radicals resulting in I/R injury.

HDL
High-density lipoprotein: Increasing concentrations of HDL particles are strongly associated with decreasing accumulation of atherosclerosis within the walls of arteries and hence lower risk of cardiovascular diseases.

HDL-C
High-density lipoprotein cholesterol: Considered as the "good" cholesterol. It absorbs cholesterol and carries it back to the liver. The liver then flushes it from the body. High levels of HDL cholesterol can lower the risk for heart disease and stroke.

Hep3B cells
Human hepatoma cells: A cellular model to study cancer biology especially, for *in vitro* liver cancer and toxicity studies.

HepG2
Hepatocarcinoma cells: An immortalized cell line, a suitable *in vitro* model system for the study of liver diseases.

HFD
High-fat diet: A suitable model for studies on impaired glucose tolerance (IGT) and early type 2 diabetes and also for examining novel therapeutic interventions.

HFF-1 cells
Human foreskin fibroblast cell line: A cellular system used as a reprogramming control alongside a specific cell type.

HFIP
Hexafluoro-2-propanol: A volatile polar solvent used in organic synthesis and for solubilizing a wide range of polymers, including those that are not soluble in the most common organic solvents.

HGF cells
Human gingival fibroblast cells: A cellular system used to assess the cytotoxicity of several dental materials.

HHC
Hexahydrocurcumin: A naturally occurring molecule present in the plants of dietary importance and also one of the phase I reductive metabolites of curcumin.

Hhcy
Hyperhomocysteinemia: A medical condition characterized by an abnormally high level of homocysteine in the blood, conventionally described as above 15 μmol/L. It may be associated with various neurologic conditions, including stroke, minimal cognitive impairment, dementia, Parkinson's disease, multiple sclerosis, epilepsy, and pregnancy.

HIF-1α
Hypoxia-inducible factor-1α: A basic helix-loop-helixPER-ARNT-SIM (PAS) domain containing protein, considered as the master transcriptional regulator of cellular and developmental response to hypoxia (a condition in which the body or a region of the body is deprived of adequate oxygen supply at the tissue level).

HIV
Human immunodeficiency virus: A retrovirus occurs as two types, HIV-1 and HIV-2 and causes HIV infection which over time develops acquired immunodeficiency syndrome (AIDS). Both types are transmitted through direct contact with HIV-infected body fluids, such as blood, semen, and vaginal fluids, or from a mother who has HIV to her child during pregnancy, labor and delivery, or breastfeeding (through breast milk).

HL-60 cells
Human acute myelogenous leukemia cells: An attractive cellular model system for studies of human myeloid cell differentiation.

HMG CoA reductase
3-Hydroxy-3-methyl-glutaryl-CoA reductase or HMGR: The rate-limiting enzyme of the mevalonate pathway, responsible for cholesterol and other isoprenoid biosynthesis.

HNE
4-hydroxy-2-nonenal: An α,β-unsaturated hydroxyalkenal produced by lipid peroxidation in cells, and most studied products of phospholipid peroxidation, owing to its reactivity and cytotoxicity.

HO-1
Heme oxygenase-1: A Nrf2-regulated gene plays a critical role in the prevention of vascular inflammation. It is the inducible isoform of HO, responsible for the oxidative cleavage of heme

GLOSSARY

groups leading to the generation of biliverdin, carbon monoxide, and release of ferrous iron.

HOMA-IR
Homeostatic model assessment of insulin resistance: A method used to quantify insulin resistance and beta-cell function.

HORAC
Hydroxyl radical averting capacity: An assay based on the oxidation of fluorescein by hydroxyl radicals via a classic hydrogen atom transfer (HAT) mechanism.

HPDL tissues
Human periodontal ligament-like tissues: Connective tissues that lie between tooth root and alveolar bone.

HPLC
High performance liquid chromatography: An analytical technique to separate, identify, and quantify components in a mixture.

HPMC K4M
Hydroxypropyl methylcellulose K4M: A semi-synthetic, inert, viscoelastic polymer used as an excipient and controlled-delivery component in oral medicaments.

HSC
Hepatic stellate cell: Key cellular element involved in the development of hepatic fibrosis.

HT-29 cells
A human colon cancer cell line used extensively in biological and cancer research.

Hydrogenation
A chemical reaction between molecular hydrogen and another compound or element, usually in the presence of a catalyst such as nickel, palladium or platinum. The process is commonly employed to reduce or saturate organic compounds.

I/R injury
Ischemia-reperfusion injury: A common feature of ischemic stroke, which occurs when blood supply is restored after a period of ischemia or lack of oxygen (anoxia or hypoxia).

IC_{50}
The half maximal inhibitory concentration is a measure of the potency of a substance in inhibiting a specific biological or biochemical function. This quantitative measure indicates how much of a drug or other substance is needed to inhibit a given biological process by half.

IκB kinase
Inhibitor of nuclear factor kappa-B kinase: An enzyme complex that is involved in propagating the cellular response to inflammation.

IκB-α
Inhibitor of nuclear factor kappa-B kinase subunit alpha: It blocks the ability of NF-κB transcription factors to bind to DNA, which is required for NF-κB's proper functioning in propagating the cellular response to inflammation.

IL
Interleukins: Cytokines expressed by white blood cells that play a very important role in all aspects of inflammation and immunity.

IL-1α & 1β
Interleukin 1α and 1β: Equally potent inflammatory cytokines that activate the inflammatory process, and their deregulated signaling causes devastating diseases manifested by severe acute or chronic inflammation.

GLOSSARY

IL-4Rα
Interleukin 4 receptor alpha: Ubiquitously expressed on both innate and adaptive immune cells, controls the signaling of archetypal type 2 immune regulators; IL-4 and IL-13.

IL-5
Interleukin-5: A growth factor and chemoattractant for eosinophils and is thought to play an essential role in allergic rhinitis, eosinophilic esophagitis and idiopathic hypereosinophilic syndrome.

IL-6
Interleukin-6: A soluble mediator with a pleiotropic effect on inflammation, immune response, and hematopoiesis.

IND
Investigational new drug: A new drug or biologic used in a clinical investigation.

iNOS
Inducible nitric oxide synthase: A key enzyme generating nitric oxide and plays an important role in numerous physiological and pathophysiological (including inflammation, infection etc.) conditions.

IOD
Integrated optical density: A quantitative analysis to evaluate chromogenic *in-situ*-hybridization (CISH) or its fluorescent counterpart (FISH) staining in tissue sections.

Islet β-cell
The insulin-secreting β-cell, one of four major types of cells in pancreatic islet, secretes the hormone insulin in response to several nutrients, hormones and nervous stimuli and plays a primary role in the maintenance of glucose homeostasis.

JAG 1 and 2
Jagged1 and jagged 2: Jagged family members, two of five cell surface proteins (ligands) interact with 4 receptors in the mammalian Notch signaling pathway.

JNK
c-Jun N-terminal kinase aka Jun amino terminal kinase: Responsible to stress stimuli and plays a role in T-cell differentiation and cellular apoptosis pathway.

Keap1
Kelch-like ECH-associated protein 1: A dimeric protein consisting of 624 amino acid residues. Keap1 has been shown to interact with Nrf2, a master regulator of the antioxidant response, which is important for the amelioration of oxidative stress.

Ki-67
Ki-67 protein: Widely used as a marker for proliferation in human tumor cells.

L02
Immortalized normal liver cells: A cell line used as normal control for the analysis of hepatocellular carcinoma.

LC3
Light chain 3: A microtubule-associated protein 1A/1B with a molecular mass of approximately 17 kDa distributed ubiquitously in mammalian tissues and cultured cells.

LC3-II/I
Conjugated forms of LC3: LC3-phosphatidylethanolamine conjugate (LC3-II/I) -Autophagy-associated protein markers.

LC-MS
Liquid chromatography–mass spectrometry: An analytical technique used in separating mixtures in accordance with their physical and chemical properties, then identifying the components within each peak and detecting based on their mass spectrum.

LC-MS/MS
Liquid chromatography with tandem mass spectrometry: A powerful analytical technique that combines the separating power of liquid chromatography with the highly sensitive and selective mass analysis capability of triple quadrupole mass spectrometry.

LD$_{50}$
Lethal dose 50%: The amount of substance expected to cause death in half (50%) of a group of a particular animal species when it enters the body by ingestion or skin absorption, generally used as an indicator to determine the substance's acute toxicity.

LDL
Low density lipoprotein: One of the five major groups of lipoproteins which when oxidized and enter the endothelium, pose a threat for cardiovascular diseases.

LDL-C
Low-density lipoprotein cholesterol: Considered the "bad" cholesterol, it reflects the amount of cholesterol carried by LDL and an important marker for the risk of developing heart disease.

LLC-PK1 cells
Renal tubular cells: An *in vitro* model for studying the renal tubular reabsorption of protein drugs.

LMTK3
Human lemur tyrosine kinase-3: An oncogenic receptor tyrosine kinase (RTK) implicated in various types of cancer.

L-NAME
N-nitro-*L*-arginine methyl ester: A nitric oxide synthase inhibitor.

LPL
Lipoprotein lipase: An enzyme present in the tissue vascular bed catalyzes the hydrolysis of plasma TAG carried in the TAG-rich lipoproteins, chylomicron, and VLDL; and the key enzyme for their metabolic clearance.

LPS
Lipopolysaccharides, also known as lipoglycans and endotoxins: Large molecules consisting of a lipid and a polysaccharide composed of O-antigen, outer core and inner core joined by a covalent bond; and the major component of outer membrane of Gram-negative bacteria.

MAO
Monoamine oxidase: An enzyme involved in the degradation process for various monoamines released by neurons and glia cells, including dopamine, serotonin and norepinephrine.

MAO-B
Monoamine oxidase-B: An enzyme on the outer mitochondrial membrane that catalyzes the oxidation of arylalkylamine neurotransmitters. Monoamine oxidase B inhibitors are typically used in the treatment of Parkinson's disease.

MAPKs
Mitogen-activated protein kinases: Serine–threonine kinases that mediate intracellular signaling involved in regulating protein and cell functioning related to membrane, intra- and intercellular processes and transformation, proliferation/growth, differentiation, survival, and death.

MCAO
Middle cerebral artery occlusion: A common cerebral hemodynamic status in patients.

MCF-7 cells
Human breast cancer cells: A cellular system used ubiquitously in research for ER-positive breast cancer cell experiments.

MDA
Malondialdehyde: An important marker for lipid peroxidation / oxidative stress.

MDA-MB-231 cells
Estrogen-receptor negative human breast cancer cell lines.

MDM2
Murine double minute 2: A protein in humans is encoded by the MDM2 gene and an important negative regulator of the p53 tumor suppressor.

MET
Mesenchymal-epithelial transition: Process observed during reprogramming of somatic cells into induced pluripotent stem cells and in disease states such as fibrosis, inflammation, and cancers.

Mfn2
A mitochondrial membrane protein participates in mitochondrial fusion and contributes to the maintenance and operation of the mitochondrial network.

MG-63 cells
A cell line derived from an osteosarcoma patient.

MI
Myocardial infarction (Heart attack): Irreversible death (necrosis) of heart muscle secondary to prolonged lack of oxygen supply (ischemia).

MIA
Monoiodoacetate: Used for joint disruption in experimental osteoarthritis models, both rats and mice.

Microsomal Enzyme
A group of enzymes associated with a certain particulate fraction of liver homogenate that plays a role in the metabolism of many drugs.

MM/PBSA
Molecular Mechanics/Poisson-Boltzmann Surface Area: An efficient method for the calculation of free energies of diverse molecular systems.

mMCB
Modified medium for colon bacteria: Supports the growth of various human colon bacteria.

MMP
Matrix metalloproteinase: Calcium dependent endopeptidase responsible for tissue remodeling and degradation of the extracellular matrix.

MPTP
1-Methyl-4-phenyl-1,2,3,6-tetrahydropyridine: A prodrug to the neurotoxin, 1-methyl-4-phenylpyridinium (MPP+), which causes permanent symptoms of Parkinson's disease by destroying dopaminergic neurons in the substantia nigra of the brain.

MS/MS
Mass spectrometry/mass spectrometry: A technology in which compounds are separated by molecular weight by one mass spectrometer, fragmented as they exit, and identified on the basis of their fragments by a second mass spectrometer.

MTHFR
Methylenetetrahydrofolate reductase: A key enzyme in the conversion to 5-methyltetrahydrofolate, the

major circulating form of folate in the body and the primary methyl donor for the methylation of homocysteine to methionine.

mTOR
Mammalian target of rapamycin: Also known as the mechanistic target of rapamycin, an atypical serine/threonine kinase that is present in two distinct complexes (mTOR complex, mTORC1 and mTORC2). Aberrant mTOR signaling is involved in many disease states including cancer, cardiovascular disease, and diabetes.

MTT assay
3-(4,5-Dimethylthiazol-2-yl)-2,5-diphenyl-tetrazolium bromide assay: A standard cell proliferation assay used to test the anti-proliferating activities *in vitro*.

NaC
Sodium curcuminate: Sodium salt of curcumin exerts higher anti-inflammatory effect than curcumin.

NADPH
Nicotinamide adenine dinucleotide phosphate: A cofactor used in anabolic reactions, such as the Calvin cycle, lipid and nucleic acid syntheses and also required for the CYP-mediated biotransformation.

NADPH: QR
NADPH-quinone reductase: An enzyme that catalyzes the chemical reaction.

NAFLD
Non-alcoholic fatty liver disease: A very common disorder refers to a group of conditions where there is accumulation of excess fat in the liver of people who drink little or no alcohol.

ND
Normal diet: A healthy food plan that includes a variety of healthy foods from all the food groups.

NEC
Nano-emulsion curcumin formulation: A specific formulation used for a particular study.

NF-κB
Nuclear Factor-kappa B: A protein complex involved in cellular response to stress and plays a central role in inflammation.

NIH 3T3 cells
Primary mouse embryonic fibroblast cells: A powerful system to test gene function due to their easy accessibility, rapid growth rates, and the possibilities of a large number of experiments.

NIX
Nip-like protein X: A typical BCL-2 homology domain 3-only proteins involved in cell death, autophagy, and programmed mitochondrial clearance.

NMR
Nuclear magnetic resonance: A physical phenomenon in which nuclei in a strong static magnetic field are perturbed by a weak oscillating magnetic field and respond by producing an electromagnetic signal with a frequency characteristic of the magnetic field at the nucleus.

NO
Nitric oxide: A reactive free radical produced by the NO synthase (NOS) family and is involved in several cellular functions, such as neuro-transmission, the regulation of vessel tone and immune response.

NOAEL
No observed adverse effect level: The highest dose at which no toxicity or adverse effect is observed.

Notch 1 & 2
Notch signalings play a key role in tumorigenesis.

Nrf2
Nuclear factor erythroid 2–related factor 2: A key regulator of the cellular antioxidant response and a crucial regulator of the cellular defense mechanisms against oxidative stress triggered by injury and inflammation.

NTBI
Non-transferrin bound iron: Free iron present in serum or plasma. NTBIs generate highly reactive free radical and known to cause an immense amount of damage to various organs of the body including heart, liver, pancreas, endocrine glands and erythroid cells etc., depending on final location of its deposition.

Nuclear p65
Nuclear factor NF-kappa-B p65 subunit: A protein that in humans is encoded by the RELA gene as a part of the NF-κB signaling pathway. It is typically involved in the body's inflammatory response.

OA
Oleic acid: A mono-unsaturated omega-9 fatty acid occurs naturally in various animal and vegetable sources and used to induce lipid accumulation, oxidative stress and insulin resistance in experimental studies to determine the underlying mechanisms of action of drug molecules.

OGTT
Oral-Glucose-Tolerance Test: A test performed for the measurement of Insulin Resistance.

OHC
Octahydrocurcumin: A naturally occurring molecule present in the plants of dietary importance and also one of the phase I reductive metabolites of curcumin.

OKT3
Muromonab-CD3 (trade name Orthoclone OKT3): A murine (mouse) monoclonal IgG2a antibody (immunosuppressant drug) used to reduce the natural immunity of patients who receive organ transplants such as liver transplants.

ORAC
Oxygen Radical Absorbance Capacity: A method of measuring antioxidant capacities in biological samples *in vitro*.

OVX rats
Ovariectomized obese rats: Female rats whose ovaries have been removed and used as a model in investigations of osteoporosis and osteoporotic therapies.

p21
A potent cyclin-dependent kinase inhibitor (CKI) and tumor suppressor protein that protects from DNA damage.

p38 MAPK
Mitogen activated protein kinase p38: An important intracellular kinase activated by cellular stress.

p47phox
A 47-kilodalton protein that in humans is encoded by neutrophil cytosolic factor 1 (NCF1) gene, heavily phosphorylated and plays a vital role in the activation of NADPH oxidase.

p53
A tumor suppressor protein that protects from DNA damage.

p62
A multifunctional cytoplasmic protein that is an important regulatory molecule linking ubiquitinated protein to autophagy.

GLOSSARY

p-ACC
Phospho-Acetyl-CoA Carboxylase (Ser79): A biotin-containing enzyme catalyzes the carboxylation of acetyl-CoA to malonyl-CoA. It is the key enzyme in the biosynthesis and oxidation of fatty acids.

pAKT
Phosphorylated Protein kinase B: A protein kinase that plays a key role in multiple cellular processes.

p-AMPK
5' Adenosine monophosphate activated protein kinase: A member of a metabolite-sensing protein kinase family that functions as a metabolic 'fuel gauge' in skeletal muscle.

PARP
Poly (ADP-ribose) polymerase: A family of proteins involved in a number of cellular processes such as DNA repair, genomic stability, and programmed cell death.

PB
Phenylbutazone: An effective drug used for the treatment of rheumatic and arthritic diseases.

PBMCs
Peripheral blood mononuclear cells: A critical component in the immune system to fight infection, adapt to intruders and defined as any blood cell with a round nucleus (i.e. a lymphocyte, a monocyte, or a macrophage). They are widely used in research and clinical applications.

PCNA
Proliferative cell nuclear antigen: A nuclear protein that acts as a cofactor of DNA polymerase δ and is involved in DNA repair. It is known as a molecular marker for proliferation given its role in replication.

PCV
Packed cell volume: A measurement of the proportion of blood that is made up of cells.

PD
Parkinson's disease: A progressive nervous system disorder that affects predominantly dopamine-producing ("dopaminergic") neurons in a specific area of the brain called substantia nigra.

Pd/C
Palladium on carbon, often referred to as Pd/C: A catalyst used in organic synthesis.

PE
Phenylephrine: A decongestant that shrinks blood vessels in the nasal passages.

PGE2
Prostaglandin E2: An essential homeostatic factor that is released in response to infection or inflammation.

Phase I metabolites
These are broadly grouped into three categories, oxidative, reductive, and hydrolyzed metabolites.

Phase II metabolites
These are formed as result of conjugation reactions and are catalyzed by enzymes mainly transferases.

PI3K
Phosphoinositide 3-kinases: The lipid kinases that phosphorylate the 3'-hydroxyl group of the inositol ring on phosphatidylinositol.

PKC
Protein kinase C: A key family of enzymes involved in signaling pathways that specifically phosphorylates substrates at serine/threonine residues.

GLOSSARY

PKG
Protein kinase G: A serine/threonine-specific protein kinases which is dependent on cyclic GMP and catalyzes the phosphorylation of serine or threonine residues of proteins.

PLA2
Phospholipase A2: Designated class of enzymes that hydrolyze the *sn*-2 ester of glycerophospholipids to produce a fatty acid and a lysophospholipid.

Pls
Phospholipids: A class of lipids present as main component of all cell membrane.

PMA
Phorbal-12-myristate-13-acetate (an activator of protein kinase C): A phorbol ester works as a tumor promoter and is involved in gene transcription, cell growth, differentiation, programmed cell death, immune pathway and receptor desensitization via protein kinase C (PKC) signaling pathways.

p-mTOR
Phosphorylated mammalian target of rapamycin: A valuable prognostic factor for poor survival of cancer patients, especially esophageal and gastric cancer.

PNPLA3
Patatin-like phospholipase domain containing 3: Associated with nonalcoholic fatty liver disease, steatosis, fibrosis/cirrhosis, and hepatocellular carcinoma on a background of metabolic, alcoholic, and viral insults.

PPAR
Peroxisome proliferator-activated receptors: A group of nuclear receptor proteins that function as transcription factors regulating the expression of genes. PPARs play essential roles in the regulation of cellular differentiation, development, and metabolism of higher organisms.

PPARα
Peroxisome proliferator-activated receptor alpha: A nuclear receptor expressed in tissues with high oxidative activity that plays a central role in metabolism of potential drug target for non-alcoholic fatty liver disease (NAFLD).

PTHrP
Parathyroid hormone-related protein: An important driver of cancer bone metastasis.

QRT-PCR
Quantitative real-time polymerase chain reaction: A method widely used in molecular biology to make many copies of a specific DNA segment.

RBC
Red Blood Cell: Common type of blood cells responsible for oxygen delivery to body tissues.

RBL-2H3 cells
Rat basophilic leukemia cells used in inflammation, allergy and immunological research.

RIPT Test
Repeat insult patch test: A test to determine the irritation and/or sensitization potential of a test material(s).

ROS
Reactive oxygen species: Chemically reactive molecules containing oxygen that are formed as a natural by-product of the normal metabolism of oxygen and have an important role in cell signaling and homeostasis.

RT-PCR
Reverse transcription polymerase chain reaction: A laboratory technique frequently used to detect and quantify RNA expression.

GLOSSARY

RTV
Relative tumor volume: A ratio of the final tumor volume for the control and the treatment cases.

SabiWhite®
A registered product, Tetrahydrocurcumin Ultra-Pure, of Sabinsa.

SD rats
Sprague-Dawley rats: An outbred multipurpose breed of albino rat with an elongated head and a tail that is longer than its body used extensively in medical and nutritional research.

SGOT
Serum glutamic-oxaloacetic transaminase - Aka aspartate aminotransferase (AST): A test to evaluate the liver enzyme in the blood.

SGPT
Serum glutamic-pyruvic transaminase - Aka alanine aminotransferase (ALT): An initial screening for liver disease.

SIRT1
Sirtuin 1: A NAD^+-dependent deacetylase (NDAC) that functions as a key metabolic/energy sensor and mediates homeostatic responses to nutrient availability.

SIRT2
Sirtuin 2: A NAD^+-dependent deacetylase (NDAC) is associated with various physiological processes, including adipogenesis, fatty acid oxidation, gluconeogenesis, and insulin sensitivity and possible role in metabolic disorders.

SMEDDS
Selfmicroemulsifying drug delivery systems: A drug delivery system that uses a microemulsion achieved by chemical rather than mechanical means.

SOD
Superoxide dismutase: An enzyme found in all living cells that catalyzes the destruction of the oxygen free radical and thus protects oxygen metabolizing cells against harmful effects of superoxide free-radicals.

SREBP-1C
Sterol regulatory element binding protein-1C: A metabolic-syndrome-associated transcription factor that controls fatty acid biosynthesis under glucose/insulin stimulation.

STAT6
Signal transducer and activator of transcription 6: A protein coding gene. Diseases associated with STAT6 include hemangiopericytoma, malignancy and nut allergy.

Strain K-12
A substrain of *Escherichia coli* H10B isolated from human feces that has the capacity to metabolize curcumin.

STZ-NA
Streptozotocin and nicotinamide are often used in animal studies concerning various aspects of diabetes.

SW480 cells
Colorectal adenocarcinoma cell line: A cell line that is used as a representative model to study metastatic cancer.

TAK1
Transforming growth factor beta-activated kinase 1: An indispensable signaling intermediate in tumor necrosis factor (TNF), interleukin 1, and Toll-like receptor signaling pathways. It is a central regulator of cell death and is activated through a diverse set of intra- and extracellular stimuli.

GLOSSARY

T-AOC
Total antioxidant capacity: A measurement of the amount of free radicals scavenged by the test solution.

TBARS
Thiobarbituric acid like reactive substance: The most widely used assays for measuring lipid peroxidation end product malondialdehyde, a reactive aldehyde produced by lipid peroxidation of polyunsaturated fatty acids.

TBI
Traumatic brain injury - also known as intracranial injury: A complex brain injury with a broad spectrum of symptoms and disabilities.

TCHO
Total cholesterol: A count of overall amount of cholesterol present in blood.

TFAs
Trans-Fatty acids: Unsaturated fats found in foods obtained from ruminants, such as dairy products and meat, and in industrially produced partially hydrogenated vegetable oils.

TG
Triglyceride: An ester derived from glycerol and three fatty acids and the main constituent of body fat in humans and animals. High levels of triglycerides in the bloodstream have been linked to atherosclerosis, risk of heart disease and stroke.

TGF-β
Transforming growth factor beta: A multifunctional cytokine belonging to the transforming growth factor superfamily that includes four different isoforms (TGF-β 1 to 4). It is a multipotent growth factor affecting cell differentiation, proliferation, apoptosis and matrix production.

TGF-β1
Transforming growth factor beta 1: A polypeptide member of the transforming growth factor beta superfamily of cytokines. It plays an important role in myocardial fibrosis.

THBDMC
Tetrahydrobisdemethoxycurcumin: One of the reductive metabolites of curcumin.

THC
Tetrahydrocurcumin: A naturally occurring molecule present in the plants of dietary importance and also one of the phase I reductive metabolites of curcumin.

THDMC
Tetrahydrodemethoxycurcumin: One of the reductive metabolites of curcumin.

TLC
Thin-layer chromatography: A commonly used chromatographic technique for identifying compounds and determining their purity.

TNF-α
Tumor Necrosis Factor-alpha: An inflammatory cytokine produced by macrophages/monocytes during acute inflammation and is responsible for a diverse range of signaling events within cells and mediates necrosis or apoptosis. A cytokine (small protein) that causes programmed cell death.

Trolox
A cell-permeable, water-soluble derivative of vitamin E with potent antioxidant properties. It is commonly used as a standard or positive control in antioxidant assays.

GLOSSARY

U-2OS cells
Human osteosarcoma cell line: A cell line that is used as a representative model to study the human diseases.

UGT
Uridine 5'-diphospho-glucuronosyltransferase: A cytosolic enzyme that catalyzes the biotransformation of curcumin to its metabolites after oral injections.

UHPLC-QTOF-MS/MS
Ultra-high-performance liquid chromatography-quadrupole time of flight tandem mass spectrometry: Used in the qualitative and quantitative analyses for complex samples because of its high separation efficiency, accurate mass accuracy and excellent sensitivity.

uPA
Urokinase plasminogen activator: Central to a spectrum of biologic processes including fibrinolysis, inflammation, atherosclerotic plaque formation, matrix remodeling during wound healing, tumor invasion, angiogenesis, and metastasis.

UV
Ultraviolet: A band of the electromagnetic spectrum with wavelength from 10 nm to 400 nm, shorter than visible light but longer than X-rays.

UVB
Ultraviolet B radiation: A band of the electromagnetic spectrum with wavelength from 280 nm to 315 nm that causes sunburn, darkening, and thickening of the outer layer of the skin.

Vanillin
A naturally occurring molecule and also one of the minor degradation products of curcumin.

VAS score
Visual analogue score: The leading outcome measures to quantify pain and function in patients.

VEGF
Vascular endothelial growth factor: A signal protein that promotes the growth of new blood vessels to restore blood supply to cells and tissues.

VLDL
Very low-density lipoprotein: A protein that contains triglyceride oils and fats, that are shuttled to body cells that use them as energy or to fat cells that store them. High levels of VLDL cholesterol and triglycerides are at risk for CVD. People who are obese also have higher levels of VLDL cholesterol.

X-ray crystallography
A scientific method used for determining the precise positions/arrangements of atoms in a crystal.

ZMapp™
An experimental treatment for Ebola viral disease which consists of monoclonal antibodies that serve as antiviral therapy.